# AGING
*Volume 32*

---

# AGING AND THE BRAIN

# Aging Series

Aging
*Volume 32*

---

# Aging and the Brain

Editor

## Robert D. Terry, M.D.

*Department of Neurosciences*
*School of Medicine*
*University of California, San Diego*
*La Jolla, California*

Raven Press ⚮ New York

**Raven Press, 1185 Avenue of the Americas, New York, New York 10036**

Made in the United States of America

**Library of Congress Cataloging-in-Publication Data**

Aging and the brain.

    (Aging : v. 32)
    Based on an international symposium sponsored by the Princesse Liliane Foundation of Belgium in Oct. 1986.
    Includes bibliographies and index.
    1. Alzheimer's disease—Congresses.  2. Brain—Aging—Congresses.  I. Terry, Robert D.  II. Foundation Princesse Liliane.  III. Series.
[DNLM:  1. Aging—congresses.  2. Alzheimer's Disease—congresses.  3. Brain—physiopathology—congresses.  4. Dementia, Senile—congresses.
[W1 AG342E v. 32 / WT 150 A2669  1986]
RC523.A35    1988    618.87'683    87-42553
ISBN 0-88167-329-3

9 8 7 6 5 4 3 2 1

# Preface

The modern era of research on Alzheimer disease began about 25 years ago with ultrastructural studies of the cortical lesions. Interest accelerated with the discovery 10 years ago of quantitative deficiencies of specific neurotransmitters. Now the work is entering a third phase—one of molecular investigation. Other major disorders of the elderly are also being vigorously attacked, and new concepts of neurobiology and technology are being applied to those diseases and to the problems of normal aging. Some of the questions we have been asking during the past quarter century begin to be answered, and some of the discords are at least clarified in this book. New questions and new disagreements arise, but the research quickens and final answers surely approach.

We hope that this book will be of interest to other students of the disease, to gerontologists, geriatricians, clinical psychologists, neuropathologists, and neurologists.

*Robert D. Terry, M.D.*

# Acknowledgments

In October 1986 the Princesse Liliane Foundation of Belgium sponsored an international symposium on brain aging and certain related diseases. We met in the Royal Academy of Medicine in Brussels, and this volume represents the proceedings.

On behalf of all the contributors, the editor would like to thank the Foundation, especially Princesse Liliane herself, Professor van Ypersele, and Dr. Antonio Gotto for their support and organization.

*Robert D. Terry, M.D.*

On behalf of my colleagues of the International Scientific Council of the Foundation Cardiologique Princesse Liliane, I want to express gratitude to Dr. Robert D. Terry for organizing this symposium on aging and the brain. The topic of the conference was one of immense importance to twentieth century man. The International Scientific Council and the Foundation are most grateful to all the speakers for their excellent participation and for preparation of their manuscripts, thereby providing a means for sharing this symposium with other scientific colleagues. The annual symposia of the Foundation have been kept small in order to promote intimate discussion between the participants. Another hallmark of the meetings is the hospitality of Her Royal Highness, Princess Liliane of Belgium, which contributes greatly to the pleasure of all the participants. Speaking for the International Scientific Council, I express our gratitude for the philanthropy of the Foundation that makes it possible to hold and report these meetings. HRH Princess Liliane of Belgium is the creator and sustainer of the Foundation, without whom none of its work would be possible. The Council also thanks Baron Snoy et d'Oppuers, President of the Board, the distinguished members of the Foundation's Board, and the Belgium Advisory Medical Committee for their support.

*Antonio M. Gotto, Jr., M.D.*

# Contents

*ix*

# Contributors

**Stanley H. Appel**
Department of Neurology
Baylor College of Medicine
Houston, Texas 77030

**M. Flint Beal**
Neurology Service and Department of
    Neurology
Massachusetts General Hospital
    and Harvard Medical School
Boston, Massachusetts 02114

**Nancy Bernstein**
Department of Neurosciences
School of Medicine
University of California, San Diego
La Jolla, California 92093

**Konrad Beyreuther**
Institute of Genetics
University of Cologne
D-5000 Cologne 41, Federal Republic
    of Germany

**Anders Björklund**
Department of Histology
University of Lund
S-223 62 Lund, Sweden

**J. Robert Bostwick**
Department of Neurology
Baylor College of Medicine
Houston, Texas 77030

**D. M. Bowen**
Miriam Marks Department of
    Neurochemistry
Institute of Neurology
University of London
London WC1N 1PJ, United Kingdom

**Eileen M. Bryant**
Department of Pathology
Alzheimer Disease Research Center
University of Washington
Seattle, Washington 98195

**Nelson Butters**
Psychology Service
San Diego Veterans Administration
    Medical Center
La Jolla, California 92161, and
Departments of Psychiatry and
    Neurosciences
School of Medicine
University of California, San Diego
La Jolla, California 92093

**Garrett Crawford**
Department of Neurology
Baylor College of Medicine
Houston, Texas 77030

**Richard S. J. Frackowiak**
MRC Cyclotron Unit
Hammersmith Hospital
    and National Hospital for Nervous
    Diseases
London W12 OHS, United Kingdom

**P. T. Francis**
Miriam Marks Department of
    Neurochemistry
Institute of Neurology
University of London
London WC1N 1PJ, United Kingdom

**Fred H. Gage**
Department of Neurosciences
School of Medicine
University of California, San Diego
La Jolla, California 92093

**Eric Granholm**
Psychology Service
San Diego Veterans Administration
  Medical Center
La Jolla, California 92161, and
Departments of Psychiatry and
  Neurosciences
School of Medicine
University of California, San Diego
La Jolla, California 92093


**John W. Griffin**
Departments of Neurology and
  Neuroscience
The Johns Hopkins School of Medicine
Baltimore, Maryland 21205


**John H. Growdon**
Neurology Service and Department of
  Neurology
Massachusetts General Hospital
  and Harvard Medical School
Boston, Massachusetts 02114


**Lawrence A. Hansen**
Department of Neurosciences
School of Medicine
University of California, San Diego
La Jolla, California 92093


**William Heindel**
Psychology Service
San Diego Veterans Administration
  Medical Center
La Jolla, California 92161, and
Departments of Psychiatry and
  Neurosciences
School of Medicine
University of California, San Diego
La Jolla, California 92093


**Paul N. Hoffman**
Departments of Ophthalmology and
  Neurology
The Johns Hopkins School of Medicine
Baltimore, Maryland 21205

**Robert Katzman**
Department of Neurosciences
School of Medicine
University of California, San Diego
La Jolla, California 92093


**Edward H. Koo**
Department of Pathology
The Johns Hopkins School of Medicine
Baltimore, Maryland 21205


**Neil W. Kowall**
Neurology Service and Department of
  Neurology
Massachusetts General Hospital
  and Harvard Medical School
Boston, Massachusetts 02114


**J. William Langston**
Institute for Medical Research
San Jose, California 95128


**Bruce Lasker**
Department of Neurosciences
School of Medicine
University of California, San Diego
La Jolla, California 92093


**S. L. Lowe**
Miriam Marks Department of
  Neurochemistry
Institute of Neurology
University of London
London WC1N 1PJ, United Kingdom


**Marston Manthorpe**
Department of Biology
School of Medicine
University of California, San Diego
La Jolla, California 92093


**George M. Martin**
Department of Pathology
Alzheimer Disease Research Center
University of Washington
Seattle, Washington 98195

**Joseph B. Martin**
*Neurology Service and Department of
   Neurology
Massachusetts General Hospital
   and Harvard Medical School
Boston, Massachusetts 02114*


**Colin L. Masters**
*Neuromuscular Research Institute
Department of Pathology
University of Western Australia
Western Australia 6009, and
Department of Neuropathology
Royal Perth Hospital
Perth, Western Australia 6001*


**Michael Mazurek**
*Neurology Service and Department of
   Neurology
Massachusetts General Hospital
   and Harvard Medical School
Boston, Massachusetts 02114*


**James L. McManaman**
*Department of Neurology
Baylor College of Medicine
Houston, Texas 77030*


**Nancy A. Muma**
*Department of Pathology
The Johns Hopkins School of Medicine
Baltimore, Maryland 21205*


**A. M. Palmer**
*Miriam Marks Department of
   Neurochemistry
Institute of Neurology
University of London
London WC1N 1PJ, United Kingdom*


**Donald L. Price**
*Departments of Pathology, Neurology,
   and Neuroscience
The Johns Hopkins School of Medicine
Baltimore, Maryland 21205*


**A. W. Procter**
*Miriam Marks Department of
   Neurochemistry
Institute of Neurology
University of London
London WC1N 1PJ, United Kingdom*


**Stanley B. Prusiner**
*Departments of Neurology and of
   Biochemistry and Biophysics
University of California
San Francisco, California 94143*


**David P. Salmon**
*Psychology Service
San Diego Veterans Administration
   Medical Center
La Jolla, California 92161, and
Departments of Psychiatry and
   Neurosciences
School of Medicine
University of California, San Diego
La Jolla, California 92093*


**Dennis J. Selkoe**
*Department of Neurology
   (Neuroscience)
Harvard Medical School, and
Center for Neurologic Diseases
Brigham and Women's Hospital
Boston, Massachusetts 02115*


**Robert D. Terry**
*Department of Neurosciences
School of Medicine
University of California, San Diego
La Jolla, California 92093*


**Silvio Varon**
*Department of Biology
School of Medicine
University of California, San Diego
La Jolla, California 92093*


**Lawrence R. Williams**
*Department of Neurosciences
School of Medicine
University of California, San Diego
La Jolla, California 92093*

*Aging and the Brain,* edited by R. D. Terry.
Raven Press, New York © 1988.

# Genetics of Aging and of Disease Models

## George M. Martin and Eileen M. Bryant

*Department of Pathology, Alzheimer Disease Research Center, University of
Washington, Seattle, Washington 98195*

Our objectives in this review are twofold. In the first part we give an
overview of some genetic aspects of the biology of aging. In the second part
we consider genetic models of dominantly inherited genetic disease, including
some hypotheses concerning potential mechanisms of gene action in familial
dementia of the Alzheimer type, which in some pedigrees is thought to be
associated with an autosomal dominant mutation.

### GENETICS OF AGING

There are a number of compelling rationales for a genetic approach to the
study of aging. As with the investigation of other problems in biology, genetics has the potential to get at first principles, revealing primary factors that
determine differential times of onset and/or rates of development of particular
processes of aging or of particular age-related disorders. It is well known, of
course, that the average and median life spans of populations of organisms
within a species can vary substantially as a function of environment, but there
is little evidence that environmental influences can enhance the maximum life
span potential of the species. The latter appears to be a constitutional feature
of speciation. In other words, when a new species evolves, one consequence
may be a genetically determined permissiveness of a new characteristic maximum life span potential. Among mammalian species, a figure of 30- to 40-fold
is usually cited as the range of maximum life span potentials (45), but there is
considerable uncertainty about such figures. At the upper end of the scale
(the circa 115–120 years maximum life span potential for *Homo sapiens*) (8)
the data base is vast. At the lower end, however, there is still much uncertainty. Thus one should maintain considerable caution before concluding that
the regimen of dietary restriction in rodents greatly increases the maximum
life span of the *species* in contrast to the maximum life span of the *cohort* that
is investigated (52). Now that the National Institute on Aging has subsidized
the production of tens of thousands of aging mice, we are beginning to get
some surprising longevity records. A number of mice are living substantially
beyond 3 to 4 years (R. C. Sprott, *personal communication*, 1986). Until

*1*

recently this life span was considered to be the maximum potential for *Mus musculus domesticus*.

When considering the nature of gene action in aging, it is important to distinguish between two fundamentally distinct reproductive strategies. The life spans of organisms that exhibit a single and typically massive reproductive effort appear to be highly determinative or programmed. Examples include flowering plants, migrating Pacific salmon, and certain species of marsupial mice (23). This life style of reproduction has been referred to as "big bang" reproduction (10), but the proper biological term is semelparous (23).

In contrast, most mammalian species and all eutherian mammals have evolved an iteroparous reproductive strategy, with many rounds of reproduction following sexual maturation. In such organisms there appears to be more opportunity for stochastic mechanisms of aging. To illustrate this point, Fig. 1 shows a survival curve developed in our laboratory for a cohort of 202 AB6F1 hybrid male mice that were maintained under specific pathogen-free conditions (51). As for the case of humans, a number of these animals developed a variety of neoplasms as they aged. In contrast to humans, however, these animals were genetically identical and had nearly identical environments. Nevertheless, some animals succumbed, e.g., with lymphoma, at about 18 months, whereas others did not develop a lymphoma until about 36 months of age or developed other types of neoplastic or nonneoplastic disease. Our current notions of the pathogenesis of neoplasia suggests that a number of independent somatic mutational steps are necessary for the full expression of cancer. Rounds of selection appear to follow random chromosomal and point mutations. We can assume that the probability of such postmaturational mutational events vary among species and are perhaps determined by loci controlling the efficiency of DNA repair, free-radical scavenging, the fidelity of chromosomal segregation, etc. Such genes may be said to act in the domain of the maintenance of macromolecular integrity. It is reasonable to assume that they have important roles to play in all tissues, including the brain.

It is not to say, however, that there is not an important role in aging for genes that act in the domain of development. Turning from the example of possible interspecific differences in gene action setting the stage for different rates of development of neoplasia, let us consider a hypothetical genetic difference among individuals within a species that might be relevant to the age-related phenotype of a neurodegenerative disorder, Parkinson disease. It must be the case that there are genes that regulate the rates of amplification of stem cell pools as well as their rates of migration, clonal attenuation, and differentiation. Thus it is possible that allelic variations at such loci might result in varying numbers at birth of subsets of dopaminergic neurons within the substantia nigra. This situation could set the stage for different probabilities, years later, of reaching some critical threshold of neuronal depletion leading to the clinical expression of Parkinson disease. Differential rates of postmaturational aging could also contribute to varying the time of onset of

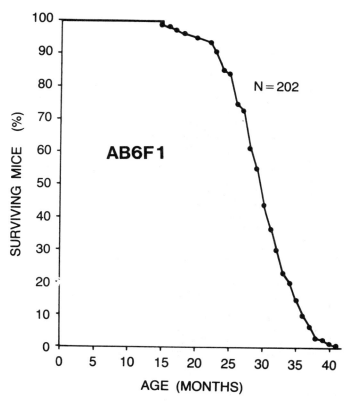

**FIG. 1.** Survival curve for a cohort of 202 male AB6F1 mice maintained under specific pathogen-free conditions. For further details, see Wolf et al. (51).

clinical expression (12). It is worthwhile noting that both autosomal dominant and X-linked recessive pedigrees have been described that contain individuals affected with idiopathic paralysis agitans in whom cerebral arteriosclerosis and encephalitis were considered to be unlikely factors in the pathogenesis (30).

Martin (27) identified some 55 genetic syndromes characterized by dementia, certain types of relevant degenerative neuropathology, or both; they are listed in Table 1. This list was selected from among 2,336 loci listed in the 4th edition of McKusick's catalogue (29). The proportion of such loci, which were thought to have potential relevance to aging of the central nervous system, was therefore 55 of 2,336 (2.35%). Assuming an upper limit of 100,000 genes in man (29), this number would give as many as 2,350 genes, allelic variation at which could potentially modulate—for better or for worse—how our brains age. Even assuming that only 1% or about 23 loci, are of major significance to how most of us age, it still gives an opportunity for an enormous amount of

TABLE 1. *Genetic syndromes characterized by dementia and/or degenerative neuropathology of relevance to the pathobiology of aging*[a]

**Autosomal dominant syndromes**

| | |
|---|---|
| *10050 | Acanthocytosis with neurologic disease |
| 10310 | Adie syndrome |
| 10430 | Alzheimer disease of brain |
| 10480 | Amyloidosis I (Andrade or Portuguese type) |
| *10490 | Amyloidosis II (Indiana or Rukavina type) |
| *10510 | Amyloidosis IV (Iowa or Van Allen type) |
| *10512 | Amyloidosis V (Finland or Merotoju type) |
| *10540 | Amyotrophic lateral sclerosis |
| 10550 | Amyotrophic lateral sclerosis—parkinsonism dementia complex of Guam |
| 10845 | Ataxia, late onset, with glucose intolerance |
| *11740 | Cerebelloparenchymal disorder I |
| ?11785 | Cervical lipodysplasia, familial |
| *12340 | Creutzfeldt-Jakob disease |
| *14310 | Huntington chorea |
| *15850 | Muscular atrophy, ataxia, retinitis pigmentosa, diabetes mellitus |
| 15870 | Muscular atrophy, progressive |
| *16235 | Neuronal ceroid-lipofuscinosis, dominant or Parry type |
| *16860 | Parkinsonism |
| 16870 | Parkinsonism dementia |
| 17250 | Photomyoclonus, diabetes mellitus, deafness, nephropathy, and cerebral dysfunction |
| *17270 | Pick disease of brain (lobar atrophy) |
| 17650 | Presenile dementia with spastic paralysis |
| 17660 | Presenile dementia, Kraepelin type |
| 19020 | Tremor of intention, ataxia and lipofuscinosis |

**Autosomal recessive syndromes**

| | |
|---|---|
| *20010 | Abetalipoproteinemia (acanthocytosis) |
| *20015 | Acanthocytosis |
| *20420 | Amaurotic family idiocy, juvenile type |
| *20510 | Amyotrophic lateral sclerosis, juvenile |
| 20520 | Amyotrophic lateral sclerosis, juvenile, with dementia |
| 20870 | Ataxia with myoclonus epilepsy and presenile dementia |
| *20890 | Ataxia telangiectasia |
| *21310 | Cerebelloparenchymal disorder II, late onset |
| 21360 | Cerebral calcification, nonarteriosclerotic (Fahr disease) |
| *21370 | Cerebral cholesterosis |
| *21640 | Cockayne syndrome |
| *22930 | Friedreich ataxia |
| 23960 | Hyperserotonemia |
| 24530 | Kuru |
| *24580 | Laurence-Moon syndrome |
| *24880 | Marinesco-Sjögren syndrome |
| *24890 | Mast syndrome (recessive presenile dementia) |
| *25773 | Neuronal ceroid lipofuscinosis, infantile, Finnish type |
| *26970 | Seip syndrome |
| 26980 | Senile plaque formation |
| *27800 | Wolman disease |
| ?27870 | Xeroderma pigmentosum |
| ?27871 | Xeroderma pigmentosum II |
| ?27872 | Xeroderma pigmentosum III |
| ?27875 | Xeroderma pigmentosum with normal excision repair rate |
| *27880 | Xeroderma idiocy of De Sanctis and Cacchione |

TABLE 1. (*continued*)

**X-linked recessive syndromes**

| | |
|---|---|
| *30010 | Addison diseases and cerebral sclerosis |
| 30740 | Hypogonadism, male, and ataxia |
| *30940 | Menkes syndrome (kinky hair disease) |
| *31150 | Parkinsonism |
| *31160 | Pelizaeus-Merzbacher disease |
| | Down syndrome |

*a*Numerical code of McKusick (29).
*Mode of inheritance thought to be certain.
After Martin (27).

genetic heterogeneity within our population. The number 23 is convenient for purposes of doing some simple calculations of the extent of such genetic heterogeneity, as it corresponds to the haploid chromosome number in man. Let us assume that these loci are distributed throughout the genome, perhaps with one locus on each of the 23 chromosomes. Given the simplest case of a two-allele system, it would produce 223, or 8,388,608 different kinds of sperm or egg. Some of the loci are likely to be highly polymorphic, however, with many more than two alleles. Crossing over during meiosis could of course give vastly more variation of gametes with respect to neighboring genes and segments of DNA on the same chromosomes, some of which might influence the expression of the relevant loci, e.g., via position effects. Thus one can conclude that each of us is probably unique with respect to how our nervous system is genetically buffered against neurodegenerative processes.

## DISEASE MODELS

The various neurodegenerative genetic syndromes listed in Table 1 represent experiments of nature, a number of which might prove to be exceedingly valuable in the elucidation of mechanisms of aging in the brain. There are at least two promising directions for future research on such spontaneous mutations in the human population. The first involves a search for the expression of a phenotype in cultivated nonneuronal somatic cells. It would open the door to a variety of biochemical genetic and somatic cell genetic experiments aimed at defining the genetic aberration, including the isolation of mutant and corresponding wild-type genes. Perhaps the most famous and successful example of this approach is the work of Goldstein and Brown on familial hypercholesterolemia that led to the identification of a series of mutations in the gene coding for the low density lipoprotein (LDL) receptor (6). One should recall that the original series of crucial experiments were not performed with cells from the principal target tissues of this disease, the arteries. Instead, fibroblast-like cells from the dermal skin were employed to establish cultures from affected and control individuals.

There is another important lesson that has developed from that line of research. We now know that genetic variation at a number of independent genetic loci can substantially influence atherogenesis (35,50,53). Even for the case of the now classical LDL receptor locus, a series of distinctive mutations have been found, including compound heterozygotes (6).

Expression of a phenotype in cultivated somatic cells opens the door to somatic cell genetic experiments aimed at the direct identification of the mutant locus. For recessive disorders, e.g., ataxia telangiectasia and the Cockayne syndrome, there is the possibility of complementing the defective genes via DNA transfection. The latter is probably best carried out via retroviral vectors with dominant selectable markers (31). Such vectors exhibit extraordinarily high efficiencies of transfection for cultures of normal diploid human fibroblasts, which are comparatively difficult to transfect; efficiencies of more than 50% have been obtained (36). Because the genes of human and other eukaryotes have large numbers of introns, transfections using a cDNA library rather than a genomic DNA library would be most feasible for such experiments. A major limitation of this approach, however, is that an unknown proportion of successful transfectants could result from complementation via suppressor loci rather than via the corresponding wild-type locus.

For dominant mutations, e.g., Huntington disease, one could, in principle, transfect a cDNA library from a cell line from such a patient to a normal recipient line and, via either selective techniques or replicate plating, identify clones having a phenotype comparable to the Huntington phenotype. It remains to be seen, however, how many such neurodegenerative disorders do in fact exhibit a phenotype, or can be *induced* to exhibit a phenotype, in cultivated nonneuronal somatic cells. Expression in "immortalized" cell lines would likely be required. Euploid or near-euploid immortalized lines, e.g., Epstein-Barr (EB) virus-transformed lymphoblastoid cell lines, would be especially favorable materials.

A second new direction for research on the genetically determined neurodegenerative disorders is the application of the rapidly mounting numbers of DNA probes for restriction fragment length polymorphisms and the more traditional genetic markers for purposes of linkage analyses. Given suitably large kindreds, including many living affected subjects, it has been calculated that as few as 200 probes evenly spaced over the genome would suffice to assign a given gene to a region within a particular chromosome (4). The prototype for such research has been established by Gusella and his colleagues for the case of Huntington disease. By a combination of such family studies and the use of somatic cell hybrid segregational analysis of an anonymous DNA probe, they were able to map the Huntington gene to the short arm of chromosome 4 (15). In view of the rapid technical progress in chromosome "walking" and "hopping" (39), it is a reasonable expectation that the Huntington gene itself will be isolated and sequenced.

A caveat in this second approach is the difficulty of finding suitably large kindreds and the dangers of pooling results from multiple, independent smaller pedigrees. As in the case of atherosclerosis, certain of the more common neurodegenerative disorders, e.g., familial dementia of the Alzheimer type, are likely to be heterogeneous in terms of underlying genetic susceptibility factors and pathogenesis.

The subject of familial Alzheimer disease is examined later, but we first want to illustrate some examples of important genetic approaches to aging research that do not rely on spontaneous genetic variation in human subjects.

Although neurological colleagues are likely to maintain a healthy skepticism, it can be argued that the lowly bread mold *Neurospora crassa* might tell us something important about the aging of neurons. Like many fungi, *Neurospora* can reproduce sexually via ascospores and asexually via proliferating mycelia or vegetative spores called conidia. Like neurons, conidia are somatic, postreplicative cells that retain a complete set of genetic information and that are subject to a gradual decrease in viability. Unlike neurons, however, given suitable conditions conidia can germinate to establish new colonies, thus providing a powerful bioassay of survivorship. A series of mutants have been isolated by Munkres and his colleagues that result in either diminished or enhanced longevities of conidia, over almost a 10-fold range (33). A large set of these mutants have been mapped to a single major gene complex on one arm of one of the seven chromosomes of *N. crassa*. Biochemical studies have revealed a high positive correlation of conidial longevity with the specific activities of a cyanide-resistant, mitochondrial form of superoxide dismutase, catalase, and glutathione peroxidase. These results could be interpreted as support for a free-radical theory of cellular aging.

The nematode *Caenorhabditis elegans* is a multicellular organism that provides great opportunities for a biochemical genetical analysis of cellular aging, including that of the nervous system. Its entire somatic cell lineage from the one-cell zygote to the 959-cell young adult hermaphrodite has been described (49) and is being utilized for the analysis of the programmed cell death that accompanies development (11). Although the pathogenesis of the presumably stochastic cell degeneration and cell death that accompanies postmaturational aging in certain regions of the human brain is likely to be different, we are certain to learn a great deal about the basic mechanisms leading to irreversible cell alteration by investigating such models.

At the whole organism level, Johnson has made much progress in demonstrating the importance of genes in modulating life span. With one approach he has recombined and randomly segregated the genomes of two parental strains having comparable life spans (17,19). Unlike mammalian inbred parental lines, such crosses do not exhibit a heterosis effect (hybrid vigor) in F1 hybrids. In the recombinant inbred lines derived from such crosses, however, there was about a fourfold range of life spans, including maximum life spans substantially greater than that of either parental line. It provides powerful material for a biochemical genetic analysis of life span.

In a second approach Johnson has investigated single-gene mutants that differ in life span, and he described one mutant, originally isolated by Klass, that exhibits an enhanced maximum life span (18). Unfortunately, we know comparatively little about the optimal husbandry and pathophysiology of the aging of *C. elegans.* It is conceivable that some genes may be acting to enhance life span in comparatively trivial ways.

A good deal more is known about specific pathogen-free conditions for raising mice, and a variety of inflammatory, degenerative, and neoplastic disorders can be readily detected and diagnosed. Thus it would be desirable to carry out innovative studies of the role of genetics in the aging of *Mus musculus domesticus.* An example being pursued in a few laboratories is investigation of the effects of exogenous genetic material introduced into the male pronucleus of the fertilized egg, resulting in "transgenic" mice (14). Another is the utilization of cultivated euploid lines of multipotent embryonal cells (42) for the isolation of mutants (1) as well as for the introduction of new genetic material. Such multipotent cells, when injected into blastocysts, can form chimeric mice, from which germ line segregation of the newly engineered genome can occur (5).

Finally, to return to man, let us consider the case for a genetic approach to the study of dementia of the Alzheimer type. There are at least six lines of evidence that support such an approach (Table 2).

The first approach, pioneered by the late Franz Kallmann (20), compares the frequency of concordance for expression of the disease in identical versus nonidentical twins. A definitive large-scale study of this question with rigorous evidence of monozygosity, differentiation of early- and late-onset disease, autopsy proof of the disease, and such niceties as comparison of twins raised apart with those raised together has yet to be reported. The current evidence is consistent, however, with an important genetic component, although the occasional observations of striking differences in time of expression also point to important environmental factors. In studies of "senile psychosis" (21), there was an 8.0% concordance rate for dizygotic twins and a 42.8% concordance rate for monozygotic twins. These concordance rates must be regarded as minimal estimates, because in many instances a twin died from other causes before there was an opportunity for expression of the disease. For the

TABLE 2. *Lines of evidence supporting a genetic approach
to research on the pathogenesis of dementia
of Alzheimer type*

---

Twin studies
Population studies
Pedigree analysis
Genetic marker associations
Trisomy 21
Cell culture studies

---

interpretation of such data, one should also be aware of the fact that monozygotic female twins are less identical than monozygotic male twins. It is because female twins are somatic mosaics with respect to genes in the X chromosome, as a result of random inactivation of paternally derived versus maternally derived X chromosomes in different subsets of cells during early development. If there were genes on the X chromosome that have the potential to modulate the expression of Alzheimer disease, one would expect to observe a lesser degree of concordance among monozygotic female twin pairs compared to monozygotic male twin pairs.

The second line of evidence was pioneered by Professor Leonard Heston and his colleagues at the University of Minnesota. Some of their results are plotted on Fig. 2, which shows the cumulative risk of developing Alzheimer disease as a function of age for several populations. Probands were identified from among a series of 2,000 autopsies. The highest-risk populations consisted of siblings of autopsied Alzheimer patients who (a) had had a comparatively early age of onset and (b) shared with that patient a mother or a father who also had Alzheimer disease. Provided the siblings live long enough, the cumulative risk for this group is 50:50. In contrast, the lowest-risk population consisted in siblings whose brothers or sisters developed Alzheimer disease after the age of 70 and who did *not* have a parent with Alzheimer disease. Between these extremes were siblings whose brothers or sisters developed early-onset disease but who did not have an affected parent.

The fourth line of evidence is illustrated by Fig. 3, which shows one of a number of pedigrees under investigation at the University of Washington's Alzheimer Disease Research Center under the leadership of Thomas Bird and Gerard Schellenberg. It satisfies criteria for autosomal dominant inheritance: involvement of several sequential generations that include individuals old enough to express the disease, involvement of both male and female members in an approximately 50:50 distribution, and male to male transmission. Such pedigrees do not prove mendelian heritance, however; proof requires a linkage analysis, as discussed earlier.

The fourth item listed in Table 2 is *association* with a genetic marker, which is quite different from genetic *linkage*. Association is a term used by human geneticists to indicate the nonrandom occurrence of two genetically separate traits in a population. When two genes occur on the same chromosome within detectable distances of one another, they are said to be genetically linked. If a high frequency of a given genetic marker is found in association with a particular disease or trait, we *cannot* conclude that the gene involved in the disease and the marker gene are close together on the same chromosome. For example, persons with type O blood group are 1.8 times as likely to develop a stomach ulcer as are individuals with other blood types, but this fact does not mean there is a gene for stomach ulcer close to the ABO blood group locus. Similarly, although there is now an established genetic linkage on the long arm of chromosome 9 between the loci for the ABO blood group and the nail-patella syn-

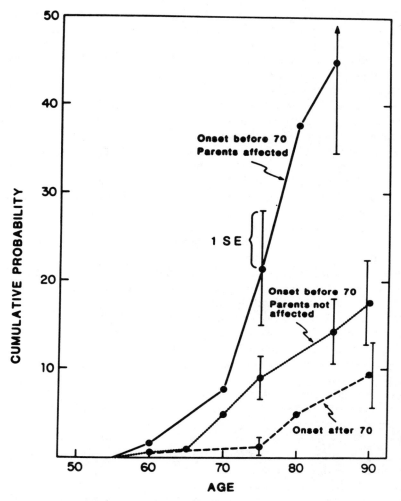

**FIG. 2.** Cumulative risks (% ± SE) for Alzheimer disease for three groups of siblings of autopsy-proved cases of the disorder. (From Heston et al., ref. 16, with permission.)

drome, it does not mean that individuals with a certain ABO blood type are more likely to develop the nail-patella syndrome, although it is a formal possibility that could result from a situation that geneticists refer to as linkage disequilibrium, a nonrandom association of alleles of each of two genes that are physically close together. Ordinarily, as a result of genetic recombination over many generations, this situation is not observed. Linkage disequilibrium can have two general causes: (a) The populations studied may have originated from a mixture of two populations having different frequencies of such alleles, and not enough time may have passed to permit complete randomization. (b) Cer-

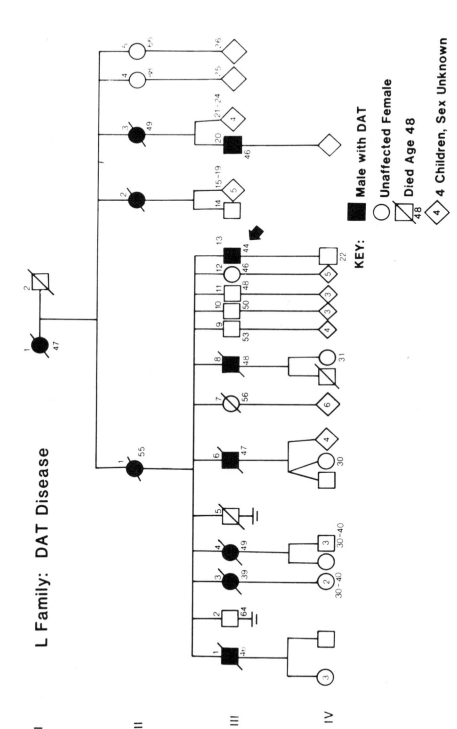

**FIG. 3.** Pedigrees of a family affected with autopsy-proved dementia of the Alzheimer type (DAT). The pattern of inheritance is consistent with the mendelian segregation of a single major autosomal dominant gene. For further details, see Schellenberg et al. (46).

tain combinations of alleles at linked loci might be maintained at high frequencies because they could confer a selective reproductive advantage to the individual, leading to a greater chance that the particular combination of alleles are passed on to subsequent generations.

Thus the demonstration of phenotypic associations raises only the *possibility* of a true genetic linkage. Such associations, in any case, point to genetic factors that modulate one's susceptibility to developing a particular disease. Are there any such associations so far established for Alzheimer disease? Although there has been little research on this question, there are already two such examples. A group at Columbia University reported an 8.8-fold increased risk of developing Alzheimer disease if the individual had the C4*B2 allele at the C4B complement locus (34). The complement system, especially C4, appears to be essential as a defense against viral infections. Thus this observation might lend support to the "slow virus" theory of the causation of dementia of the Alzheimer type. No family histories were reported in that study, so we do not know what proportion of the subjects had sporadic as opposed to familial Alzheimer disease. Genetic linkage of at least one familial form of Alzheimer disease to the chromosome (number 6) bearing the complement and HLA loci appears to have been ruled out, however (7,32).

Studies by our group in Seattle (46,47), have provided evidence of an association between familial Alzheimer disease and one of two alleles at a genetic locus, located on chromosome 19, that codes for the synthesis of apolipoprotein CII (apoCII). ApoCII is a cofactor for lipoprotein lipase. Patients who are deficient in this activity have high levels of serum triglycerides. Although there is no evidence of a connection between lipid metabolism and Alzheimer disease, one can speculate on such possible connections. One such example could be an association between an altered form of apoCII and the propensity to develop amyloid depositions, as there is evidence of such associations involving different types of apolipoprotein in research carried out in Seattle by Benditt and co-workers (2,3), and in studies by a group of investigators in Kyoto who are investigating a strain of mice that appear to age prematurely (24).

Most investigators are familiar with the fifth line of evidence—the fact that virtually all subjects with trisomy 21 (Down syndrome) who reach age 40 or so exhibit all of the known neuropathological stigmata and probably the major neurochemical stigmata of Alzheimer disease. One hypothesis that has been suggested (28) as an explanation for such a remarkable susceptibility is that there is a gene on chromosome 21 coding for one of the three subunit polypeptides that go to make up neurofilaments, structures that some investigators believe to be key participants in the genesis of neurofibrillary tangles. Such an extra dose could lead to the overproduction of that subunit, leading to the synthesis, over time, of insoluble abnormal trimers, analogous to the abnormal tetramers that one sees with certain of the hemoglobinopathies, e.g., some thalassemias. Such abnormal proteins, perhaps the neurofibrillary

TABLE 3. *Cellular sensitivity to genotoxic agents in Alzheimer disease*

| Cell type | No. of cultures tested | Agent | Sensitivity | Ref. |
|---|---|---|---|---|
| LCL | 3 | X-ray[a] | + | Robbins et al. (41) |
| LCL | 16 | X-ray[b] | + | Kidson et al. (22; *personal communication*) |
| LCL | 6 | X-ray[a] | + | Robbins et al. (40) |
| FIB | 3 | MMS[c] | + | Robison et al. (43; *personal communication*) |
| FIB | 4 | MNNG[c] | + | Li & Kaminskas (26) |
| FIB | 3 | MNNG[d] | + | Scudiero et al. (48) |
| LCL | ? | MMS[c] | ± | Robison et al. (44) |
| PBL | 6 | MMC[e] EMS | − | Das (9) |
| FIB | 4 | X-ray[d] | − | Lewis et al. (25) |

(+) significantly more sensitive than normal ($p \leq 0.02$); (−) not significantly different from normal.

EMS = ethylmethane sulfonate. FIB = skin fibroblasts. LCL = lymphoblastoid cell line. MMS = methylmethane sulfonate. MNNG = *N*-methyl-*N'*-nitro-*N*-nitrosoguanidine. PBL = peripheral blood lymphocytes.

[a]Viability ration.
[b]Multiple assays, e.g., cytogenetics.
[c]Repair replication.
[d]Colony-forming ability.
[e]Sister chromatid exchange.

tangles themselves, could interfere with axonal transport and thus cause much of the other pathology. This general notion of a primary role of abnormalities in axonal transport has been favored by Gajdusek (13). By a similar line of reasoning, a mutation at an analogous locus leading to *decreased* synthesis of one of the subunits could also lead to trimeric proteins with similar consequences. This situation is an example of how an autosomal dominant gene mutation might lead to one type of familial Alzheimer disease.

The sixth and final line of evidence is the possibility that there is phenotypic expression of the disease in cultivated nonneuronal somatic cells from patients with the familial form. So far there are only hints that it might be true. One line of research suggests an abnormality in calcium metabolism (37,38). The second line of research, involving several laboratories, but notably that of Robbins of the National Institutes of Health (NIH) (9,22,25,26,40,41,43,44,48), suggests the cultivated cells from patients are especially sensitive to certain physical and chemical agents that damage the genetic material, e.g., x-irradiation or treatment with the chemical mutagen *N*-methyl-*N'*-nitro-*N*-nitrosoguanidine. Table 3 summarizes the status of this research. We are currently investigating this problem in Seattle. The reports of hypersensitivity raise the question that, at least for some individuals or for some pedigrees with Alzheimer disease, there is an intrinsic instability of the genome of neurons. One possibility is an increased susceptibility to oxygen-mediated free-radical injury. Neurologists might therefore want to take research on the biochemical genetics of aging in bread molds more seriously.

## CONCLUSION

Genetic approaches to research on aging and age-related disease are promising. For the case of the most important age-related disorder, Alzheimer disease, it is now of the greatest importance to identify large kindreds of putative autosomal dominantly inherited disease so that a formal linkage analysis can be achieved. Because of the probability of genetic heterogeneity, it is important that a number of such kindreds be identified. In the United States the National Institute on Aging has expressed great interest in supporting such projects. One hopes that substantial sources of support for this urgent research can also be made available in Europe and Japan within the near future.

## REFERENCES

1. Aizawa, S., Ohashi, M., Loeb, L. A., and Martin, G. M. (1985): A multipotent mutator strain of mouse teratocarcinoma cells. *Somatic Cell Mol. Genet.*, 11:211–216.
2. Benditt, E. P., and Erikson, N. (1977): Amyloid protein SAA is associated with high density lipoproteins from human serum. *Proc. Natl. Acad. Sci. USA*, 74:4025–4028.
3. Benditt, E. P., Hoffman, J. S., Erikson, N., Parmelee, D. C., and Walsh, K. A. (1982): SAA, an apoprotein of HDL: its structure and function. *Ann. N.Y. Acad. Sci.*, 389:183–189.
4. Bishop, D. T., and Skolnick, M. H. (1983): Genetic markers and linkage analysis. *Banbury Rep.*, 14:251–259.
5. Bradley, A., Evans, M., Kaufman, M. H., and Robertson, E. (1984): Formation of germline chimaeras from embryo-derived teratocarcinoma cell lines. *Nature*, 309:255–256.
6. Brown, M. S., and Goldstein, J. L. (1986): A receptor-mediated pathway for cholesterol homeostasis. *Science*, 232:34–47.
7. Clemenceau, S., Foncin, J-F., Muller, J-Y., Halle, L., Hauptmann, G., Seger, J., and Salmon, C. (1986): Absence de liason entre la maladie d'Alzheimer et les marqueurs du complement. *C. R. Acad. Sci. [III]*, 303:149–154.
8. Comfort, A. (1979): *The Biology of Senescence.* Elsevier, New York.
9. Das, R. K. (1986): Mitomycin C and ethyl methanesulphonate-induced sister-chromatid exchanges in lymphocytes from individuals with Alzheimer's pre-senile dementia. *Mutat. Res.*, 173:127–130.
10. Diamond, J. M. (1982): Big-bang reproduction and ageing in male marsupial mice. *Nature*, 298:115–116.
11. Ellis, H. M., and Horvitz, H. R. (1986): Genetic control of programmed cell death in the nematode C. elegans. *Cell*, 44:817–829.
12. Finch, E. E. (1980): The relationships of aging changes in the basal ganglia to manifestations of Huntington's chorea. *Ann. Neurol.*, 7:406–411.
13. Gajdusek, D. C. (1985): Hypothesis: interference with axonal transport of neurofilament as a common pathogenetic mechanism in certain diseases of the central nervous system. *N. Engl. J. Med.*, 312:714–719.

14. Gordon, J. W. (1983): Studies of foreign genes transmitted through the germ lines of transgenic mice. *J. Exp. Zool.*, 228:313–324.
15. Gusella, J. F., Tanzi, R. E., Anderson, M. A., Hobbs, W., Gibbons, K., Raschtcheau, R., Gilliam, T. C., Wallace, M. R., Wexler, N. S., and Conneally, P. M. (1984): DNA markers for nervous system disease. *Science*, 225:1320–1326.
16. Heston, L. L., Mastri, A. R., Anderson, E., and White, J. (1981): Dementia of the Alzheimer type: clinical genetics, natural history, and associated conditions. *Arch. Gen. Psychiatry*, 38:1085–1090.
17. Johnson, T. E. (1983): Aging in Caenorhabditis elegans. *Rev. Biol. Res. Aging*, 1:37–49.
18. Johnson, T. E. (1985): Aging in Caenorhabditis elegans: update 1984. *Rev. Biol. Res. Aging*, 2:45–60.
19. Johnson, T. E., and Wood, W. B. (1982): Genetic analysis of life-span in Caenorhabditis elegans. *Proc. Natl. Acad. Sci. USA*, 79:6603–6607.
20. Kallmann, F. J. (1956): Genetic aspects of mental disorders in later life. In: *Mental Disorders in Later Life*, 2nd ed., edited by O. J. Kaplan, p. 26. Stanford University Press, Stanford.
21. Kallmann, F. J., and Jarvik, L. F. (1959): Individual differences in constitution and general background. In: *Handbook of Aging and the Individual*, edited by J. E. Birren. University of Chicago Press, Chicago.
22. Kidson, C., Chen, P., Imray, F. P., and Gipps, E. (1983): Nervous system disease associated with dominant cellular radiosensitivity. In: *Cellular Responses to DNA Damage*, edited by E. C. Friedberg and B. A. Bridges, pp. 721–729. Alan R. Liss, New York.
23. Kirkwood, T. B. L. (1985): Comparative and evolutionary aspects of longevity. In: *Handbook of the Biology of Aging*, 2nd ed., edited by C. E. Finch and E. L. Schneider, pp. 27–44. Van Nostrand Reinhold, New York.
24. Kunisada, T., Higuchi, K., Aota, S., Takeda, T., and Yamagishi, H. (1986): Molecular cloning and nucleotide sequence of cDNA for murine senile amyloid protein: nucleotide substitutions found in apolipoprotein A-II cDNA of senescence accelerated mouse (SAM). *Nucleic Acids Res.*, 14:5729–5740.
25. Lewis, P. D., Kumar, N., and Sabovljev, S. A. (1986): Normal cellular sensitivity to x-rays in Parkinson's disease and Alzheimer's disease. *J. Neurol. Neurosurg. Psychiatry*, 49:973 (abstract).
26. Li, G., and Kaminskas, E. (1985): Deficient repair of DNA lesions in Alzheimer's disease fibroblasts. *Biochem. Biophys. Res. Commun.*, 129:733–738.
27. Martin, G. M. (1978): Genetic syndromes in man with potential relevance to the pathobiology of aging. *Birth Defects*, 14:5–39.
28. Martin, G. M. (1982): Syndromes of accelerated aging. *J. Natl. Cancer Inst. Monogr.*, 60:241–247.
29. McKusick, V. A. (1975): *Mendelian Inheritance in Man*, 4th ed. Johns Hopkins University Press, Baltimore.
30. McKusick, V. A. (1983): *Mendelian Inheritance in Man*, 6th ed. Johns Hopkins University Press, Baltimore.
31. Miller, A. D., Law, M., and Verma, I. (1985): Generation of helper-free amphotropic retroviruses that transduce a dominant-acting, methotrexate-resistant dihydrofolate reductase gene. *Mol. Cell Biol.*, 5:431–437.
32. Muller, J-Y., Clemenceau, S., Foncin, J-F., Salmon, D., Halle, L., Castellano, F., and Salmon, C. (1986): Absence de liason entrola maladie d'Alzheimer et le systeme HLA. *C. R. Acad. Sci. (III)*, 303:105–109.
33. Munkres, K. D. (1985): Aging of fungi. *Rev. Biol. Res. Aging*, 2:29–43.
34. Nerl, C., Mayeux, R., and O'Neill, G. J. (1984): HLA-linked complement markers in Alzheimer's and Parkinson's disease: C4 variant (C4B2) a possible marker for senile dementia of the Alzheimer type. *Neurology*, 34:310–314.
35. Nerup, J., Mandrup-Poulsen, T., Owerbach, D., Johanson, K., Ingerslev, J., and Hansen, A. T. (1985): Association between DNA-sequences flanking the insulin gene and atherosclerosis. *Acta Endocrinol. [Suppl. 272] (Copenh.)*, 110:35–41.
36. Palmer, T. D., Hock, R. A., Osborne, W. R. A., and Miller, A. D. (1987): Efficient retrovirus mediated transfer and expression of a human adenosine deaminase gene in diploid

skin fibroblasts from an adenosine deaminase-deficient human. *Proc. Natl. Acad. Sci. USA,* 84:1055–1059.

37. Peterson, C., and Goldman, J. E. (1986): Alterations in calcium content and biochemical processes in cultured skin fibroblasts from aged and Alzheimer donors. *Proc. Natl. Acad. Sci. USA,* 83:2758–2762.

38. Peterson, C., Gibson, G. E., and Blass, J. P. (1985): Altered calcium uptake in cultured skin fibroblasts from patients with Alzheimer's disease. *N. Engl. J. Med.,* 312:1063–1065.

39. Poustka, A., Pohl, T., Frischauf, A-M., and Lehrach, H. (1987): Jumping libraries and linking libraries, a new generation of techniques in mammalian genetics (abstract). *Proc. 7th Int. Congr. Hum. Genet.* (in press).

40. Robbins, J. H., Otsuka, F., Tarone, R. E., Polinsky, R. J., Brumback, R. A., and Nee, L. E. (1985): Parkinson's disease and Alzheimer's disease: hypersensitivity to x-rays in cultured cell lines. *J. Neurol. Neurosurg. Psychiatry,* 48:916–923.

41. Robbins, J. H., Otsuka, F., Tarone, R. E., Polinsky, R. J., Brumback, R. A., Moshell, A. N., Nee, L. E., Ganges, M. B., and Cayeux, S. J. (1983): Radiosensitivity in Alzheimer disease and Parkinson disease. *Lancet,* 1:468–469.

42. Robertson, E., Bradley, A., Kuehn, M., and Evans, M. (1986): Germ-line transmission of genes introduced into cultured pluripotential cells by retroviral vector. *Nature,* 323:445–448.

43. Robison, S. H., Munzer, G. S., Tandam, R., Bradley, R., and Bradley, W. G. (1985): Repair of alkylated DNA is impaired in Alzheimer's disease cells. *Neurology,* 35:217 (abstract).

44. Robison, S. H., Polinsky, R., Kubie, S., Tandan, R., and Bradley, W. G. (1986): DNA repair in familial Alzheimer's disease. *Neurology,* 36:300 (abstract).

45. Sacher, G. A. (1972): Table of lifespans of mammals. *Handbook of Biological Data.* Federation of American Society of Experimental Biology, Washington, D.C.

46. Schellenberg, G. D., Deeb, S. S., Boehnke, M. L., Bryant, E. M., Martin, G. M., Lampe, T. H., and Bird, T. D. (1986): Association of an apolipoprotein CII allele with familial dementia of the Alzheimer type. *Am. J. Hum. Genet.,* 39 (Suppl.):A218.

47. Schellenberg, G. D., Deeb, S. S., Boehnke, M. L., Bryant, E. M., Martin, G. M., Lampe, T. H., and Bird, T. D. (1987): Association of an apolipoprotein CII allele with familial dementia of the Alzheimer type. *J. Neurogenet.,* 4:97–108.

48. Scudiero, D. A., Polinsky, R. J., Brumback, R. A., Tarone, R. E., Nee, L. E., and Robbins, J. H. (1986): Alzheimer disease fibroblasts are hypersensitive to the lethal effects of a DNA damaging chemical. *Mutat. Res.,* 159:125–131.

49. Sulston, J. E., Schierenberg, E., White, J. G., and Thomson, J. N. (1983): The embryonic cell lineage of the nematode Caenorhabditis elegans. *Dev. Biol.,* 100:64–119.

50. Williams, D. L. (1985): Molecular biology in arteriosclerosis research. *Arteriosclerosis,* 5:213–227.

51. Wolf, N. S., Giddens, W. E., and Martin, G. M. (1987): Life table analysis and pathologic observations in male mice of a long-lived hybrid strain (Af × C57Bl/6)F1. *Submitted.*

52. Yu, B. P. (1985): Recent advances in dietary restrictions and aging. *Rev. Biol. Res. Aging,* 2:435–443.

53. Zannis, V. I., and Breslow, J. L. (1985): Genetic mutations affecting human lipoprotein metabolism. *Adv. Hum. Genet.,* 14:125–215.

*Aging and the Brain*, edited by R. D. Terry.
Raven Press, New York © 1988.

# Advances in the Diagnosis of Dementia: Accuracy of Diagnosis and Consequences of Misdiagnosis of Disorders Causing Dementia[1]

Robert Katzman, Bruce Lasker, and Nancy Bernstein

*Department of Neurosciences, School of Medicine, University of California,
San Diego, La Jolla, California 92093*

It is remarkable that one of the major advances in regard to Alzheimer disease and other dementing illnesses during the past decade has been a significant improvement in the accuracy of clinical diagnosis. Whereas diagnosis was found to be in error 30% of the time in early follow-up series, there are more recent series using clinical criteria in which pathological verification confirms the diagnosis of "probable" Alzheimer disease in more than 90% of cases. Thus although there are still major gaps in our diagnostic accuracy, substantial progress has been made.

## DIAGNOSIS OF THE CLINICAL SYNDROME DEMENTIA

An important component of the advance in diagnostic accuracy has been the differentiation of the syndrome or symptom complex denoted by the term *dementia* and the diagnosis of the specific disorders that may present as dementia. It is now recognized that there are more than 70 such disorders, as shown in Tables 1 and 2. Alzheimer disease is but one of these 70; its importance is that it alone accounts for more than half, perhaps nearer 60%, of all cases of dementia. Hence the accuracy of the diagnosis of Alzheimer disease is emphasized in this report.

---

[1]This chapter is based on a report prepared for the Office of Technology Assessment, United States Congress.

TABLE 1. *Diseases presenting as dementia*

**Alzheimer disease**
  With or without vascular disease
  With or without Parkinson disease

  With or without other dementing diseases

**Other irreversible dementias**
  *Degenerative diseases*
  Pick disease
  Huntington disease
  Progressive supranuclear palsy
  Parkinson disease
  Cerebellar degenerations
  Amyotrophic lateral sclerosis (ALS)
  Parkinson–ALS–dementia complex of Guam and New Guinea
  Rare genetic and metabolic diseases (Hallervorden-Spatz, Kuf, Wilson, late-onset
    metachromatic leukodystrophy, adrenoleukodystrophy)

  *Vascular dementias*
  Multi-infarct dementia
  Cortical microinfarcts
  Lacunar dementia
  Binswanger disease
  Cerebral embolism by fat or air

  *Anoxic dementia*
  Cardiac arrest
  Cardaic failure (severe)
  Carbon monoxide

  *Traumatic*
  Dementia pugilistica (boxer's dementia)
  Head injuries (open or closed)

  *Infections*
  Acquired immunodeficiency syndrome (AIDS)
    AIDS dementia
    Opportunistic infections
  Creutzfeldt-Jakob disease (subacute spongiform encephalopathy)
  Progressive multifocal leukoencephalopathy
  Postencephalitic dementia
  Behçet syndrome

**Treatable dementias**
  *Infections*
  Herpes encephalitis
  Fungal meningitis or encephalitis
  Bacterial meningitis or encephalitis
  Parasitic encephalitis
  Brain abscess
  Neurosyphilis (general paresis)

  *Normal-pressure hydrocephalus* (communicating hydrocephalus of adults)

  *Space-occupying lesions*
  Chronic or acute subdural hematoma
  Primary brain tumor
  Metastatic tumors (carcinoma, leukemia, lymphoma, sarcoma)

  *Multiple sclerosis* (some cases)

  *Autoimmune disorders*
  Disseminated lupus erythematosus
  Vasculitis

TABLE 1. (*continued*)

*Toxic dementia*
  Alcoholic dementia
  Metallic poisons (e.g., lead, mercury, arsenic, manganese)
  Organic poisons (e.g., solvents, some insecticides)

*Other disorders*
  Epilepsy
  Concentration camp syndrome
  Whipple disease
  Heat stroke

*Note:* Many of these disorders produce dementia in a small percentage of patients (e.g., epilepsy, tumors).

TABLE 2. *Reversible causes of dementia*

*Psychiatric disorders*
  Depression
  Sensory deprivation
  Other psychoses

*Drugs*
  Sedatives
  Hypnotics
  Antianxiety agents
  Antidepressants
  Antiarrhythmics
  Antihypertensives
  Anticonvulsants
  Digitalis and derivatives
  Drugs with anticholinergic side effects
  Others (mechanism unknown)

*Nutritional disorders*
  Pellagra (vitamin $B_6$ deficiency)
  Thiamine deficiency (Wernicke syndrome, acute phase treatable)
  Cobalamin (vitamin $B_{12}$) deficiency or pernicious anemia
  Folate deficiency
  Marchiafava-Bignami disease

*Metabolic disorders*
  Hyper- and hypothyroidism (thyroid hormones)
  Hypercalcemia (calcium)
  Hyper- and hyponatremia (sodium)
  Hypoglycemia (glucose)
  Hyperlipidemia (lipids)
  Hypercapnia (carbon dioxide)
  Kidney failure
  Liver failure
  Cushing syndrome
  Addison disease
  Hypopituitarism
  Remote effect of carcinoma

*Note:* Most of these disorders produce dementia in only a small percentage of cases.

**Historical Perspective**

*Clinical and Mental Status: Changes Typical of Dementia*

Interest in the accuracy of the diagnosis of dementia is a relatively recent phenomenon. During the first half of this century medical attention about dementing illness focused on neurosyphilis. After establishment of the serological test for syphilis, the discovery of arsenical therapy by Ehrlich, and the delineation of the late brain sequelae of this spirochetal infection and methods of treating it, physicians began to specialize in syphilology, and a new medical specialty arose. Other dementing illnesses, however, were often lumped together under rubrics such as senility ("She's getting old, what do you expect") or cerebral arteriosclerosis ("It's just hardening of the arteries; the pipes get rigid you know"). From a public health point of view it seemed to make little difference. Demented patients who could not be cared for at home could be sent to state mental hospitals or to community "chronic hospitals" without regard to the diagnosis. The numbers were not overwhelming, and medical and community concern was at a minimum. The low level of medical interest was reflected in the available English language textbooks of neurology and psychiatry (there was a somewhat greater interest in the phenomenology of dementia by European psychiatrists), which gave little space to dementing illnesses.

Several events have radically changed this situation. Life expectancy, which was about 49 years at the turn of the century, will approach 79 years by the year 2000. Life expectancy of those over 60 has increased dramatically, thereby greatly increasing the numbers of individuals at risk for dementia. At the same time, the advent of potent neuroleptics and antidepressants for the treatment of schizophrenia and depression has made it possible to begin to treat such patients in the community. When economic considerations prompted many state governments to empty out state mental hospitals insofar as possible, most of the beds occupied by dementia patients were also closed. As more governmental funds were applied to medical care with the advent of Medicare and Medicaid, state regulatory agencies instituted strict regulations and eligibility criteria resulting in the closing of many "chronic" hospitals. Thus patients with dementia, increasing in total numbers at a time of hospital closings, became an increasing burden on the community and on families.

*Differentiation of Dementia from Other Syndromes*

During the 1950s intensive clinical studies of the elderly with cognitive and behavioral impairment by foresighted physicians such as Martin Roth in

Great Britain led to delineation of the clinical syndromes involved. The results of such studies made it possible to begin to diagnose the specific disorders producing these symptom complexes. During the 1960s breakthroughs in three specific disorders awakened medical interest in the diagnosis of dementia: (a) the discovery by Gajdusek and colleagues—a discovery important enough to have led to a Nobel Prize—of latent virus as the cause of Creutzfeldt-Jakob disease previously thought to be a degenerative disorder; (b) the studies by Terry and Kidd of the ultrastructural changes in the Alzheimer brain and the prospective quantitative study by Blessed, Tomlinson, and Roth relating the degree of Alzheimer pathology to the degree of dementia in the elderly, which formed the basis for the recognition of Alzheimer disease as the most common form of dementia in the elderly; (c) and perhaps the most important of all from the diagnostic point of view, the delineation of "normal-pressure hydrocephalus" by Adams and Hakim as a reversible cause of dementia. These advances were instrumental in focusing public attention on the predominant form of dementia, Alzheimer disease, and in creating recognition of the need for accurate differential diagnosis of the dementia syndrome in order to identify conditions that can be treated. A consensus statement on the importance of the diagnosis of reversible causes of dementia was developed by a work group sponsored by the National Institute on Aging (NIA) (103), and criteria for the diagnosis of Alzheimer disease were developed by a committee jointly sponsored by the National Institute of Neurological and Communicative Disorders and Stroke (NINCDS) and the Alzheimer Disease and Related Disorders Association (ADRDA)(100).

### Current Distinctions

*Definition of Dementia*

"Dementia" is the term used to describe the symptom complex of intellectual deterioration in the adult. This symptom complex may be caused by more than 70 disorders, and the most important of these is Alzheimer disease, which alone accounts for more than half of the cases. The term dementia had been used by physicians for many decades, but in 1952 the American Psychiatric Association (APA) in the first edition of its *Diagnostic and Statistical Manual of Mental Disorders* (*DSM*) did not include this term but, instead, introduced a new diagnostic term, "chronic organic brain syndrome" (2). The definition of the latter term included the requirement that the condition be progressive and irreversible. It becomes evident that many conditions that produced chronic symptoms of intellectual deterioration (e.g., normal-pressure hydrocephalus) were in fact reversible.

*Advantages Based on Phenomenology and Clear Criteria*

In 1980 the APA dropped the invented label "chronic organic brain syndrome" and reintroduced "dementia," defined in terms of observable clinical criteria (3). The criteria were based on clinical observation and judgment; no attempt was made to present specific operational criteria, e.g., scores on functional disability scales or mental status tests. Many clinicians who were not psychiatrists welcomed this approach, and the *DSM-III* definition has been widely accepted.

*Limitations*

### DSM-III

There are, however, limitations to the *DSM-III* diagnostic criteria. No definition exists of the degree of functional disability needed to qualify for the diagnosis of dementia, and there is not as yet a consensus among workers in the field as to the appropriate scale to be used in these early cases. The definition stipulates impairment in memory and in at least one other area of cognition. A small number of patients with dementing disorders have atypical presentations involving only a single area (e.g., language, visual perception, constructional ability, personality change, memory) for as long as 2 to 3 years, after which time more widespread involvement of cognitive functions becomes evident (24,68,102,112). Adherence to *DSM-III* criteria would unduly delay diagnosis in such patients. Another problem is the exclusion criteria, which tend to be recursive in *DSM-III*. Thus the *DSM-III* criteria for dementia require exclusion of such conditions as depression, but the criteria for depression in *DSM-III* require exclusion of dementia. The extent to which this problem with definition contributes to the frequent misdiagnosis of these two conditions has not been adequately explored. Finally, there is lack of agreement with the decision made in the formulation of *DSM-III* to separate the amnestic syndrome from dementia. The most common cause of the amnestic syndrome in the United States is Korsakoff's psychosis, which is related to thiamine deficiency and alcoholism. Patients with this disorder are included by many workers in their dementia series. Despite these limitations, however, experience indicates that diagnostic accuracy has been significantly advanced by the *DSM-III* definition of dementia.

*Comparison of DSM-III with alternative criteria for diagnosis of dementia*

Although the *DSM-III* criteria for diagnosis of dementia have had wide impact, several alternative diagnostic criteria have been proposed. Table 3 provides a direct comparison of these criteria. Included in this table are the *DSM-III* criteria (3), the ADRDA/NINCDS criteria (100), the NIA/AMA

TABLE 3. *Comparison of diagnostic criteria for dementia*

| Criteria | DSM-III[a] | ADRDA/ NINCDS[b] | NIA/AMA[c] | Jorm & Henderson[d] |
|---|---|---|---|---|
| Loss of intellectual abilities | R | R | R | R |
| Confirmed on mental status tests | | R | | R |
| Impaired social or occupational function | R | | | R |
| Memory impairment | R | R | R | R |
| Impairment of additional area of cognition (e.g., language, construction, praxis, or personality change) | R | + | R | + |
| State of consciousness not clouded—alert, awake | R | R | R | R |
| Evidence of organic factor or absence of conditions other than organic mental syndrome | R | | | R |

R = required. + = desirable/not required.
[a]American Psychiatric Association Task Force (3).
[b]McKhann et al. (100).
[c]Ref. 103.
[d]Ref. 59.

criteria (103), and the modification of *DSM-III* by Jorm and Henderson (59). All the 1980 and later definitions require evidence of loss of intellectual ability in a patient who is awake and alert; the ADRDA/NINCDS and the NIA/ AMA definitions do not require specific evidence of deterioration in social or occupational function, but the ADRDA/NINCDS stipulates that the intellectual dysfunction be demonstrable on a formal mental status test. Two of the sets of criteria require demonstration of memory impairment and impairment of another area of cognition; Jorm and Henderson accept either or both in this regard and hence make it possible to include the Korsakoff syndrome as a dementing disorder. Neither the ADRDA/NINCDS nor the NIA/AMA criteria require exclusion of other *DSM-III* diagnoses and therefore simplify the diagnosis of coincidental dementia and depression.

Comparison of the more recent sets of diagnostic criteria for dementia with the 1952 *DSM-I* criteria for "chronic organic brain syndrome," its designation for the dementia syndrome, reveals important differences. The *DSM-I* criteria (2) required the presence of irreversibility and chronicity, two criteria eliminated from current diagnostic approaches. The question of reversibility or irreversibility of dementia deserves comment. It has become evident that "irreversibility" is a term that may be appropriately applied to certain disorders but that its use reflects the state of ignorance of the medical profession at a given date; a condition that may be irreversible in the spring of 1987 might become reversible at a later time. There are many precedents. At the turn of the century general paresis, the form of dementia that occurred in neurosyphilis, was indeed irreversible. During the early 1900s the discovery that fever therapy would reverse many of the symptoms of this disorder was considered important enough to result in a Nobel prize; and when specific antibiotics were discovered, the entity essentially disappeared. The same story can be told for the dementia associated with pernicious anemia; when an intrinsic factor was discovered, the dementia suddenly moved from the category of irreversible to reversible; today with tests for blood levels of vitamin $B_{12}$ and with treatment with parenteral vitamin $B_{12}$ available, this disorder is among the most reversible.

Herpes simplex encephalitis, one of the most common of the viral encephalitides, only a few years ago was one of the most devastating; it is now treatable with antiviral agents if diagnosed promptly enough, and the symptoms are often reversible. Other major examples of dementias that can be reversed if diagnosed early enough include the dementia associated with normal-pressure hydrocephalus and with intracranial masses, e.g., subdural hematomas. As research progresses, it might be anticipated (or hoped) that presently irreversible conditions, e.g., Alzheimer disease, will become reversible. Moreover, it is feasible to suppose that treatments will be discovered that might reverse symptoms of dementia before the underlying condition is treatable (an example is the effect of L-DOPA in reversing the motor symptoms of Parkinson disease).

An important issue is the classification of confusional states associated with drug toxicity. In most instances such patients present acutely with some clouding of consciousness, and their condition is appropriately diagnosed as delirium. However, at times an older individual may show the typical symptoms of dementia without any clouding of consciousness; moreover, the cognitive changes may come on insidiously and continue for months as use of an apparently innocuous medication continues. Although this scenario may occur with drugs with known anticholinergic properties, it is also seen as an idiosyncratic response to beta blockers used to treat hypertension, to digitalis-related medicines, or to diazepam-related sleep medicines. Elderly individuals sometimes do not metabolize drugs in the time course expected, and consequently blood concentrations build up over days or weeks and lead to chronic symptoms. A misdiagnosis of Alzheimer disease may be made in individuals with such symptoms. Subsequent to the NIA/AMA task force on the reversible dementias, clinicians have been more aware of the possibility that drug toxicity may cause the symptoms of dementia. They are now more likely to recommend a therapeutic trial consisting in symptomatic elimination or replacement of each medication that might be at fault. In addition, such a procedure often reveals cases in which a medicine is not responsible by itself for the dementia symptoms but has added to the cognitive impairment, an instance of a treatable "excess disability."

## Problem Areas

### Depression and dementia

An important diagnostic problem area is the differentiation of depression and dementia. The significance of the role of depression in the misdiagnosis of dementia was brought to the fore by the study of Ron et al. (122). This study was of particular interest because it was carried out at Maudsley Hospital, the premiere pyschiatric hospital in London. These investigators reported that on a 4-year follow-up 31% of the patients who had been diagnosed between 1963 and 1972 as having presenile dementia were in fact misdiagnosed and that the most common misdiagnosis occurred in patients who were depressed and had associated memory complaints. Subsequent series (Table 4) appeared to confirm the frequency of misdiagnosis.

The relation of depression and dementia is a complex one. Individuals with typical manic-depressive disorders (bipolar affective disorder) or recurrent depressions (unipolar affective disorder) may, with aging, develop memory and other cognitive changes in association with their affective disorder. Folstein et al. (37) reported that aggressive treatment of the depression (often with electroconvulsive therapy) in such patients resulted in improvement of

TABLE 4. *Diagnosis of dementia syndrome: misclassification based on follow-up studies*

| Study | Total No. | Original diagnosis | | Outcome diagnosis | | Misclass- ification | |
|---|---|---|---|---|---|---|---|
| | | Demented | Non- demented | Demented | Non- demented | No. | % |
| Kendell, 1974 (74) | 98 | 98 | 0 | 75 | 23 | 16 | 23 |
| Ron et al., 1979 (122) | 51 | 51 | 0 | 35 | 16 | 16 | 31 |
| Smith & Kiloh, 1981 (130) | 200 | 200 | 0 | 164 | 36 | 36 | 18 |
| Rabins, 1981 (114) | 41 | 41 | 0 | 37 | 4 | 4 | 10 |
| Reding et al., 1984 (118) | 56 | 56 | 0 | 55 | 1 | 1 | < 2 |
| Larson et al., 1985 (85) | 200 | 200 | 0 | 198 | 2 | 2 | 1 |

cognition. These investigators found that a history of depression, a subacute onset, and typical depressive vegetative signs and self-reports of depressed mood identified these patients. Rabins et al. (115) have reported a 2-year follow-up of patients meeting these criteria showing continued improvement in memory and cognition, confirming the initial diagnosis of depression.

Depression presenting as dementia has been called "pseudodementia" by Kiloh (77), a term that has been considered inappropriate by other authors (e.g., 89,119). Folstein and McHugh (36) suggested that "dementia in depression" was a more appropriate term. Depression and dementia may coexist, and in such patients treatment of depression may alleviate the affective symptoms without altering the dementing process (30,119).

The relation of dementia and depression may be even more complex. McCallister and Price (97), Kral (81), and Reding et al. (117) have identified patients who initially met criteria for "pseudodementia" and later developed a frank dementia. There are several possible explanations. Perhaps dementia presents as depression in some patients, a conclusion endorsed by Reding et al. (117); or the diagnostic criteria for dementia used in their clinic were too strict. In favor of this possibility is the fact that a relatively insensitive mental status test, the Mental Status Questionnaire (MSQ), was in routine use. Alternatively, perhaps the biological bases of depression and dementia are entwined in a manner not presently understood. The apparently complex relation of depression and dementia has been explored in a useful editorial by Mahendra (90) who pointed out the "considerable challenge to his [the diagnostician's] prowess." Clearly we are faced with a limitation in our understanding of the relations between these two conditions, a limitation that hinders our ability to make accurate diagnoses and that may lead to significant errors in predictions.

*Normal age changes and dementia*

The definition of the boundary between normal changes and dementia is the most difficult and perhaps insurmountable aspect of the diagnosis of dementia. On the one hand, changes in memory often accompany normal aging, an aspect that has been extensively studied by psychologists [see review by Katzman and Terry (71)]. On the other hand, the onset of certain of the dementias, particularly Alzheimer disease, is insidious. At the time of the first clinical examination, family members may disagree among themselves whether the first changes occurred 6 months or 3 years earlier. Kral and Muller (80,82) used the term "benign senescent forgetfulness" to describe individuals with memory changes who were still functional, but there is evidence that such memory changes are not always benign. In patients with mild cognitive changes one cannot make an exact diagnosis even with the best neuropsychological tests available; only the likelihood of developing dementia can be estimated. In a prospective study of 488 volunteers, age 75 to 85 years, who were nondemented on initial examination, approximately 50 developed an unequivocal dementia over a 3-year period (R. Katzman et al., *unpublished:* Bronx Aging Study). Extensive neuropsychological tests had been carried out annually; the best predictor of dementia was the score on the Blessed mental status test. Subjects who initially made 0 to 2 errors (of 33 possible errors) on this mental status examination developed dementia at a rate of less than 1% per year; those who made 5 to 8 errors developed dementia at a rate of more than 10% per year, but only one-third of those who made 5 to 8 errors have developed dementia as yet. The latter subset of subjects may be best described as an "at risk" group.

## Dementia and delirium

Delirium is a traditional medical term that was introduced as a diagnostic category by *DSM-III*. Delirium is a symptom complex used to describe global intellectual impairment associated with a clouded state of awareness. This syndrome was called "acute brain syndrome" in *DMS-I*. This phrase encompassed other terms, such as "acute confusional state," "toxic psychosis," and "metabolic encephalopathy." As indicated by these descriptions, delirium is often associated with metabolic or toxic conditions and most often is acute in onset and short in duration, but these features are not necessary criteria. Memory, orientation, and other cognitive areas are involved, and mental status tests are abnormal; the condition is differentiated from dementia on the basis of a fluctuating level of awareness. Delirium can accompany a high fever, pneumonia, cardiac failure, alcohol intake, alcohol withdrawal, high doses of psychoactive medications, and liver or kidney failure—in fact a wide spectrum of systemic, metabolic, and toxic disorders. Although focal intracranial processes (e.g., stroke) usually present with focal features (e.g., hemiparesis), such disorders may also be accompanied by delirium. Thus delirium often represents a medical emergency and is most often diagnosed in emergency rooms; the treatment of the delirium is the treatment of the causative condition. Therefore in most instances delirium is easily differentiated from dementia.

There are two instances in which a diagnostic problem may arise. Although delirium can occur in a person at any age if the metabolic insult is sufficiently great, it occurs more often in older patients and in those with preexisting dementia, perhaps because there is less "cerebral reserve." If delirium due to an intercurrent infection occurs in a patient with an undiagnosed dementia, for example, there may be temporary diagnostic difficulty until the two conditions are sorted out. A second situation in which there is diagnostic difficulty occurs when the delirium is due to chronic exposure to a toxic source; for example, an older patient does not metabolize adequately a sleeping medication, the level of which then builds up, leading to a persistent daytime confusional state. In such situations delirium is not short-lived if the patient takes the medication on a regular basis. In this particular instance it is not critical whether the label is delirium or dementia so long as the physician recognizes the cause and takes the patient off the precipitating medicine.

### Validity of diagnostic series

When is the diagnosis of dementia to be considered correct? The difficulty in differentiating dementia and depression raises the question of what criteria for the validity of the diagnosis of dementia can be used. In the extensive literature on the diagnosis of dementia three implicit criteria have been employed. The first might be called the "authoritative opinion": A patient is referred to an academic center where an extensive examination is carried out and, often after a group discussion, a diagnosis is made. If this diagnosis differs from that of the referring or primary care physician, an error in the latter's diagnosis is assumed. Thus the initial series of Marsden and Harrison (92), Garcia et al. (45), and others are based on a thorough but one-time evaluation. The problem with this approach has been demonstrated by the work of Reding et al. (118), described above, who found that half the patients reported by Garcia et al. (45) as examples of "pseudodementia" later developed frank dementia.

A second approach is to base diagnosis on a 1- to many-year follow-up. Most dementing illnesses progress. As a dementia progresses and cognitive loss becomes more evident, there is less uncertainty of diagnosis. If after several years cognitive impairment has not progressed or has improved, the diagnosis of dementia can be questioned. This follow-up strategy was used, for example, by Reding et al. (117,118), Lijtmaer et al. (87), and others. Diagnosis by follow-up is clearly valid in terms of the question of whether dementia is present when the cognitive state has clearly gotten significantly better or worse. However, this approach must be used cautiously in patients whose deficit has remained static, because a subset of Alzheimer patients have periods of 2 years or more during which their disease does not progress, a so-called plateau period.

The greatest validity would be achieved if the clinical diagnoses were compared to predicted cerebral biopsy or autopsy diagnoses. Such comparisons are at present available only for a subset of dementia patients who have met research diagnostic criteria for Alzheimer disease.

### Tools/Technologies/Strategies to Improve Diagnosis of Dementia

The *DSM-III* diagnosis of dementia requires evidence of both cognitive and functional loss, although cognitive loss alone satisfies other criteria (Table 3). Both forms of impairment may become readily apparent when the history is first taken. Intellectual changes involving several areas of cognition may be described, including repetitiousness, forgetting names and appointments, losing a chain of thought, difficulty finding the right word, losing one's way, and losing objects. These symptoms are experienced occasionally by normal individuals but are exaggerated in dementia. Functional impairment may present as poor performance on the job, difficulty managing the household, or withdrawal from hobbies or social activities; the most sensitive indicator of change in cognitive performance is often difficulty coping with fiscal affairs, e.g., the checkbook or tax form.

However, such symptoms may not be readily apparent early in the course of a dementia. Social conversation may be normal. The physician may not become aware of impairment during the usual course of history taking. However, impairment becomes evident if specific probing of mental status is undertaken. Medical students are taught to do a mental status examination. This area is reinforced during specialty training of neurologists, psychiatrists, and geriatricians. In practice, many primary care physicians do not routinely carry out an adequate mental status examination, and specialists may put it aside if another complaint appears dominant. For example, McCartney and Palmateer (98) found that mental status examinations had been carried out on only 4 of 165 patients over the age of 65 admitted to the general medical services of a major teaching hospital. As a consequence, 50 patients with cognitive impairment were missed. Other instances of significant underdiagnosis of cognitive impairment have been found not only in general medical settings but also on neurologic (35), psychiatric (54), and rehabilitation (45) services, where such mistakes might not have been anticipated.

Thus the mental status examination remains the key to the diagnosis of dementia. The mental status examination as currently used was developed over decades of experience. Mayer-Gross and Guttmann (94,95) and other European psychiatrists were interested in identifying aspects of examination that distinguished generalized affections of the brain (i.e., dementia and delirium) from local disorders (e.g., aphasias or language disorders produced by strokes or tumors localized to the temporal lobe of the dominant hemisphere). After Mayer-Gross migrated to Great Britain during the 1930s, several of his British students (Roth among them) began to formulate specific test items to formalize the mental status examination; a large number of individual items were subsequently examined in terms of their specificity (126), and following these studies items were combined to develop effective instruments. The two mental status tests now in widest use are the information-concentration-orientation test of Blessed et al. (16) and the Mini-Mental State (MMS) examination of Folstein et al. (37). The test of Blessed et al. is the most sensitive (two test items—the memory phrase and the months of the year backward—are more difficult than items on other tests) and therefore of greatest use in very early cases; it has the added advantage that it has been validated in two autopsy series, with the error score on the test correlating with a quantitative measure of pathology, i.e., the number of neuritic plaques per microscopic field in cases of Alzheimer disease

(16,70). The Blessed et al. test, however, is entirely verbal and measures recent and past memory, orientation, and concentration. The Mini-Mental State examination of Folstein et al. is broader in that it also tests language, writing, and drawing. These two tests have been brought together in a combined instrument that is being systematically tested. The Mental Status Questionnaire (60) is contained within this combined test and can be scored separately. This combined test may be useful as a public health tool; it is, however, inappropriate to use this test with individuals who are mentally retarded or who have had a poor educational background. Also the tests are not appropriate for persons who are not fluent in English and for persons with different cultural backgrounds. Alternative tests need to be developed for such groups.

The use of other diagnostic tools in the differentiation of dementia and the differential diagnosis of dementia and depression has been suggested. Thus Ron et al. (122) in their retrospective follow-up study found that both slowing on the electroencephalogram (EEG) and neuropsychological test scores (the difference between WAIS verbal and performance scores) helped differentiate patients with presenile dementia from those whose cognitive impairment was attributed to depression. The dexamethasone test has not been found useful in differentiating dementia and depression (6,18,63,99).

Some physicians implicitly use the presence of atrophy on computed tomography (CT) scans as a criterion of dementia. Such use of CT is inappropriate. Dementia is a clinical syndrome that can be present in patients without atrophy on CT. Although cerebral atrophy is a common characteristic of Alzheimer disease, some Alzheimer patients do not have evidence of atrophy on CT; conversely, many individuals during normal aging show a moderate degree of atrophy; consequently, the Alzheimer process and normal aging overlap in this regard, although group differences are real. However, in patients under age 60 significant atrophy on CT may be a useful indicator of a dementing process.

## Misdiagnosis of Dementia

### Diagnostic errors in general medical settings

*Underdiagnosis* of cognitive impairment occurs in general medical settings in situations where the cognitive impairment is not the presenting complaint. Cognitive impairment (both dementia and delirium) was found in more than one-fourth of the general medical inpatients at The Johns Hopkins Medical Institutions but had not been recognized by staff in most of these patients (78); similar results were found on a neurology service (29) and in a rehabilitation hospital (45) (Table 4). Underdiagnosis in these series occurs because of failure by the physicians to carry out systematic mental status examinations.

*Diagnostic errors in specialized medical settings*

Underdiagnosis also occurs in the setting of specialized dementia clinics. Kral (81) reported a 4- to 18-year follow-up of 22 patients with an initial diagnosis of pseudodementia. Twenty of these 22 patients had gone on to develop progressive dementia of the Alzheimer type. It might be argued that the diagnostic criteria (pre-*DSM-III*) initially used in this study were inadequate. Reding et al. (117) reported similar results in a 2-year follow-up of a series of patients in whom diagnoses had been based on the *DSM-III* criteria. Thirty-one of the 225 subjects referred to their dementia clinic were initially diagnosed as having depression rather than dementia. On follow-up, however, 16 of the patients diagnosed as depressed and nondemented went on to develop frank dementia. The diagnoses in these 16 patients included Alzheimer-type dementia, multi-infarct state, Parkinson disease, progressive supranuclear palsy, and spinocerebellar disorders.

In contrast, *overdiagnosis* of dementia in patients referred to dementia clinics or referral practices has been reported to range from 10 to 50% (44). An example is the report of Hoffman (54), which indicates that the diagnosis of dementia was changed in 40% of the patients admitted to a medical-psychiatric inpatient service, and that in two-thirds of those with an altered diagnosis a reversible condition was found. It is important to note, however, whether the report of misdiagnosis is based simply on a single evaluation—no matter how complete—or on follow-up, as there is a significant error rate in the former group. It is also important to recognize that the nature of the patient referrals in these reports leads automatically to over- rather than to underdiagnosis errors because the patient had been referred for suspected dementia. Examples of overdiagnosis reported in series in which follow-up ascertainment has been used are shown in Table 4. It is striking that the rate of overdiagnosis has fallen dramatically in the two most recent series, both begun after *DSM-III* criteria became available.

## ACCURACY OF DIFFERENTIAL DIAGNOSIS OF DEMENTING DISORDERS

### Diseases that Present as Dementia

*Clinical and Pathological Series*

A number of published studies have reported the frequency of various disorders in patients presenting with the dementia syndrome. Several of these clinical series are summarized in Table 5; pathological series are in Table 6. Diagnoses on more than 700 clinical cases and 1,100 pathological cases are presented in these tables. In both clinical and pathological series, Alzheimer disease (or a synonymous diagnosis such as degenerative dementia) accounts

TABLE 5. *Disorders producing dementia: diagnoses in nine clinical series*[a]

| Diagnosis | No. | % |
|---|---|---|
| *Alzheimer* | 499 | |
|   + Parkinson | 10 | |
|   + Vascular | 8 | |
| Total | 517 | 65.9 |
| *Other irreversible dementias* | | |
|   Vascular (MID)[b] | 85 | |
|   Parkinson | 10 | |
|   Huntington | 15 | |
|   Progressive supranuclear palsy | 3 | |
|   Amyotropic lateral sclerosis | 1 | |
|   Kufs disease | 1 | |
|   Postanoxic/CO | 5 | |
|   Posttraumatic | 8 | |
|   Postencephalitic | 3 | |
|   Creutzfeldt-Jakob | 3 | |
| Total | 134 | 17.1 |
| *Treatable dementias* | | |
|   Neurosyphilis | 2 | |
|   Fungal infections | 2 | |
|   Tumor | 22 | |
|   Alcohol | 22 | |
|   Subdural | 4 | |
|   Hydrocephalus | 27 | |
|   Epilepsy | 3 | |
| Total | 82 | 10.5 |
| *Reversible dementias* | | |
|   Drug toxicity | 21 | |
|   Metabolic | 16 | |
|     Hepatic | 1 | |
|     Hyponatremia | 1 | |
|     Calcium/PTH | 4 | |
|     Vitamin $B_{12}$ | 2 | |
|     Thyroid | 7 | |
|     Hypoglycemia | 1 | |
| Total | 37 | 4.7 |
| *Cause uncertain* | 14 | 1.8 |
| *Total No.* | 784 | 100 |

[a]Series include studies by Marsden and Harrison (92), Freeman and Rudd (39), Coblentz et al. (21), Smith and Kiloh (130), Rabins (114), Delaney (28), Garcia et al. (44), Larson et al. (85), and Katzman et al. (*unpublished*).
[b]Multi-infarct dementia.

TABLE 6. *Pathological diagnoses in dementia*

| Diagnosis | Age < 70 years | | Age > 70 years | |
|---|---|---|---|---|
| | No. | % | No. | % |
| Alzheimer atrophy | 73 | 44.8 | 502 | 52.7 |
| Vascular | 25 | 15.4 | 214 | 22.5 |
| Mixed vascular/Alzheimer | 1 | 0.6 | 148 | 15.2 |
| Pick | 15 | 9.2 | 8 | 0.8 |
| Parkinson | 3 | 1.8 | 10 | 1.0 |
| Olivo-ponto-cerebellar | 3 | 1.8 | 1 | 0.1 |
| Wernicke encephalopathy | 6 | 3.7 | 6 | 0.6 |
| Postanoxic | — | | 2 | 0.2 |
| Posttraumatic | — | | 5 | 0.5 |
| Hydrocephalus | 9 | 5.5 | 5 | 0.5 |
| Tumor | 14 | 8.6 | 34 | 3.5 |
| Creutzfeldt-Jakob | 5 | 3.1 | 4 | 0.4 |
| Inflammatory (MS/general paresis) | 9 | 5.5 | 6 | 0.6 |
| Unclassified or normal | — | | 8 | 0.8 |
| Total No. | 163 | | 953 | |

Data from Jellinger (58), Tomlinson (139), and R. Terry (*personal communication,* 1985).

for more than half of the cases. The clinical and pathological series diverge, however, in several aspects: Clinical series report cases of toxic and metabolic dementias; these causes are not associated with diagnostic histologic changes and hence are not included in the pathological series. Pathological series include a much higher percentage of vascular dementia than do most clinical series. This increase probably represents the sampling biases inherent in clinical series in which patients had been evaluated in a geriatric or dementia clinic or in a geriatric hospital. Thus patients who develop overt strokes may have been treated in an acute care hospital and not sent to a dementia referral center. In support of this assumption is the fact that clinical studies based on community sampling include a higher proportion of cases of vascular dementia [(35); R. Katzman et al., *unpublished:* Bronx Aging Study]. Not all disorders that have been reported to present as dementia (53,67,69) appear in published series. This finding reflects both the relative infrequency of some of the disorders and the sampling bias that has occurred. Thus both factors may explain why dementia pugilistica (punch drunk syndrome) is not included in any of the published series. Series are gathered over years, and therefore newly discovered entities (e.g., AIDS virus encephalopathy, which may become the third most common cause of dementia within the next 3 years) are not yet found in available series.

*Age Versus Frequency of Disorders that Produce Dementia*

An important factor that must be taken into account in regard to the relative frequency of disorders that produce dementia is age. This factor significantly affects the public health consequences of misdiagnosis. The incidence and prevalence of Alzheimer disease increase exponentially with age at least to age 85. The incidence and prevalence of stroke also increase with age in an exponential fashion (66,83). In contrast, other disorders that produce dementia may be age-independent or peak during middle age (Table 6). Huntington disease is one obvious example. An important reversible dementia that peaks during middle age is normal-pressure hydrocephalus (perhaps better called adult communicating hydrocephalus). In a review Katzman (65) noted that most reported cases were in individuals in their fifties and sixties. An autopsy series of dementia patients reported by Jellinger (58) confirmed that most hydrocephalus patients were under age 70, accounting for 5% of dementia cases under age 70 and only 0.3% of cases over age 70. However, these "treatable" conditions do occur in persons whose first symptoms occur past the age of 75, as shown in the Bronx Aging Study (described above) in which one case of hydrocephalus and one of brain tumor (glioma) were among the first 35 cases of dementia to develop.

**Components of Diagnostic Work-up**

*Current Work-up; Technical Limits: Risks, Benefits, Costs (1986)*

*Clinical evaluation*

The clinical evaluation, i.e., history, mental status, and physical and neurological examinations, is central to the diagnosis of dementia and to the differential diagnosis of dementing illness. There is considerable variation as to how this clinical examination is carried out. Thus at one extreme, in a dementia clinic associated with a geriatric evaluation clinic and supported in part by a state grant, each patient is seen by an internist, neurologist, and psychiatrist; mental status tests and a neuropsychological battery are administered by a neuropsychologist; a nurse practitioner visits the home; a CT scan, blood tests, and other procedures needed are carried out; and a diagnosis is made at a consensus conference. At the other extreme, some patient families report that they have been told that their relative has Alzheimer disease by a busy practitioner, based apparently on a 10-min examination and a CT scan. There is evidence that the first type of evaluation can result in a high level of accuracy in diagnosis, as shown by the autopsy follow-up of Larson et al. (85), described below. The cost of such an evaluation in one specialized clinic that accepts Medicare reimbursement is $644 for the clinical and psychiatric evaluations and $718 for the laboratory tests, for a total of $1,362.

It is important to point out the impact of current federal policy on the work-up of a dementia patient. The combination of a complete history and physical and neurological examinations with, for example, a mental status examination (at a minimum the combined Blessed and MMS), and a discussion of the problem with the family takes at least 1 hr 15 min by an experienced physician. Current Medicare payment does not provide reimbursement for the additional time spent on a dementia patient, time that is almost certainly the most cost-effective part of the entire work-up.

*CT scan*

The CT scan is universally accepted as an essential component of the diagnostic work-up. It is required for the diagnosis of hydrocephalus and mass lesions in the brain, including brain tumors and subdural hematomas. Dementia secondary to hydrocephalus and subdural hematoma can be arrested and sometimes reversed by prompt intervention; occasional benign brain tumors (e.g., pituitary adenomas, meningiomas) can be removed and symptoms arrested or reversed; other brain tumors, such as astrocytomas and microgliomas (primary brain reticulum cell sarcomas), may be usefully treated. Typical patterns of atrophy are sometimes diagnostic of Huntington disease and Pick disease. The CT scan of Binswanger disease is also characteristic (124). Although generalized cortical atrophy is not in itself diagnostic of Alzheimer disease, the loss of tissue measured by combining cortical atrophy and ventricular enlargement is a useful adjunct in diagnosis (42). The cost of a noncontrast CT scan varies from about $225 to about $450 in different localities and with scanners of different resolution; we use a figure of $341 for our estimates. The advantages of high-resolution scans include their capacity for identifying many vascular lesions, infarcts, and white matter changes that are missed on lower-resolution scans.

*Blood tests—systemic and metabolic disorders*

Although systemic and metabolic disorders account for only 1% of patients presenting with symptoms of dementia, their identification is critical because progression of cognitive impairment can be arrested and sometimes function restored by treatment. Automated analytical systems make it possible to obtain 18 to 20 blood chemistries for less than $10, and a complete blood count adds only a few dollars. Unfortunately, tests of thyroid function, serum vitamin $B_{12}$ and folate levels, and syphilis detection are not included in available automated runs, and their addition increases the cost to about $80. HTLV III antibody tests would increase the costs further. A modest federal effort to reward development of automation of these tests would be a cost-effective expenditure.

*Chest radiograph and electrocardiogram*

The chest x-ray film and electrocardiogram (ECG) are traditional parts of the routine annual examination and are included in most work-ups for dementia. There are no studies justifying their cost-effectiveness as part of the dementia work-up, but information as to the presence of a tumor or infection in the lung or if there has been a silent myocardial infarct is often useful. The cost for these two procedures varies; current Medicare reimbursement levels in California are $84 and $53 for chest radiograph and ECG, respectively.

*EEG*

The EEG reflects the activity of the cerebral cortex and might be assumed to be a useful diagnostic tool. In patients with Alzheimer disease and other forms of dementia, the typical 8- to 12-Hz occipital alpha rhythm may slow in frequency and disappear and the slower 4- to 7-Hz theta rhythm become predominant. Ron et al. (122) found that the EEG did help discriminate between dementia and depression. The EEG is of specific use in a small subset of patients in whom cognitive impairment is the expression of seizure activity, particularly temporal lobe seizures, and in patients with Creutzfeldt-Jakob disease, who may develop a striking periodic rhythm. Although such patients constitute fewer than 1% of the dementia patients, the condition is treatable and would justify the cost. The cost of an EEG varies from $100 to $160.

*Neuropsychological evaluation*

The neuropsychological evaluation is not universally recommended as an essential part of the dementia work-up and its cost-effectiveness has not been determined. Many investigators, however, find neuropsychological testing to be useful in confirming the presence of dementia and in identifying in a semiquantitative fashion the kinds of impaired function. It is valuable in distinguishing between dementia and depression (e.g., 122) and between so-called cortical dementia (e.g., Alzheimer disease) and subcortical dementias (e.g., progressive supranuclear palsy) (25). Additionally, neuropsychological evaluation provides a precise way to follow changes in cognition. Neuropsychological evaluations often take a number of hours and hence are labor-intensive. Costs range up to $500. Medicare reimbursement, however, is limited to about $200.

The tests listed above constitute the core of the dementia work-up. These tests are essentially risk-free; the small amount of x-ray exposure resulting from the CT and chest radiograph has little effect in the older patient. Several other tests, described below, may be needed in special circumstances.

*Lumbar puncture*

Lumbar puncture (LP) with analysis of the cerebrospinal fluid (CSF) had been traditionally included in the routine dementia work-up and is needed to diagnose such treatable causes of dementia as neurosyphilis and chronic fungal meningitis. Infectious etiologies of dementia, however, have been found to be uncommon. In a retrospective study of the results of lumbar puncture in 402 patients hospitalized in two major teaching hospitals for the evaluation of dementia, four patients with central nervous system infections were found, two with fungus infections (due to *Cryptococcus*), one with tuberculosis, and one with *Staphylococcus* infection (9). In all these patients there was a subacute onset of a change in mental status, and all had either fever or signs of meningeal irritation (i.e., a stiff neck). The authors concluded that, in the absence of such signs, "LP and CSF analysis should not be part of the routine evaluation of patients with dementia." A new category of patients in whom LP is needed are those with cognitive changes who have AIDS because the dementia in AIDS can be due to either coincident opportunistic infections or primary AIDS virus infection; the presence of the virus can now be demonstrated in CSF. The risk associated with an LP is the post-LP headache which, however, is less frequent in older patients. Post-LP infection is a theoretical risk but is not seen in routine practice. The cost of CSF analysis is about $70.

*Tests of CSF circulation*

In patients in whom the CT scan suggests the presence of hydrocephalus, special procedures such as isotope cisternography or infusion test may be necessary before surgical shunting. In patients with suspected vascular dementia a search for etiology, e.g., carotid artery or cardiac sources of embolization, is often carried out. Although this practice is accepted and rational, its diagnostic value has not been adequately studied (e.g., 113).

There are several tests which measure functions that are altered in dementia but that are not diagnostic; these tests can be considered to be of research interest but have no proved value in the clinical diagnosis of dementia. They include measurements of cerebral blood flow with the xenon inhalation technique and measurements of evoked potentials.

## Cerebral Biopsy

At the present time and in the absence of specific biochemical markers, the definitive diagnosis of Alzheimer disease, Pick disease, and Creutzfeldt-Jakob disease depends on confirmation by microscopic examination of the presence of characteristic changes in neurons of the cerebral cortex: in the case of Alzheimer disease, the presence of abnormal foci of degenerating nerve endings, termed a neuritic plaque, and the presence of neurofibrillary tangles, abnormal nerve cells containing accumulations of submicroscopic fibrils; in the case of Pick disease, abnormal inclusions in neurons, termed Pick bodies; in the case of Creutzfeldt-Jakob disease, the spongy appearance of the cortex resulting from a particular pattern of nerve cell dropout and gliosis. Thus during life one can achieve a definitive diagnosis for these conditions only by the use of cerebral biopsy, i.e., by the surgical removal of a small piece of cerebral cortex with subsequent histological examination supplemented by electron microscopic examination and biochemical and virological studies. In addition to its critical role in diagnosis, cerebral biopsy has played a central role in advancing the understanding of these diseases. The classical electron microscopic Alzheimer disease studies by Terry and co-workers (134,135) and Kidd (76) depended on the availability of brain biopsy; the studies of Bowen et al. (17) demonstrating the involvement of the cholinergic system during the first year of symptoms in Alzheimer disease depended on the availability of biopsy specimens; the demonstration that Creutzfeldt-Jakob disease is transmissible to chimpanzees primarily, but not exclusively, involved implantation of biopsy specimens into chimpanzee brain. Yet the cerebral biopsy procedure is used in much fewer than 1% of dementia patients in the United States, although it is used more commonly in Great Britain. Is this conservative approach justified by the risks of biopsy? How frequently do biopsies give unequivocal answers?

There are two surgical approaches to brain biopsy: (a) Open surgery with removal of a piece of cerebral cortex under direct visualization. If the presentation is that of a diffuse disease, the biopsy is carried out in the right frontal lobe (in right-handed patients) as there is no apparent neurological defect that results from removal of a small amount of cortex in this "silent" area. (b) Needle biopsy under stereotactic or CT guidance. In the first procedure a 1-cm$^3$ block of tissue is removed; in the second a small core of tissue the diameter of a needle is removed. In practice, the first procedure is used when disease of the cerebral cortex, e.g., the dementias, is present because this procedure preserves the architecture of the cortex, which may be important in diagnosis; in addition, the gram of tissue usually removed makes it possible to carry out special staining procedures needed for diagnosis of dementias and illnesses (e.g., silver or thioflavin stains for neurofibrillary tangles); also this amount of tissue permits biochemical analysis (e.g., for markers of the cholinergic system) and immunohistochemistry to be carried out, thereby increasing the chance of specific diagnosis. In practice, the second procedure is used if a lesion is deep to the cortex, particularly if it is a suspected tumor or inflammatory lesion. Needle biopsies have been used extensively to confirm the diagnosis of herpes encephalitis, which affects the medial temporal region. This condition is the only one that regularly presents with mental status changes in which needle biopsy is performed.

Needle biopsies were seldom carried out for diagnostic purposes in subjects with symptoms of diffuse cerebral disease prior to the availability of antibiotics. Cerebral biopsy, however, came into use, particularly in Europe, during the late 1950s and early 1960s. We have been able to identify 11 series (Table 7) with diagnostic and/or risk data encompassing 587 patients. Most of the patients reported were children in whom diagnoses of recessive metabolic disorder (e.g., Tay-Sachs disease) was sought. Because most of the recessive metabolic disorders can now be diagnosed using skin cultures or other peripheral tissues, such biopsies are not so common today. There are four series (132 cases) that focus on adult patients with symptoms of dementia.

*Diagnostic accuracy*

In the five general series (encompassing 419 patients, predominantly children), cerebral biopsy yielded a specific diagnosis in 40.0%; 34.5% of the biopsies were abnormal but not diagnostic, and 25.5% were normal [(4,14, 32,48); all were summarized by Blackwood (13) and Kaufman and Catalano (72)]. Autopsy data were reported in 46 cases. In the autopsied cases all specific diagnoses were confirmed (26 cases); two of four cases reported as normal on biopsy were found to be normal at autopsy; in one case there was an active meningoencephalitis that had been missed and in the other case cerebellar atrophy. The significant problem was the 16 cases in which biopsies were abnormal but not specific. At autopsy, four continued to show nonspecific findings, and there was one case of white matter (Schilder) disease. Tumors were present in five cases, all of which were seen pre-CT scan and probably would be diagnosed by imaging. There were also four cases with diffuse diseases not diagnosed on biopsy, including two cases of lipidosis and two of Creutzfeldt-Jakob disease. Hence in terms of specific diffuse diseases, there were no false positives, but there were 5 of 46, or about 11%, false negatives and another 10% without specific diagnoses even at autopsy.

Directly pertinent to the question of the usefulness of cerebral biopsy in patients with dementia are the four series that concentrated on such cases. Green et al. (46) reported the results of biopsies of 15 patients with presenile dementia. There were 7 cases of Alzheimer disease, 1 case of Pick disease, and 7 cases showing nonspecific changes. In the series of 59 biopsies in patients with presenile dementia reported by Smith et al. (131), there were 34 cases of Alzheimer, 1 combined case of Alzheimer and Pick, 2 Pick, 2 vascular, 2 chronic meningoencephalitis, and 1 Creutzfeldt-Jakob. Seventeen (29%) biopsies showed no specific changes. Bowen et al. (17) reported 36 brain biopsy samples; Alzheimer disease accounted for 23, Creutzfeldt-Jakob disease for 1, vascular disease for 2, leukodystrophy for 1, and microglioma for 1; 8 cases had no diagnostic changes. A 23-case series of Katzman and associates (21,24,61, 79) included 11 Alzheimer, 1 Pick, 2 microinfarcts, 1 normal-pressure hydrocephalus with meningeal thickening, 2 Creutzfeldt-Jakob, 1 chronic meningitis, 1 vasculitis, and 4 nonspecific. We are aware of eight autopsies; six confirmed specific diagnoses. One of the patients who had nonspecific changes on biopsy turned out to have motor neuron disease on autopsy; the other had a

TABLE 7. *Diagnostic cerebral biopsies*

| Studies | No. of cases | Diagnostic | Abnormal but not diagnostic | No specific changes | Deaths | Morbidity |
|---|---|---|---|---|---|---|
| General series | | | | | | |
| Antunes (4) | 28 | 15 | 6 | 7 | | |
| Eadie (32) | 50 | 15 | 14 | 21 | | |
| Blackwood & Cumings (14) | 178 | 77 | 66 | 35 | 0 | 0 |
| Groves & Møller (48) | 117 | 44 | 37 | 36 | 1[a] | 1[b] |
| Kaufman & Catalano (72) | 46 | 17 | 22 | 7 | 1[c] | 5[d] |
| Total No. | 419 | 168 | 145 | 106 | | |
| % | | 40 | 34.5 | 25.5 | | |
| Dementia series | | | | | | |
| Green et al. (46) | 15 | 8 | | 7 | 0 | 1[e] |
| Smith et al. (131) | 59 | 42 | | 17 | 1[f] | 0 |
| Bowen et al. (17) | 36 | 28 | | 8 | —[g] | —[g] |
| Katzman et al.[h] | 23 | 19 | | 4 | 0 | 2 |
| Fox et al. (38) | 11 | 11 | | — | 0 | 0 |
| Neary et al. (104) | 24 | 18 | | 6 | 0 | 1 |
| Total | 168 | 126 | | 42 | 1 | 4 |
| % | | 75 | | 25 | | |

[a]Cardiac arrest, 15 months.
[b]Hemiparesis, cleared.
[c]Aspiration.
[d]Three pneumonia, one pulmonary embolus, one focal epilepsy.
[e]Postoperative.
[f]Subdural hematoma with pneumonia.
[g]No report.
[h]Update and series. Also Coblentz et al. (21), Kaplan et al. (61), Crystal et al. (24), and Koto et al. (79).

lacunar state. Thus in the earlier series of Green et al. (46) and Smith et al. (131), 24 of 74 biopsies were nonspecific and failed to provide a diagnosis. In contrast, in the series of Bowen et al. and Katzman et al. the number of nondiagnostic biopsies fell to 21%. This drop may be attributed in part to the improved diagnosis of subcortical diseases by use of modern imaging methods and in part to improved understanding of diseases that produce dementia. Specifically the changes in the brain characteristic of Creutzfeldt-Jakob disease were not yet appreciated at the time of the Green et al. and Smith et al. series, nor had the syndromes of normal-pressure hydrocephalus and multi-infarct dementia been defined at the time of those two series. Overall, however, in these four series 73% of the biopsies gave a specific diagnosis.

## Risks of biopsy

Risk data are not available for the important biopsy series of Bowen et al. (17). Data are, however, available for six series that include 437 cases. These data are heavily skewed by the Blackwood and Cumings (14) series of 178 biopsies; these authors stated: "There has been no evidence at all that the patients have suffered in any way. There was neither immediate clinical deterioration nor was there post-operative death in any case. There was no evidence of post-operative epilepsy or haemorrhage, or infection." Perhaps this salutary experience explains why biopsies are more readily carried out in Great Britain. In the remaining 259 cases [series of Green et al. (46), Groves and Møller (48), Smith et al. (131), Kaufman and Catalano (72), and Katzman et al.] (Table 7) there were three postoperative deaths (two associated with postoperative hemorrhage, one a cardiac arrest in a 15-month-old who also underwent ventriculography), and there were 10 instances of morbidity, none resulting in permanent neurological deficit. Among the entire 437 cases the overall mortality was 0.75% and the morbidity 2%. If one considers only the three dementia series included, there was one death in 96 biopsies, or about a 1% mortality rate, and three instances of postoperative morbidity, a 3% rate. If in fact there has been no morbidity in the Bowen series, these percentages would be reduced by about one-third.

An additional risk not to be found in these statistics is that of spreading infection of the latent virus disorder, Creutzfeldt-Jakob disease. Instances of spread by improperly sterilized instruments that are used in subsequent brain operations has been documented (11). However, the parameters for adequate chemical as well as heat sterilization have now been established and are used in most neurosurgical operating rooms (1,43,140).

## Role of biopsy

Cerebral biopsy has played a critical role in advancing knowledge of dementias. The classical description of the ultrastructural changes in Alzheimer disease during the early 1960s by Terry (134) and Kidd (76) required the availability of fresh tissue obtained at cerebral autopsy. The extensive bio-chemical studies of Bowen and colleagues that have established the changes in the acetylcholine and other neurotransmitter systems early in the course of Alzheimer disease required biopsy tissue. In the immediate future, Alzheimer biopsy material may be needed for adequate study of the molecular biology of the disease and for determining what genes are expressed in the diseased brain—information that is necessary for an understanding of pathogenesis and that may help in determining etiology. In addition, cerebral biopsy has led to delineation of the pathology characteristic of several unusual but important disorders that present with dementia.

The use of cerebral biopsy for diagnosis has been more controversial. One concern is that 20 to 25% of the biopsies do not produce a specific diagnosis. In most instances when an autopsy has been carried out in patients with nonspecific diagnoses, unusual disorders have been found that reflect the selected nature of patients being referred for this procedure. Although the numbers are small in these series, there was no instance of a case in which the biopsy was nondiagnostic and the autopsy showed Alzheimer disease. In our experience, histological changes on biopsy are often dramatic, even in early cases. Thus the procedure does have significant diagnostic usefulness. One could raise the issue of whether it would be a cost-effective approach. A second concern is the risk; this factor has been extraordinarily variable among series and undoubtedly increases in relation to the degree of cognitive impairment of the patient. In our own series two of the three instances of postoperative morbidity were due to bleeding at the operative site resulting in subdural hematomas. In both instances the patients had advanced dementia and large ventricles and were being considered for ventricular shunts; as indications have changed, they would no longer be considered suitable candidates for ventricular shunting; nor would they have been considered to be suitable candidates for diagnostic biopsy alone. The third instance of postoperative morbidity was a prolonged bout of aseptic meningitis in a patient with isolated primary cerebral vasculitis. The three deaths that were reported in the series of 437 biopsies were all from the 1960s or earlier. It seems reasonable in the absence of large recent series to assume a mortality of about 0.5%. Under these circumstances it is likely that diagnostic biopsies at present will be used sparsely in the United States and reserved for cases that are difficult to diagnose. The situation will change radically if a therapy with efficacy but significant side effects were developed (an example would be a drug that had to be administered by intraventricular cannula); then the risk of biopsy would be quite reasonable. Until that occurs, Biemond's criteria (12) still hold: When the patient has a progressive disorder with dementia and "all other possible diagnostic methods have already been tried and failed to provide sufficient diagnostic certainty; the general condition of the patient permits it . . ." Biemond also recommended that "modern diagnostic possibilities are exploited to the fullest in the examination of the material obtained."

## Limits of Autopsy Certainty

Alzheimer was both psychiatrist and anatomist, and his description of the case that proved to be the prototype of Alzheimer disease included a description of symptoms and changes in brain tissue. A 1984 NIA conference on the diagnosis of dementia emphasized that Alzheimer disease is truly a clinical pathological diagnosis dependent on the presence during life of dementia and on the typical pathology (silver-staining neurofibrillary tangles and neuritic plaques) at biopsy or autopsy (75). In most autopsied cases the pathological changes are so evident that there would be full agreement among pathologists concerning the diagnosis. However, in a few cases pathological changes are mild. This finding creates uncertainty because the brains of nondemented elderly (139,141) may show a few neurofibrillary tangles in the hippocampus or amygdala or an occasional neuritic plaque in the cerebral cortex. The NIA conference (75) recommended specific autopsy criteria for the diagnosis of Alzheimer disease. Samples for microscopy should be stained with the Bielschowsky silver technique, thioflavin S method (with ultraviolet illumination), or the Congo red technique (polarized light), as these methods are highly sensitive. To compensate for an inadequate history and to ensure a separation greater than 95% of Alzheimer disease from normal aging changes, the panel recommended that the diagnosis be made if the number of neuritic plaques exceed $15/mm^2$ of microscopic field in patients older than 75, $10/mm^2$ in patients between 65 and 74 years old, $8/mm^2$ in patients between the ages of 50 and 64, and $2/mm^2$ in patients under 50. In addition, neurofibrillary tangles anywhere in the neocortex should not be present in patients under age 75. The report stated: "In the presence of a positive clinical history of [Alzheimer disease] these criteria should be revised downward, although to what extent remains to be determined by future research. One suggestion was that one might only need 50% as many lesions in neocortical samples to retain a high confidence for the histological diagnosis."

Another limitation of autopsy accuracy occurs because of a small percentage of cases—perhaps about 5% in the typical series—in which there is an absence of pathological change in the brains of patients known to be demented during life. Such cases are represented in 4% of autopsies of the Tomlinson (139) series, 11% of the Sulkava et al. (132) series, and 6% of the Terry et al. series (R. Terry, *personal communication,* 1985). In the latter series, 6 of 101 autopsies of quite elderly (average age 85) nursing home patients belonged in this category. The traditional neuropathological studies were supplemented with quantitative counts of nerve cells remaining in cerebral cortex and with measurements of markers of the cholinergic system and the somatostatin system. All were within limits of normal relative to age-matched brains. Such cases may represent neurodegenerative disorders whose pathology cannot be demonstrated by the typical stains (which, in the case of the Terry et al. series, include hematoxylin and eosin, silver, and thioflavin stains) or biochemical measurements. However, it is also possible that at least some of these cases represent metabolic or toxic dementias that were potentially reversible and were not diagnosed during life. Thus the existence of such cases reflects the limitations of current diagnostic accuracy.

## New Technologies

### Magnetic resonance imaging

Magnetic resonance imaging (MRI) was approved for reimbursement by Medicare on January 1, 1986. MRI images are spectacular in the amount of anatomical detail that can be visualized. It is possible that MRI will eventually replace CT as the primary imaging technique, but there is not yet sufficient experience to warrant this change.

Magnetic resonance imaging may be especially effective in the diagnosis of multi-infarct dementia, lacunar states, and Binswanger disease, all forms of vascular dementia, because it is so sensitive to alterations in tissue structure produced by vascular lesions. In fact, the current problem is that vascular and white matter changes are seen in some asymptomatic persons, and limits of normal have yet to be defined. MRI correlation with autopsy findings is needed. The vascular etiology of dementia may become an MRI diagnosis. The current cost of an MRI is about $700.

### Positron emission tomography and single photon emission computed tomography

The development of positron emission tomography (PET) using a fluorine-18-labeled cogen of glucose has made it possible to examine brain metabolism in specific brain regions during life. This dramatic new technology has been used to examine Alzheimer patients at different stages of their disease. There is evidence that memory changes may precede measurable metabolic changes (26, 27). However, it has been found that in relatively early cases an asymmetrical but bilateral reduction in metabolism in parietal cortex is present (40,41); later there is a dramatic reduction in metabolism throughout the cerebral hemispheres. Experience is still too limited to know how useful the biparietal pattern may be in diagnosis. The potential usefulness of PET as a clinical diagnostic tool is limited by the short half-life of positron-emitting isotopes (about 90 min for fluorine-18) and the need for a local cyclotron with a team of physicists and radiochemists. Single photon emission CT (SPECT), however, has been touted as a "poor man's PET." SPECT cannot be used at present for metabolic measures, but it can be used to measure truly regional blood flow accurately using iodine-123-labeled compounds that are commercially available. SPECT equipment is within the range of capital expenditures that most hospitals can make; moreover, there are many nuclear medicine specialists capable of using SPECT whose skills are underutilized because CT and MRI have displaced isotope scanning in many instances (for example, the brain scan is no longer used). Hence there is great interest on the part of such specialists in this new technique. Nevertheless, there is need for great caution. The sensitivity and specificity of SPECT measurements of blood flow in the diagnosis of dementia has not been determined. This matter is of public health interest because the total expenditure for SPECT might be large at a time when justification of its use is in doubt.

### Biological markers

The identification of a specific biological marker of Alzheimer disease that can be used clinically would be an important advance in the diagnosis of this disorder. This area has attracted the attention of many sophisticated laboratories. Two major types of marker are being investigated: (a) CSF changes reflecting altered brain neurotransmitters or abnormal proteins; (b) peripheral markers, reflecting changes in skin or blood cells. The first is straightforward conceptually, but so far disappointing. The second approach is based on the assumption that systemic changes occur in Alzheimer disease, changes that have not been demonstrated pathologically or biochemically. A number of reputable investigators have claimed success in finding such peripheral markers; but most attempts have not yet been replicated, and there is no consensus as to their potential usefulness as diagnostic markers. Specifically, none of the changes reported have been shown to differentiate normal patients from Alzheimer patients early in the course of the disease. Nor is it certain that any proposed marker distinguishes Alzheimer disease from other brain disorders.

*Markers reflecting brain changes.* Thal (136) and Thienhaus et al. (137) have reviewed the extensive data available on CSF changes in dementia. The enzyme acetylcholinesterase is decreased in cerebral cortex; some investigators have found it decreased in CSF, and others have not. Thal suggested that the apparent decrease in some studies may be a dilutional effect secondary to ventricular enlargement. Even if this is not the explanation, however, decreases in the dopamine metabolite homovanillic acid (HVA), which have been found to be consistent in a subgroup of patients and appear to be related to the severity of dementia, are also found in other disorders, notably Parkinson disease. The neuropeptide somatostatin is markedly reduced in the cerebral cortex in Alzheimer disease; in CSF it has been found to be decreased in some patients but not in others. Norepinephrine is often decreased in the brain of Alzheimer patients but is increased in the CSF (116). At present, changes in neurotransmitters or their metabolites in the CSF do not appear to be likely diagnostic markers.

An interesting area still to be explored is if one or more of the abnormal brain proteins associated with Alzheimer disease can be found in CSF or serum. Proteins of interest include paired helical filament protein, amyloid protein, and Alzheimer-specific nucleus basalis antigen (145). At present none of the antibodies to these proteins has served to identify the minute quantities of these abnormal proteins that may escape from the brain. Nonetheless, the effort certainly seems worthwhile.

*Peripheral markers.* Possible changes in peripheral cholinergic markers have interested a number of investigators. There have been reports of changes in red blood cell and plasma choline levels and influxes in Alzheimer patients, but others have either not been able to confirm these changes or have found statistical changes that are not useful as diagnostic tests (15,47,52). Changes in pseudocholinesterase and in red blood cell acetylcholinesterase that sometimes occur are not diagnostic (19,109,129). One group of investigators found that sodium-lithium countertransport rates in red blood cells were elevated in Alzheimer disease, but the number of subjects was small and this finding has not been replicated (31). The susceptibility of persons with Down syndrome to Alzheimer disease has led many workers to seek evidence of abnormal chromosomes in lymphocytes from Alzheimer patients. Although several investigators have reported increased chromosomal fragmentation or aneuploidy in cultured cells, others have not been able to confirm it (91,93,106,133,144). Cook-Deegan and Austin (22) found that the DNA content in noncultured lymphocytes was not altered in familial or sporadic Alzheimer disease, making chromosomal aberration unlikely.

*Olfactory deficits.* Demonstration of biochemical and pathological changes in the olfactory bulb and olfactory cortex in Alzheimer patients encourages investigation of olfaction in Alzheimer patients (5,34,127). Several investigators have now found that there are deficits in olfactory recognition as well as olfactory threshold in the Alzheimer patient. Thus Peabody and Tinklenberg (107) found that 8 of 18 patients had olfactory deficits, but only 1 of 26 controls. Corwin et al. (23) also reported difficulty in olfactory recognition that did not appear to be related to the degree of dementia. Further investigation is needed to determine the optimum testing procedure for discriminating Alzheimer patients from normals. It is uncertain at this time whether such tests will improve the accuracy of diagnosis.

The most intriguing work at the present is represented by reports of alteration of function of cultured Alzheimer fibroblasts. Changes reported to occur include increased $CO_2$ production (128), increased superoxide dismutase (138), decreased calcium uptake (111) but increased intracellular calcium (110), and reduced DNA repair (121). Some of these reported changes are quite striking; for example, Bradley and co-workers (121) found no overlap between the rates of DNA repair obtained in Alzheimer cultures compared to control cultures; a change in DNA repair was also reported by Li and Kaminskas (86). All of these reports are preliminary, and one can point to possible methodological flaws. (For example, some of the Alzheimer patients may have received neuroleptics, whereas controls have not; some of the Alzheimer patients may have become cachetic and the controls not; additional control groups are needed, including cells from patients with other neurological diseases; some of the studies have used fibroblasts from the NIA repository, cells obtained from highly selected families who may be atypical.) Nevertheless, the changes reported are sufficiently dramatic to warrant a high-priority pursuit of these findings. If one of these changes turns out to be specific for Alzheimer patients, it would not only be an important diagnostic marker but might also provide a clue as to etiology.

Another important approach is the search for genetic markers for Alzheimer disease. Based on studies of families in which Alzheimer disease has appeared for several generations, it is assumed that a dominant autosomal gene predisposing to this disorder is present. Several groups are now attempting to use the sophisticated methodology currently available for locating genes [employing restriction fragment length polymorphisms (RFLPs)], the methodology that was so successful in locating the Huntington gene, to study Alzheimer disease. This approach may not work if several genes produce Alzheimer disease; moreover, it may be quite difficult because of the late age of onset of Alzheimer disease, creating uncertainty as to which living members of a family are really free of disease. The use of subtraction libraries containing DNA and cDNA clones may provide alternate approaches to the molecular genetics of Alzheimer disease.

## Diagnostic Criteria

Specific criteria that have been developed for the diagnosis of Alzheimer disease and multi-infarct dementia have contributed to an improvement in diagnostic accuracy. Two widely used sets of criteria for the diagnosis of Alzheimer disease are compared in Table 8: (a) the *DSM-III* (3) criteria for the diagnosis of "primary degenerative dementia" (PDD) [which are similar to those suggested by Eisdorfer and Cohen (33)]; and (b) the ADRDA-NINCDS criteria for the probable, possible, and definite diagnoses of Alzheimer disease. The introduction of the term "primary degenerative dementia" by the *DSM-III* was somewhat of an anomaly, as elsewhere in that manual specific and simple terms such as "dementia" had been substituted for cumbersome phrases such as "chronic organic brain syndrome." *DSM-III* states that PDD is intended to include Alzheimer disease, Pick disease, and dementias with nonspecific brain changes (the latter group referred to in this chapter as the "5% problem"). In fact, it has turned out that many investigators have used the *DSM-III* criteria to identify the typical case of Alzheimer disease for

TABLE 8. *Comparison of diagnostic criteria: Alzheimer and "primary degenerative dementia"*

| Criteria | DSM-III/PPD[a] | ADRDA/NINCDS[b] | | |
|---|---|---|---|---|
| | | Alzheimer probable | Alzheimer possible | Alzheimer definite |
| Dementia present | | | | |
|   Clinical evaluation | R | R | R | R |
|   Mental status tests | | R | R | |
| Cognitive deficit in two or more areas | R | R | + | |
| Impairment of function | R | + | + | |
| Onset age 40–90 | | R | + | |
| Insidious onset | R | + | + | |
| Progressive course | R | R[c] | R[c] | |
| Exclusive of systemic or brain disorders that may produce dementia | R | R | + | |
| Exclusive of depression and other psychiatric disorders | R | | | |
| Tests | | | | |
|   Normal LP | | + | + | |
|   EEG normal or slowing | | + | + | |
|   CT atrophy | | + | + | |
| Absence of focal motor or sensory changes | | + | + | |
| Histological changes characteristic of Alzheimer | | | | R |

R = required. + = desirable/not required.
[a]American Psychiatric Association Task Force (3).
[b]McKhann et al. (100).
[c]Accepts plateaus.

research purposes; autopsy studies have shown that more than 90% of patients who meet *DSM-III* criteria for PDD have Alzheimer disease. Most clinicians hope that in the next edition of its diagnostic and statistical manual the American Psychiatric Association will drop the term primary degenerative dementia and use the term Alzheimer disease. *DSM-III* criteria for PDD include the *DSM-III* criteria for dementia with "an insidious onset with uniformly progressive deterioration course . . . exclusion of all other specific causes of dementia by history, physical examination, and laboratory tests" (3). The ADRDA/NINCDS criteria for probable Alzheimer disease are similar to the *DSM-III* criteria but are more detailed; the ADRDA/NINCDS also allows for more variation in course, recognizing, for example, that the course is not always progressive and that plateaus may occur. Both sets of criteria are restrictive, however. Karasu (62) noted: "Essentially *DSM-III* is a research oriented instrument, which requires that there be a minimum of false-positive diagnoses in order to obtain a homogeneous sample and to keep any distortion or dilution of statistical data at the lowest possible level." This goal it succeeds in accomplishing with its criteria for PDD/Alzheimer disease. Karasu continued: "In contrast, clinical practice must insist on a minimum of false-negative diagnoses."

The latter statement is appropriately applied to the *DSM-III* criteria for Alzheimer disease because there are many patients with autopsy- or biopsy-proved Alzheimer disease who do not meet the criteria. For example, some patients present with impairment of only one area of cognition (e.g., memory, language, or right parietal lobe deficit) (24,68). Not infrequently an Alzheimer patient may have a coexistent disorder that by itself may produce dementia (e.g., hypothyroidism), but treatment is found not to slow the progression of the cognitive loss. The report of the ADRDA/NINCDS committee on the diagnosis of Alzheimer disease recommended that patients with an atypical course, findings, or coexistent disease be diagnosed as "possible Alzheimer" (100). Because the designation of possible Alzheimer disease is so recent, there are as yet no follow-up reports on its validity. This same report reserved the designation of "definite Alzheimer" for cases with biopsy or autopsy confirmation. The ADRDA/NINCDS reports used the term "probable Alzheimer" for patients who meet criteria similar to those of *DSM-III*.

*DSM-III* also included criteria for the diagnosis of multi-infarct dementia. These criteria include the presence of dementia, "a stepwise deteriorating course [i.e., not uniformly progressive] with 'patchy' distribution of deficits early in the course . . . focal neurological signs and symptoms . . . evidence . . . of significant cerebrovascular disease" (3). Relatively few patients are found to meet these criteria exactly. It has been found that scoring systems, introduced by Hachinski (51) and modified by Rosen et al. (123), have been of much greater utility for diagnostic purposes. However, these "ischemic scores" have so far been validated only retrospectively, and a prospective autopsy series needs to be carried out. A defect of these scoring systems is that patients with pure multi-infarct dementia as well as patients with combined multi-infarct dementia and Alzheimer disease score similarly. Also, clinicians now find that evidence of infarct or lacunes [a lacune is a small hole in the brain—less than 15 mm in diameter—resulting from destruction of a small region of brain tissue due to the occlusion of a small artery deep in the white matter or adjacent nuclei (gray matter), a region where there is inadequate collateral circulation and many small arteries are "end-arteries"] on CT scan is helpful in the diagnosis, and MRI may provide specific laboratory confirmation of multi-infarct dementia, although not differentiating patients with multi-infarct dementia and Alzheimer disease. New criteria taking into account these techniques need to be formulated. At present the accuracy of the diagnosis of multi-infarct dementia cannot be determined.

### Diagnostic Errors: Current Status

There is every indication that the current work-up combined with the use of specific diagnostic criteria has greatly improved the clinical differential diagnosis of dementing disorders in the middle or later stages of these disorders. Larson et al. (85) reported confirmation of specific clinical diagnoses by autopsy data obtained during a retrospective study of 200 patients with suspected dementia who had been referred to a specialized geriatric outpatient evaluation clinic. Each patient underwent an intensive evaluation including the diagnostic work-up described above, and a consensus diagnosis was obtained on each. There were 37 deaths and 17 autopsies. Fifteen patients diagnosed clinically as having Alzheimer disease had the diagnosis confirmed; 3 of the 15 patients had pathological evidence of Parkinson disease in addition to Alzheimer disease; the coexistence of Alzheimer and Parkinson diseases had been recognized in two of these patients during life. Correct diagnoses were also made in the remaining two patients, one with changes consistent with alcoholism, the other with Parkinson disease without Alzheimer disease. These data are encouraging. Unfortunately, the results cannot yet be generalized. These patients were evaluated after 3.5 years of symptoms, and they demonstrated scores on the MMSE in the moderately impaired range. Hence the data may not be applicable to the early diagnosis of mildly impaired patients. Moreover, there is an evident selection bias in this sample. There was a paucity of patients with diagnoses seen in other series; specifically, only 1% of the cases had multi-infarct dementia, there were no cases of normal-pressure hydrocephalus or brain tumor, and no indication of cases of Creutzfeldt-Jakob disease or Huntington chorea, all of which are present in prospective series and in large autopsy series. Perhaps diagnoses of such conditions had been made by other physicians, reducing the likelihood of the families of patients with predominantly neurological conditions seeking the services of this clinic.

There are additional autopsy data in regard to the accuracy of the diagnosis of Alzheimer disease or "primary degenerative dementia" (*DSM-III* equivalent of Alzheimer) in patients who meet research diagnostic criteria. In three prospective series, such patients have been followed to autopsy; in the Berg et al. (10) series 6 of 6 diagnoses were confirmed at autopsy, in the Raskind (*personal communication*) series 13 of 14 diagnoses were confirmed, and in the Sulkava et al. series (133) 22 of 27 were found to have Alzheimer disease. The missed diagnoses include Creutzfeldt-Jakob disease and Parkinson disease, as well as two instances of subcortical gliosis and two without specific changes. This increased accuracy of clinical diagnosis is also reflected in current biopsy series; 7 of 7 confirmed in the Fox et al. series (38) and 18 of 24 in the Neary et al. series (104). If generally applicable, this experience indicates that clinical diagnoses carried out under these optimal conditions approach a 90% level of accuracy, a level that probably exceeds that reached by physicians for most diseases. This 90% level of diagnostic accuracy is particularly striking when compared to that reported by Jellinger (58) from the Neurological Institute of the University of Vienna. Jellinger had obtained 1,009 autopsies in patients who had been found to be demented during life. Clinical diagnoses of these patients during life included presenile (163 cases) and senile (286 cases) dementia and cerebral atherosclerosis (560 cases); when compared to the pathological diagnoses, 45.3% of the clinical diagnoses of presenile dementia (including pathologically Alzheimer and combined Alzheimer and multi-infarct dementia cases) were correct, 77.6% of the diagnoses of senile dementia were correct, and 49.9% of the diagnoses of cerebral atherosclerosis were correct (here accepting combined Alzheimer and multi-infarct dementia cases as correct diagnoses) so that the overall accuracy was 65.3%. One can speculate that the availability of specific criteria and increasing clinical awareness of the differential diagnosis of dementia has greatly improved diagnostic accuracy.

## PROGNOSIS AND PROGNOSTIC ACCURACY

That the course of dementing illnesses is progressive and malignant, leading to early death, has been recognized for more than three decades and has formed part of the argument for differentiating dementing illness from other behavioral afflictions of the elderly (64,125,143).

### Estimates of Life Expectancy and Mortality

Wang (143) compared the duration of disease and survival reported in several pathological series during the 1960s to survival anticipated from life tables: Patients with senile dementia (mean age of onset 71.3 years) survived on the average 6.0 years, half of the expected survival of 11.1 years; patients with presenile dementia (mean age of onset 53.8 years) survived 6.9 years against an expected survival (based on the life statistics of an age- and sex-matched group) of 22.3 years; and patients with vascular dementia (mean age of onset 66.8 years) survived 3.8 years with an expected survival of 13.4 years. In the most recently published series, Barclay et al. (7,8) reported a mean survival time in Alzheimer patients of 8.1 years and 6.7 years in patients with multi-infarct dementia. Life expectancy in men is particularly affected. Barclay et al. found that at 5 years after diagnosis of Alzheimer disease the actual survival relative to the anticipated survival of an age- and sex-matched group is about 60% in women and about 25% in men. This low rate of survival of men with dementia may in part account for mortality differences between Alzheimer and multi-infarct patients because there is a higher proportion of men in the multi-infarct dementia group. The fact that mean survival was increased in Barclay's 1985 series compared to Wang's 1960s series is consistent with the improved life expectancy of the elderly and better care for dementia patients, a phenomenon that Gruenberg has termed "the failures of success" (49,50).

## Predictors of Mortality

It is evident from these studies that dementia is a predictor of death, and this fact has been confirmed in a variety of reports. Nielsen et al. (105), who carried out a 15-year follow-up of the entire population of a Danish island, found that those with severe dementia at the beginning of the study were all dead within 5 years, and that survival was significantly shorter for both men and women with dementia. Similar results were obtained in a study of a large (500-bed) nursing home by Peck et al. (108). In the same nursing home, Vitaliano et al. (142), using a dichotomous (branching, two-choice) model, found that the presence of dementia, an age over 80, and being male predicted mortality. In the Vitaliano et al. study, functional status (also treated dichotomously) was not a predictor of death; T. Brown et al. (*unpublished*) found, on the contrary, that the Blessed et al. (16) functional scale was the best predictor of mortality. Additional studies using sensitive functional scales are needed in this regard.

Bronchopneumonia was the major cause of death in dementia patients in the nursing home study, an observation previously noted by Kay (73). Peck et al. (108) noted that: "Inability to communicate one's medical and nursing needs diminishes the prospect of being treated adequately by others, professionals and nonprofessionals."

## Functional Decline

### Course

Alzheimer disease is characterized by progressive cognitive and functional decline. The disease may progress from a point where there are only mild cognitive deficits in a still functioning individual to the stage where the patient becomes mute, incontinent, and must be dressed, bathed, and fed. The decline is more or less continuous although quite variable between individuals. This variability must be emphasized. An early edition of Merrit's *A Textbook of Neurology* (101) described the course of the disorder as between 1 and 20 years. We have documented individuals with autopsy-proved Alzheimer disease who have gone from mild forgetfulness to inability to give their name in 1 year and individuals with autopsy-proved Alzheimer disease and mild dementia who showed no change on mental status scores over a 2-year period. In most individuals cognition and function decrease together, but there are again significant individual differences; for example, one occasionally finds patients whose measured cognitive impairment is so great that they cannot give their own name yet are able to care for most activities of daily living without help.

## Stages

Despite the variability in rate of progression and in individual cognitive functional components, it is sometimes convenient to characterize "stages" of the disorder. The most commonly used classifications are the Clinical Dementia Rating (CDR) devised at Washington University (55) and the Global Deterioration Scale (GDS) devised by Reisberg et al. (120).

Are there predictors (other than age and sex) of the rate of functional decrease and of mortality? The data available from longitudinal studies are scanty. Information from the Duke longitudinal study suggested that changes in EEG occipital domain frequency, the WAIS deterioration quotient, and neurological changes were predictive (143). Berg et al. (10) did not find EEG predictive, nor were changes on the CT scan or visual evoked responses predictive; the best predictors in their study were WAIS subtest scores, especially the digit symbol subtest, and an aphasia battery. Both Chui et al. (20) and Mayeux et al. (96) found that the presence of myoclonus and extrapyramidal signs unrelated to medication indicated poor prognosis.

Reisberg et al. (120) reported a follow-up study of 41 community-residing Alzheimer patients. Although the numbers are small, the data may be of some practical use. Six patients died, and six were institutionalized over an average 2-year period. Patients with only subtle clinical evidence of a decrement in cognitive performance (GDS scores of 2 and 3) could be expected to be alive and residing in the community over a 2-year period. Patients who had begun to show functional deficits in such areas as shopping and handling their own financial affairs had a "guarded" prognosis: more than one-fourth of such patients either died or required institutionalization.

Although there is a paucity of information regarding the course and prognosis of Alzheimer disease, longitudinal data concerning other dementias are almost nonexistent. Barclay et al. (7,8) found that patients with Alzheimer disease and those with multi-infarct dementia had comparable progression of behavioral and cognitive impairment and need for home care or institutionalization. This fact is in accord with findings in the Bronx Aging Study and in our own experience. We reviewed the extensive literature available on the results of placement of shunts in patients with normal-pressure hydrocephalus (65). Approximately 55% of patients showed significant improvement after surgery, but it was in part offset by a 40% complication rate. As far as we are aware, there has been no long-term follow-up of such patients. Even more striking is the lack of data concerning patients with other forms of "reversible" dementia. We have already described evidence suggesting that some of the patients diagnosed as having pseudodementia later presented with a frank dementia presumably of the Alzheimer type. Larson et al. (84) diagnosed reversible dementias in 15 of 107 dementia patients. Eleven of these 15 showed initial improvement when treated. However, only three patients with potentially reversible dementia became completely normal; their diagnoses included subdural hematoma, medication toxicity, and rheumatoid vasculitis. Particularly discouraging was the finding that 8 of the 15 patients with reversible dementia followed for more than 2 years developed progressive deterioration consistent with an Alzheimer-type dementia. The initial diagnoses of these patients included hypothyroidism ($n = 3$), subdural hematoma ($n = 1$), and medication toxicity ($n = 4$). Thus it appears that patients with subclinical Alzheimer disease may be more likely to develop excess disability with coincident metabolic or intracranial processes. However, even if improvement is short-lived, diagnosis and treatment are certainly desirable.

## Excess Disability

Yesavage (146) has emphasized the importance of excess disability that may occur when a patient with Alzheimer or multi-infarct dementia has a concurrent depression, infection, or other medical condition. Larson et al. (84), in their follow-up of 107 dementia patients, noted five patients with the diagnosis of irreversible dementia who improved cognitively when coexistent diseases including congestive heart failure, depression, anemia, and Parkinson disease were treated. These five patients remained demented, but improved cognition was measurable on the Mini-Mental State examination and the dementia rating scale. Removal of excess disability is important in improving function, but there is no evidence that it alters the overall course of these disorders.

## Predictors of Institutionalization

In considering predictors of institutionalization, one must distinguish between patients who live essentially alone in society—a significant proportion of the elderly—and those who live with family, one of whom acts as caregiver. The isolated patient may quickly reach a point where he or she cannot cope with such exigencies as shopping for food and so requires help either from a companion or attendant or by being placed in a nonmedical facility, such as a board and care unit. Dementia patients with caregivers often remain at home until quite late stages of the disorder. The caregiver of a dementia patient is often a husband, wife, sister, daughter, or occasionally a friend or son. The high level of devotion that characterizes home care is suggested by the title of the standard manual, aptly titled *The 36-Hour Day* (88). The predictors of nursing home placement in such circumstances are not the degree of cognitive impairment but the behavioral changes that result from the impairment and, more so, the ability of the family or other caregivers to cope. Thus in a study of 14 married male patients with Alzheimer disease, the items most closely associated with nursing home placement were incontinence of bladder and bowel, inability to speak coherently, and inability to bathe and groom oneself (56).

## SUMMARY

Dementia represents a symptom complex that may be caused by many disorders. Criteria for the diagnosis of this symptom complex have been well specified in the American Psychiatric Association's *Diagnostic and Statistical Manual of Mental Disorders,* third revision (3). Failure to determine that dementia is present is a greater source of misdiagnosis than are errors in the differential diagnoses of the individual conditions that produce dementia. Typically the presence of dementia is overlooked in patients who present in acute or chronic hospitals with other principal complaints because of the failure to carry out a systematic mental status examination. On the other hand, dementia is often overdiagnosed in older patients who complain of—or whose families complain of—beginning memory impairment. In a significant number of cases a treatable depression has been misdiagnosed as dementia under these circumstances. Although this situation has improved with the availability of *DSM-III* criteria for dementia and depression, serious problems remain in differentiating early dementia from depression in patients who show both mild cognitive impairment and depressive symptoms. Nor has the border-line between memory changes that occur in normal aging and beginning impairment in dementia been adequately defined. Very likely the latter boundary can be established only on a probability basis and a cohort of patients "at risk" for dementia identified. Subsequent to a diagnosis of dementia the responsibility of the physician is to identify which of the 70-plus conditions that may cause dementia is present. There is now a consensus that an adequate differential diagnosis requires a careful and thorough clinical evaluation, CT scan, and blood tests; in special circumstances a variety of other procedures, including lumbar puncture, electroencephalogram, and other tests, may be needed. On the other hand, there are other procedures that are interesting from a research perspective but whose diagnostic use has not yet been justified, e.g., measurement of cerebral blood flow and positron emission tomography.

A major thrust of this work-up is to identify potentially reversible or treatable conditions. The clinical work-up of the patient may cost somewhat more than $1,000; however, the diagnostic work-up is cost-effective (before consideration of the enormous impact on patient and family) if the result is identification of those patients with treatable and reversible causes.

The most important conditions that produce dementia are Alzheimer disease, which accounts for more than one-half of the cases, and vascular or multi-infarct dementia, which accounts for another 10 to 20% of the cases. Specific clinical criteria have proved to be useful in improving the diagnoses of these conditions; thus autopsy studies have shown a 90% clinical diagnostic accuracy in cases in which *DSM-III* criteria are met. There are, however, many patients with Alzheimer disease who do not meet these diagnostic criteria. Also, it is difficult at our present state of knowledge to correctly identify patients who have both Alzheimer disease and another dementing condition, particularly multi-infarct dementia or Parkinson disease. In each of these situations a peripheral marker for Alzheimer disease would be useful. The search for such markers should have a high priority.

## ACKNOWLEDGMENT

We gratefully acknowledge Robert W. Davignon for his excellent assistance both in preparing the original report for the Office of Technology Assessment and for the present revision.

## REFERENCES

1. American Neurological Association, Committee on Health Care Issues (ANA) (1986): Precautions in handling tissues, fluids, and other contaminated materials from patients with documented or suspected Creutzfeldt-Jakob disease. *Ann. Neurol.*, 19:75–77.
2. American Psychiatric Association Task Force on Nomenclature and Statistics (1952): *Diagnostic and Statistical Manual of Mental Disorders* (*DSM-I*), 1st ed. American Psychiatric Association, Washington, D.C.
3. American Psychiatric Association Task Force on Nomenclature and Statistics (1980): *Diagnostic and Statistical Manual of Mental Disorders* (*DSM-III*), 3rd ed., pp. 124–126. American Psychiatric Association, Washington, D.C.
4. Antunes, L. (1963): Nossa experientis actual da biopsia do cortex no diagnostico neuropsiquiatrico. *Gaz. Med. Port.*, 16:474–476.
5. Averback, P. (1983): Two new lesions in Alzheimer's disease. *Lancet*, 2:1203.
6. Balldin, J., Gottfries, C-G., Karlsson, I., Lindstedt, G., Langstrom, G., and Walinder, J. (1983): Dexamethasone suppression test and serum prolactin in dementia disorders. *Br. J. Psychiatry*, 143:277–281.
7. Barclay, L. L., Zemcov, A., Blass J. P., and McDowell, F. H. (1985): Factors associated with duration of survival in Alzheimer's disease. *Biol. Psychiatry*, 20:86–93.
8. Barclay, L. L., Zemcov, A., Blass, J. P., and Sansone, J. (1985): Survival in Alzheimer's disease and vascular dementias. *Neurology*, 35:834–840.
9. Becker, P. M., Freussner, J. R., Mulrow, C. D., Williams, B. C., and Vokaty, K. A. (1985): The role of lumbar puncture in the evaluation of dementia. *J. Am. Geriatr. Soc.*, 33:392–396.
10. Berg, L., Danziger, W. L., Storandt, M., Cobern, L. A., Gado, M., Knesevich, J. W., and Botwinick, J. (1984): Predictive features in mild senile dementia of the Alzheimer type. *Neurology*, 34:563–569.
11. Bernoulli, C., Siegfried, J., Baumgartner, G., Regli, F., Rabinowicz, T., Gajdusek, D. C., and Gibbs, C. J., Jr. (1977): Danger of accidental person-to-person transmission of Creutzfeldt-Jakob disease by surgery. *Lancet*, 1:478–479.
12. Biemond, A. (1966): Indications, legal and moral aspects of cerebral biopsies. In: *Proceed-*

ings 5th International Congress of Neuropathology, Zurich, 1965, pp. 372–375. Excerpta Medica, Amsterdam.

13. Blackwood, W. (1971): Cerebral biopsy. In: *Handbook of Neurology*, Vol. 19, pp. 680–687. Raven Press, New York.

14. Blackwood, W., and Cumings, J. N. (1966): The combined histological and chemical aspects of cerebral biopsies. In: *Proceedings 5th International Congress of Neuropathology, Zurich, 1965*, pp. 364–371. Excerpta Medica, Amsterdam.

15. Blass, J. P., Hanin, I., Barclay, L., Koop, U., and Reding, M. J. (1985): Red blood cell abnormalities in Alzheimer disease. *J. Am. Geriatr. Soc.*, 33:401–405.

16. Blessed, G., Tomlinson, B. E., and Roth, M. (1968): The association between quantitative measures of dementia and of senile change in the cerebral gray matter of elderly subjects. *Br. J. Psychiatry*, 114:797–811.

17. Bowen, D. M., Sims, N. R., Benton, S., Haan, E. A., Smith, C. C. T., Neary, D., Thomas, D. J., and Davison, A. N. (1982): Biochemical changes in cortical brain biopsies from demented patients in relation to morphological findings and pathogenesis. In: *Aging, Vol. 9: Alzheimer's Disease: A Report of Progress*, edited by S. Corkin, K. L. Davis, J. H. Growdon, et al. Raven Press, New York.

18. Carnes, M., Smith, J. C., Kalin, N. H., and Bauwnes, S. F. (1983): Effects of chronic medical illness and dementia on the dexamethasone suppression test. *J. Am. Geriatr. Soc.*, 31:269–271.

19. Chipperfield, B., Newman, P. M., and Moyes, I. C. A. (1981): Decreased erythrocyte cholinesterase activity in dementia. *Lancet*, 2:199.

20. Chui, H. C., Teng, E. L., Henderson, V. W., and Moy, A. C. (1985): Clinical subtypes of dementia of the Alzheimer type. *Neurology*, 35:1544–1550.

21. Coblentz, J. M., Mattis, S., Zingesser, L. H., Kasoff, S. S., Wisniewski, H. M., and Katzman, R. (1973): Presenile dementia: clinical aspects and evaluations of cerebral spinal fluid dynamics. *Arch. Neurol.*, 29:299–308.

22. Cook-Deegan, R. M., and Austin, J. H. (1983): Implications of normal lymphocyte DNA content in familial Alzheimer disease. *Am. J. Med. Genet.*, 15:511.

23. Corwin, J., Serby, M., Conrad, P., and Rotrosen, J. (1985): Olfactory recognition deficit in Alzheimer's and parkinsonian dementias. *IRCS Med. Sci. Biochem.*, 13:260.

24. Crystal, H. A., Horoupian, D. S., Katzman, R., and Jotkowitz, S. (1982): Biopsy proven Alzheimer's disease presenting as a right parietal lobe syndrome. *Ann. Neurol.*, 12:186–188.

25. Cummings, J. L., and Benson, D. F. (1984): Subcortical dementia: review of an emerging concept. *Arch. Neurol.*, 41:874–879.

26. Cutler, N.R., Duara, R., Creasey, H., Grady, C. L., Haxby, J. V., Schapiro, M. B., and Rapoport, S. I. (1984): Brain imaging: aging and dementia. *Ann. Intern. Med.*, 101:355–369.

27. Cutler, N. R., Haxby, J. V., Duara, R., et al. (1985): Brain metabolism as measured with positron emission tomography: serial assessment in a patient with familial Alzheimer's disease. *Neurology*, 35:1556–1561.

28. Delaney, P. (1982): Dementia: the search for treatable causes. *South. Med. J.*, 75:707–709.

29. DePaulo, J. R., Jr., and Folstein, M. F. (1978): Psychiatric disturbances in neurological patients: detection, recognition, and hospital course. *Ann. Neurol.*, 4:225–228.

30. Devanand, D. P., and Nelson, J. C. (1985): Concurrent depression and dementia: implications for diagnosis and treatment. *J. Clin. Psychiatry*, 46:389–392.

31. Diamond, J. M., Matsuyama, S. S., Meier, K., and Jarvik, L. F. (1983): Elevation of erythrocyte countertransport rates in Alzheimer's dementia. *N. Engl. J. Med.*, 309:1061–1062.

32. Eadie, M. (1964): Experience with cortical biopsy. *Proc. Aust. Assoc. Neurol.*, 2:59–63.

33. Eisdorfer, C., and Cohen, D. (1980): Diagnostic criteria for primary neuronal degeneration of the Alzheimer's type. *J. Fam. Pract.*, 11:553–557.

34. Esiri, M. M., and Wilcock, G. K. (1984): The olfactory bulbs in Alzheimer disease. *J. Neurol. Neurosurg. Psychiatry*, 47:56–60.

35. Folstein, M., Anthony, J. C., Parhad, I., Duffy B., and Gruenberg, E. M. (1985): The meaning of cognitive impairment in the elderly. *J. Am. Geriatr. Soc.*, 33:228–235.

36. Folstein, M. F., and McHugh, P. R. (1978): Dementia syndrome of depression. In: *Aging,*

*Vol. 7: Alzheimer's Disease: Senile Dementia and Related Disorders,* edited by R. Katzman, R. D. Terry, and K. L. Bick, pp. 87–93. Raven Press, New York.

37. Folstein, M. F., Folstein, S. E., and McHugh, P. R. (1975): "Mini-mental state": a practical method for grading the cognitive state of patients for the clinician. *J. Psychiatr. Res.,* 12:189–198.

38. Fox, J. H., Penn, R., Clasen, R., Martin, E., Wilson, R., and Savoy, S. (1985): Pathological diagnosis in clinically typical Alzheimer's disease. *N. Engl. J. Med.,* 313:1419–1420 (letter).

39. Freemon, F. R., and Rudd, S. M. (1982): Clinical features that predict potentially reversible progressive intellectual deterioration. *J. Am. Geriatr. Soc.,* 33:449–451.

40. Friedland, R. P., Brun, A., and Budinger, T. F. (1985): Pathological and positron emission tomographic correlations in Alzheimer's disease. *Lancet,* 1:228.

41. Friedland, R. P., Budinger, T. F., Koss, E., and Ober, B. A. (1985): Alzheimer's disease: anterior-posterior and lateral hemispheric alterations in cortical glucose utilization. *Neurosci. Lett.,* 53:235–240.

42. Gado, M., Hughes, C. P., Danziger, W., Chi, D., Jost, G., and Berg, L. (1982): Volumetric measurements of the cerebrospinal fluid spaces in demented subjects and controls. *Radiology,* 144:535–538.

43. Gajdusek, D. C., Gibbs, C. J., Jr., Asher, D. M., Brown, P., Diwan, A., Hoffman, P., Nemo, G., Rohwer, R., and White, L. (1977): Precautions in medical care of, and in handling materials from patients with transmissible virus dementia (Creutzfeldt-Jakob disease). *N. Engl. J. Med.,* 297:1253–1258.

44. Garcia, C. A., Reding, M. J., and Blass, J. P. (1981): Overdiagnosis of dementia. *J. Am. Geriatr. Soc.,* 29:407–410.

45. Garcia, C. A., Tweedy, J. R., and Blass, J. P. (1984): Underdiagnosis of cognitive impairment in a rehabilitation setting. *J. Am. Geriatr. Soc.,* 32:339–342.

46. Green, M. A., Stevenson, L. D., Fonseca, J. E., and Wortis, S. B. (1952): Cerebral biopsy in patients with presenile dementia. *Dis. Nerv. Syst.,* 13:303–307.

47. Greenwald, B. S., Edasery, J., Mohs, R. C., Shah, N., Trigos, G. G., and Davis, K. L. (1985): Red blood cell choline. I. Choline in Alzheimer's disease. *Biol. Psychiatry,* 20:367–374.

48. Groves, R., and Møller, J. (1966): The value of the cerebral cortical biopsy. *Acta Neurol. Scand.,* 42:477–482.

49. Gruenberg, E. M. (1976): Epidemiology of senile dementia. In: *Neurological Epidemiology: Principles and Clinical Application,* edited by B. S. Schoenberg. Raven Press, New York.

50. Gruenberg, E. M. (1977): The failures of success. *Milband Mem. Fund. Q.,* 55:3–24.

51. Hachinski, V. (1978): Cerebral blood flow differentiation of Alzheimer's disease from multi-infarct dementia. In: *Aging, Vol. 7: Alzheimer's Disease: Senile Dementia and Related Disorders,* edited by R. Katzman, R. D. Terry, and K. L. Bick, pp. 97–103. Raven Press, New York.

52. Hanin, I., Reynolds, C. F., III, Kupfer, D. J., et al. (1984): Elevated red blood cell/plasma choline ratio in dementia of the Alzheimer type: clinical and polysomnographic correlates. *Psychiatry Res.,* 13:167–173.

53. Hasse, G. R. (1977): Diseases presenting as dementia. In: *Dementia,* 2nd ed., edited by C. E. Wells. Davis, Philadelphia.

54. Hoffman, R. S. (1982): Diagnostic errors in the evaluation of behavioral disorders. *JAMA,* 248:964–967.

55. Hughes, C. P., Berg, L., Danziger, W. L., Coben, L. A., and Martin, R. L. (1982): A new clinical scale for the staging of dementia. *Br. J. Psychiatry,* 140:566–572.

56. Hutton, J. T., Dippel, R. L., Loewenson, R. B., Mortimer, J. A., and Christians, B. L. (1985): Predictors of nursing home placement of patients with Alzheimer's disease. *Tex. Med.,* 81:40–43.

57. Jarvik, L. F. (1980): Diagnosis of dementia in the elderly: a 1980 perspective. In: *Annual Review of Gerontology and Geriatrics,* Vol. 1, edited by C. Eisdorfer. Springer, New York.

58. Jellinger, K. (1976): Neuropathological aspects of dementias resulting from abnormal blood and cerebrospinal fluid dynamics. *Acta Neurol. Belg.,* 76:83–102.

59. Jorm, A. F., and Henderson, A. S. (1985). Possible improvement to the diagnostic criteria for dementia in DSM-III. *Br. J. Psychiatry,* 147:394–399.

60. Kahn, R. L., Goldfarb, A. I., Pollack, M., and Peck, A. (1960): Brief objective measures for the determination of mental status in the aged. *Am. J. Psychiatry*, 117:326.
61. Kaplan, J. G., Katzman, R., Horoupian, D. S., Fuld, P. A., Mayeux, R., and Hays, A. P. (1985): Progressive dementia, visual deficits, amyotrophy and microinfarcts. *Neurology*, 35:788–796.
62. Karasu, T. B. (1986): Economic realities force psychiatrists to reevaluate all kinds of psychotherapies. *Clin. Psychiatry News*, 14:1, 27.
63. Katona, C. L. E., and Aldridge, C. R. (1985): The dexamethasone suppression test and depressive signs in dementia. *J. Affective Disord.*, 8:83–89.
64. Katzman, R. (1976): The prevalence and malignancy of Alzheimer disease; a major killer. *Arch. Neurol.*, 33:217–218.
65. Katzman, R. (1977): Normal pressure hydrocephalus. In: *Dementia*, 2nd ed., edited by C. E. Wells. Davis, Philadelphia.
66. Katzman, R. (1983): Vascular disease and dementia. In: *H. Houston Merrit Memorial Volume*, edited by M. D. Yahr. Raven Press, New York.
67. Katzman, R. (1984): Dementia. In: *Current Neurology*, Vol. 5, edited by S. H. Appel. Wiley, New York.
68. Katzman, R. (1985): Clinical presentation of the course of Alzheimer's disease: the atypical patient. *Interdiscipl. Topics Gerontol.*, 20:12–18.
69. Katzman, R. (1986): Dementia. In: *Diseases of the Nervous System*, edited by A. K. Asbury, G. M. McKhann, and W. I. McDonald, pp. 890–896. Heinemann, London.
70. Katzman, R., Brown, T., Fuld, P., Peck, A., Schechter, R., and Schimmel, H. (1983): Validation of a short orientation-memory-concentration test of cognitive impairment. *Am. J. Psychiatry*, 140:734–739.
71. Katzman, R., and Terry, R. D. (1983): *Neurology of Aging*, pp. 15–50. Davis, Philadelphia.
72. Kaufman, H., and Catalano, L. W., Jr. (1979): Diagnostic brain biopsy: a series of 50 cases and a review. *Neurosurgery*, 4:129–136.
73. Kay, D. (1962): Outcome and cause of death in mental disorders in old age. *Acta Psychiatr. Scand.*, 38:249.
74. Kendell, R. E. (1974): The stability of psychiatric diagnoses. *Br. J. Psychiatry*, 124:352–356.
75. Khachaturian, Z. S. (1985): Diagnosis of Alzheimer's disease. *Arch. Neurol.*, 42:1097–1105.
76. Kidd, M. (1964): Alzheimer's disease, an electron microscopic study. *Brain*, 87:303–320.
77. Kiloh, L. G. (1961): Pseudodementia. *Acta Psychiatr. Scand.*, 37:336–351.
78. Knights, E. G., and Folstein, M. F. (1977): Unsuspected emotional and cognitive disturbances in medical patients. *Ann. Intern. Med.*, 87:723.
79. Koto, A., Rosenberg, G., Zingesser, L. H., Horoupian, D., and Katzman, R. (1977): Syndrome of normal pressure hydrocephalus: possible relationship to hypertensive and arteriosclerotic vasculopathy. *J. Neurol. Neurosurg. Psychiatry*, 40:73–79.
80. Kral, V. A. (1978): Benign senescent forgetfulness. In: *Aging, Vol. 7: Alzheimer's Disease: Senile Dementia and Related Disorders*, edited by R. Katzman, R. D. Terry, and K. L. Bick, pp. 47–51. Raven Press, New York.
81. Kral, V. A. (1983): The relationship between senile dementia (Alzheimer type) and depression. *Can. J. Psychiatry*, 28:304–306.
82. Kral, V. A., and Muller, H. (1966): Memory dysfunction: a prognostic indicator in geriatric patients. *Can. Psychiatr. Assoc.*, 11:343–349.
83. Kurtzke, J. F. (1969): *Epidemiology of Cerebrovascular Disease*. Springer-Verlag, Berlin.
84. Larson, E. B., Burton, M. P. H., Reifler, V., Featherstone, H. J., and English, D. R. (1984): Dementia in elderly outpatients: a prospective study. *Ann. Intern. Med.*, 100:417–423.
85. Larson, E. B., Reifler, B. V., Sumi, S. M., Canfield, C. G., and Chinn, N. M. (1985): Diagnostic evaluation of 200 elderly outpatients with suspected dementia. *J. Gerontol.*, 40:536–543.
86. Li, J. C., and Kaminskas, E. (1985): Deficient repair of DNA lesions in Alzheimer's disease fibroblasts. *Biochem. Biophys. Res. Commun.*, 129:733–738.
87. Lijtmaer, H., Fuld, P. A., and Katzman, R. (1976): Prevalence and malignancy of Alzheimer's disease. *Arch. Neurol.*, 33:304.
88. Mace, N. L., and Rabins, P. V. (1981): *The 36-Hour Day*. Johns Hopkins Press, Baltimore.

89. Mahendra, B. (1983): "Pseudodementia": an illogical and misleading concept. *Br. J. Psychiatry*, 143:202.
90. Mahendra, B. (1985): Depression and dementia: the multi-faceted relationship. *Psychol. Med.*, 15:227–236.
91. Mark, J., and Brun, A. (1973): Chromosomal deviations in Alzheimer's disease compared to those in senescence and dementia. *Gerontol. Clin.*, 15:253.
92. Marsden, C., and Harrison, M. (1972): Outcome of investigation of patients with presenile dementia. *Br. Med. J.*, 2:249.
93. Martin, J. M., Kellet, J. M., and Kahn, J. (1981): Aneuploidy in cultured human lymphocytes. II. A comparison between senescence and dementia. *Age Ageing*, 10:24.
94. Mayer-Gross, W. (1931): Some symptoms of organic brain disease. *Arch. Psychiatr. Nervenkr.*, 9:433–618.
95. Mayer-Gross, W., and Guttmann, E. (1937): Schema for the examination of organic cases. *J. Ment. Sci.*, 83:440–448.
96. Mayeux, R., Stern, Y., and Spanton, S. (1985): Heterogeneity in dementia of the Alzheimer type: evidence of subgroups. *Neurology*, 35:453–461.
97. McCallister, T. W., and Price, T. R. P. (1982): Severe depressive pseudodementia with and without dementia. *Am. J. Psychiatry*, 139:5.
98. McCartney, J. R., and Palmateer, L. M. (1985): Assessment of cognitive deficit in geriatric patients: a study of physician behavior. *J. Am. Geriatr. Soc.*, 33:467–471.
99. McKeith, I. G. (1984): Clinical use of the DST in a psychogeriatric population. *Br. J. Psychiatry*, 145:389–393.
100. McKhann, G., Drachman, D., Folstein, M., Katzman, R., Price, D., and Stadlar, E. M. (1984): Clinical diagnosis of Alzheimer's disease: report of the NINCDS-ADRDA work groups under the auspices of Department of Health and Human Services Task Force on Alzheimer's disease. *Neurology*, 34:939–944.
101. Merrit, H. H. (1973): *A Textbook of Neurology*, 5th ed. Lea & Febiger, Philadelphia.
102. Mesulam, M-M. (1982): Slowly progressive aphasia without generalized dementia. *Ann. Neurol.*, 11:592–598.
103. National Institute on Aging Task Force (NIA) (1980): Senility reconsidered: treatment possibilities for mental impairment in the elderly. *JAMA*, 244:259–263.
104. Neary, D., Snowden, J. S., Mann, D. M. A., Bowen, D. M., Sims, N. R., Northen, B., Yates, P. O., and Davison, A. N. (1986): Alzheimer's disease: a correlative study. *J. Neurol. Neurosurg. Psychiatry*, 49:229–237.
105. Nielsen, J., Homma, A., and Biorn-Henricksen, T. (1977): Follow-up 15 years after a geronto-psychiatric prevalence study—conditions concerning death, cause of death, and life expectancy in relation to psychiatric diagnosis. *J. Gerontol.*, 32:554–561.
106. Nordenson, I., Adolfsson, R., Beckman, G., Bucht, G., and Winblad, B. (1980): Chromosomal abnormality in dementia of Alzheimer type. *Lancet*, 1:481–482.
107. Peabody, C. A., and Tinklenberg, J. R. (1985): Olfactory deficits and primary degenerative dementia. *Am. J. Psychiatry*, 142:524–525.
108. Peck, A., Wolloch, L., and Rodstein, M. (1978): Mortality of the aged with chronic brain syndrome II. In: *Aging, Vol. 7: Alzheimer's Disease: Senile Dementia and Related Disorders*, edited by R. Katzman, R. D. Terry, and K. L. Bick, pp. 299–308. Raven Press, New York.
109. Perry, R. H., Wilson, I. D., Bober, M. J., Atack, J., Blessed, G., Tomlinson, B., and Perry, E. (1982): Plasma and erythrocyte acetylcholinesterase in senile dementia of Alzheimer type. *Lancet*, 1:174–175.
110. Peterson, C., and Goldman, J. E. (1986): Alteration in calcium content and biochemical processes in cultured skin fibroblasts from aged and Alzheimer donors. *Proc. Natl. Acad. Sci. USA*, 83:2758–2762.
111. Peterson, C., Gibson, G. E., and Blass, J. P. (1985): Altered calcium uptake in cultured skin fibroblasts from patients with Alzheimer's disease. *N. Engl. J. Med.*, 312:1063–1065.
112. Pogacar, S., and Williams, R. S. (1984): Alzheimer's disease presenting as slowly progressing aphasia. *R.I. Med. J.*, 67:181–185.
113. Postiglione, A., Grossi, D., Faccenda, F., Cicerano, U., Chiacchio, L., Rubba, P., and Campanella, G. (1985): Non invasive study of carotid arteries by echo-doppler and metabolic abnormalities in patients with dementia. *Angiology*, 36:160–164.

114. Rabins, P. V. (1981): The prevalence of reversible dementia in a psychiatric hospital. *Hosp. Commun. Psychiatry*, 32:490–492.
115. Rabins, P. V., Merchant, A., and Nestadt, G. (1984): Criteria for diagnosing reversible dementia caused by depressions: validation by 2-year follow-up. *Br. J. Psychiatry*, 144:488–492.
116. Raskind, M. A., Peskind, E. R., Halter, J. B., and Jimerson, D. C. (1984): Norepinephrine and MHPG levels in CSF and plasma in Alzheimer's disease. *Arch. Gen. Psychiatry*, 41:343–346.
117. Reding, M., Haycox, J., and Blass, J. (1985): Depression in patients referred to a dementia clinic: a three-year prospective study. *Arch. Neurol.*, 42:894–896.
118. Reding, M., Haycox, J., Wigforss, K., Brush, D., and Blass, J. (1984): Follow-up of patients referred to a dementia service. *J. Am. Geriatr. Soc.*, 32:265–268.
119. Reifler, B. V. (1982): Arguments for abandoning the term pseudodementia. *J. Am. Geriatr. Soc.*, 30:665–668.
120. Reisberg, B., Shulman, E., Ferris, S. H., de Leon, M. J., and Geibel, V. (1983): Clinical assessment of age-associated cognitive decline and primary degenerative dementia: prognostic concomitants. *Psychopharmacol. Bull.*, 19:734–739.
121. Robison, S. H., Munzer, J. S., Tandan, R., Bradley, R., and Bradley, W. G. (1985): Repair of alkylated DNA is impaired in Alzheimer's disease cells. *Neurology*, 35(Suppl. 1):217–218.
122. Ron, M. A., Toone, B. K., Garralda, M. E., and Lishman, W. A. (1979): Diagnostic accuracy in presenile dementia. *Br. J. Psychiatry*, 134:161–168.
123. Rosen, W. G., Terry, R. D., Fuld, P. A., Katzman, R., and Peck, A. (1980): Pathological verification of ischemic score in differentiation of dementias. *Ann. Neurol.*, 7:486–488.
124. Rosenberg, G. A., Kornfeld, M., Stovring, J., and Bicknell, J. M. (1979): Subcortical arteriosclerotic encephalopathy (Binswanger): computerized tomography. *Neurology*, 29:1102–1106.
125. Roth, M. (1955): The natural history of mental disorder in old age. *Br. J. Psychiatry*, 101:281–301.
126. Shapiro, M. B., Post, F., Lofbing, B., and Inglis, J. (1956): Memory function in psychiatric patients over 60: some methodological and diagnostic implications. *J. Mental Sci.*, 102:233–246.
127. Simpson, J., Yates, C. M., Gordon, A., and St. Clair, D. M. (1984): Olfactory tubercle choline acetyltransferase activity in Alzheimer-type dementia, Down's syndrome and Huntington's disease. *J. Neurol. Neurosurg. Psychiatry*, 47:1138–1140.
128. Sims, N. R., Finegan, J. M., and Blass, J. P. (1985): Altered glucose metabolism in fibroblasts from patients with Alzheimer's disease. *N. Engl. J. Med.*, 313:638–639.
129. Smith, R. C., Ho, B. T., Hsu, L., Vroulis, G., Claghorn, J., and Schoolar, J. (1982): Cholinesterase enzymes in the blood of patients with Alzheimer's disease. *Life Sci.*, 30:543–546.
130. Smith, J. S., and Kiloh, L. G. (1981): The investigation of dementia: results in 200 consecutive admissions. *Lancet*, 1:824–827.
131. Smith, T., Turner, E., and Sim, M. (1966): Cerebral biopsy in the investigation of presenile dementia. II. Pathologic aspects. *Br. J. Psychiatry*, 112:127–133.
132. Sulkava, R., Haltia, M., Paetau, A., Wikstrom, J., and Palo, J. (1983): Accuracy of clinical diagnosis primary degenerative dementia: correlation with neuropathological findings. *J. Neurol. Neurosurg. Psychiatry*, 46:9–13.
133. Sulkava, R., Rossi, L., and Knuutia, S. (1979): No elevated sister chromatid exchange in Alzheimer's disease. *Acta Neurol. Scand.*, 59:156.
134. Terry, R. D. (1963): Neurofibrillary tangles in Alzheimer's disease. *J. Neuropathol. Exp. Neurol.*, 22:629–642.
135. Terry, R. D., Gonatas, N. K., and Weiss, M. (1964): Ultrastructural studies in Alzheimer's presenile dementia. *Am. J. Pathol.*, 44:269.
136. Thal, L. J. (1985): Changes in cerebrospinal fluid associated with dementia. In: *Memory Dysfunction*, edited by D. Olton, S. Corkin, E. Gamzu, et al., pp. 235–241. New York Academy of Sciences, New York.
137. Thienhaus, O. J., Hartford, J. T., Skelly, M. F., and Bosmann, H. B. (1985): Biological markers in Alzheimer's disease. *J. Am. Geriatr. Soc.*, 33:715–726.

138. Thienhaus, O. J., Price, C. A., and Bosmann, H. B. (1984): Superoxide dismutase (SOD) in Alzheimer fibroblasts. *Pharmacologist,* 26:219.
139. Tomlinson, B. E. (1977): Morphological changes in dementia in old age. In: *Aging and Dementia,* edited by W. L. Smith and M. Kinsbourne. Spectrum, New York.
140. Traub, R. D., Gajdusek, D. C., and Gibbs, C. J., Jr. (1974): Precautions in conducting biopsies and autopsies on patients with presenile dementia. *J. Neurosurg.,* 41:394–395.
141. Ulrich, J. (1985): Alzheimer changes in nondemented patients younger than sixty-five: possible early stages of Alzheimer's disease and senile dementia of Alzheimer type. *Ann. Neurol.,* 17:273–277.
142. Vitaliano, P. P., Peck, A., Johnson, D. A., Prinz, P. N., and Eisdorfer, C. (1981): Dementia and other competing risks for mortality in the institutionalized aged. *J. Am. Geriatr. Soc.,* 29:513–519.
143. Wang, H. S. (1978): Prognosis in dementia and related disorders in the aged. In: *Aging, Vol. 7: Alzheimer's Disease: Senile Dementia and Related Disorders,* edited by R. Katzman, R. D. Terry, and K. L. Bick, pp. 309–313. Raven Press, New York.
144. Ward, B. E., Cook, R. H., Robinson, A., and Austin, J. H. (1979): Increased aneuploidy in Alzheimer disease. *Am. J. Med. Genet.,* 3:137.
145. Wolozin, B. L., Pruchnicki, A., Dickson, D. W., and Davies, P. (1986): A neuronal antigen in the brains of Alzheimer patients. *Science,* 232:648–650.
146. Yesavage, J. A. (1985): Testimony at Alzheimer's Disease Task Force, State of California, UCLA.

*Aging and the Brain*, edited by R. D. Terry.
Raven Press, New York © 1988.

# Episodic, Semantic, and Procedural Memory: Some Comparisons of Alzheimer and Huntington Disease Patients

Nelson Butters, David P. Salmon, William Heindel,
and Eric Granholm

*Psychology Service, San Diego Veterans Administration Medical Center,
La Jolla, California 92161; and Psychiatry and Neurosciences Departments, School of
Medicine, University of California, San Diego, La Jolla, California 92093*

The potential contributions of experimental studies of amnesia and dementia to the clinical understanding of these disorders were discussed in an earlier report (5). It was noted that little had been learned about the nature of the memory impairments of amnesic and demented patients via the use of standardized tests such as the Wechsler Memory Scale (WMS). Patients with alcoholic Korsakoff syndrome (AK), Huntington disease (HD), and dementia of the Alzheimer type (DAT) often earned similar Memory Quotients (MQs) despite obvious differences in their encoding, storage, and retrieval deficiencies. Our knowledge as to how these patient populations processed new information had originated primarily from the application of the concepts and experimental procedures of cognitive psychology to the assessment of severely defective memories. Butters (5) concluded that a symbiotic relation between clinical neuropsychology and cognitive psychology should be encouraged if the evaluation of patients was to advance beyond superficial statements concerning lesion sites and severity of deficiency. Any hope of a successful extension of clinical neuropsychology into the realm of pharmacological therapies and rehabilitation would depend on additional knowledge of the processes underlying defective achievement.

To exemplify the utility of cognitive psychology to the study of impaired memory, Butters (5) reviewed a series of studies comparing the memory disorders of patients with diencephalic (i.e., AK patients) and basal ganglia (i.e., HD patients) damage. It was noted that the anterograde amnesia of AK patients involved a failure in storage due to an increased sensitivity to proactive interference and limited encoding, whereas the severe deficit of HD patients on recall measures of learning was related to an inability to initiate systematic retrieval processes. The memory failures of AK patients, but not those of HD patients, could be attenuated by the introduction of procedures that reduced proactive interference (e.g., distributed rather than massed learning trials). In contrast, only the HD patients performed at almost normal levels when recognition rather than recall measures of learning were employed.

In addition to this distinction between storage and retrieval impairments, AK and HD patients appeared to differ in their ability to acquire a visuomotor skill (29). Using the reading of mirror-reflected words as a measure of skill learning, Cohen and Squire (16) had shown that AK patients were capable of normal learning and retention of this skill (as measured by reduction in the temporal durations necessary to read mirror-reflected word triads) despite a total inability to recognize the specific words used to train the skill. When Martone and her colleagues (29) extended the mirror reading paradigm to HD patients, a double dissociation between recognition memory and skill learning emerged. Although AK patients performed as described by Cohen and Squire (16), the HD patients were significantly impaired in acquisition of the visuomotor skill. However, the HD patients did demonstrate normal recognition of the words employed on the test. On the basis of these findings, Martone et al. (29) suggested that the learning of motor skills and the storage of factual (i.e., data-based) materials might depend on the integrity of the basal ganglia (especially the caudate nucleus) and limbic-diencephalic regions, respectively.

Since Butters' (5) paper, several studies from this laboratory have provided additional evidence that the memory disorders of HD patients can be characterized by failure in initiating systematic retrieval strategies and in the acquisition of motor skills. In addition to comparisons between amnesic and HD patients, these investigations have also focused on the ability of Alzheimer patients to retrieve information from short-term (i.e., episodic) and long-term (i.e., semantic) memory and to acquire motor skills and what has been called "procedural" knowledge (16,46). The findings have proved to have considerable relevance for Cummings and Benson's (18) proposed distinction between "cortical" and "subcortical" dementia as well as the neuroanatomical bases of episodic, semantic, and procedural memory.

Tulving (49) has defined episodic memories as those dependent on temporal and/or spatial cues for their retrieval. For instance, attempts to recall the previous day's breakfast meal or a specific encounter with a colleague requires the use of temporal and spatial contextual cues and therefore represents retrieval from episodic memory. Most of the traditional verbal learning techniques (e.g., paired-associate learning, list learning) employed by experimental psychologists are categorized as episodic memory tasks. In contrast, semantic memories are totally independent of contextual cues for their retrieval. Various numerical (e.g., the number of feet in a yard), historical (e.g., the name of the first president of the United States, and geographical (e.g., the capital of California) facts serve as examples of semantic memories. Because of repetition and overlearning, memories that are initially episodic in nature may become context-free and part of an individual's semantic fund of knowledge.

Procedural memory refers to a class of diverse memory tasks that remain intact in amnesic patients. For example, amnesic patients can learn and retain motor skills, classically conditioned responses, and visual contour discriminations. In addition, the amnesic patients' ability to unintentionally recall words that they cannot intentionally recall or recognize has also been placed in this category of preserved memory abilities. Although Squire (45,46) has suggested that all forms of procedural memory represent the learning of general rules or procedures rather than specific facts, the enunciation of a clear operational definition of procedural memory has to date proved elusive. Also, whether the various types of procedural memory are mediated by a single or different neuroanatomical systems remains unknown.

The HD patients who participated in our studies are similar to those described by Butters (5). They have a genetically transmitted disorder resulting in progressive atrophy of the basal ganglia, especially the caudate nucleus. The most common behavioral symptoms include involuntary choreiform movements, progressive dementia, and in most cases marked personality changes (e.g., depression, increased irritability). Although the first onset of symptomatology is difficult to judge, almost all of the patients used in these investigations initially evidenced choreiform movements during the third or fourth decade of life. These HD patients had a mean age of 46 years and had been diagnosed 3 months to 19 years prior to testing. The mean full-scale IQ (WAIS-R) and MQ (WMS) scores of these patients were in the middle 80s and high 70s, respectively. Although some of the HD patients had moderate choreiform movements (i.e., many had only mild chorea), none was considered in the terminal stages of the illness.

The patients with Alzheimer disease were diagnosed using the clinical criteria developed by the National Institute on Neurological and Communicative Disorders and Stroke and the Alzheimer's Disease and Related Disorders Association (31). All patients scored at or above 104 of a possible 144 points on the Dementia Rating Scale (DRS), a mental status examination that assesses a broad spectrum of cognitive functions (30). In addition, the patients averaged 7 to 10 errors of a possible 33 errors on Fuld's (22) adaptation of the Information-Memory-Concentration Test (3), and they had 21 to 24 correct responses of a possible 30 on the Mini-Mental State examination (21).

Most of the amnesic patients in these studies were alcoholics with Korsakoff syndrome. They were male veterans with a mean age of 58 years. They all had 20- to 30-year histories of alcohol addiction accompanied by malnutrition prior to the onset of their Wernicke-Korsakoff syndrome. At the time of testing, all of the Korsakoff patients were residing in a Veterans Administration facility or nursing home. They had severe anterograde and retrograde amnesias, as measured by the WMS and on the basis of clinical assessment, but their general intellectual functioning, as measured by the WAIS (or WAIS-R), was within normal limits (mean 103). Their MQs were a minimum of 18 points lower than their full-scale IQs. Although it is generally assumed that these patients' severe amnesia is related to hemorrhagic lesions in the medial diencephalon (50), there is some evidence that AK patients, like patients with DAT, may also have a significant loss of neurons in various structures of the basal forebrain (1).

## EPISODIC AND SEMANTIC MEMORY

The dichotomy between *episodic* and *semantic* memory has been used to differentiate the impairments of amnesic and demented patients (28,51). Although both amnesic and demented patients are impaired in the acquisition and recall of materials associated with particular temporal and/or spatial contexts (i.e., episodic memory), only demented patients are severely impaired in recalling general knowledge such as rules of grammar and multiplication tables (i.e., semantic memory). In one study Weingartner and his colleagues (51) compared the performances of AK patients with those of patients with progressive dementias (presumably Alzheimer disease) on both episodic (e.g., verbal list learning) and semantic (e.g., sentence completion, verbal fluency) memory tasks. As anticipated, both the Korsakoff and demented patients were severely impaired in the acquisition of word lists and the immediate recall of short passages, whereas only the demented patients evidenced severe deficits in the completion of highly structured sentences and on a letter fluency task. Other studies utilizing verbal fluency tasks to assess semantic memory have reported significant impairments even during the early stages of Alzheimer and Huntington diseases (11,35,39).

In addition to demonstrating the existence of episodic and/or semantic memory problems in amnesic and demented patients, some investigations have focused on the processes underlying these cognitive deficiencies. Although AK patients encounter more difficulty with episodic than with semantic memory tasks, their performances on both are marked by several indices of increased sensitivity to proactive interference. For example, AK patients are highly prone to prior-item (list, passage) intrusions on short-term memory tasks (8), verbal paired-associate learning (52), recall of short passages (12), and verbal fluency tests (12). In comparison to AK patients, demented HD patients appear to be severely impaired on both episodic and semantic memory tasks due to a general retrieval problem. On list learning tests and tasks involving memory of prose passages HD patients perform as poorly as do AK patients when recall measures are employed, but the HD patients are superior to amnesic patients if recognition tests are introduced (12,13). On letter fluency tasks, HD patients generate fewer correct responses (as well as perseverative errors) than do AK patients. This double dissociation between

HD and AK patients on verbal recognition and verbal fluency tests has been cited as evidence that HD patients are impaired in the initiation of systematic strategies for searching both episodic and semantic memory (12). More specifically, as the retrieval demands are reduced (e.g., the use of recognition rather than recall memory tests) or increased (e.g., letter fluency test), the performances of HD patients change dramatically in comparison to those of amnesic subjects.

One of our most recent investigations (10) has extended these analyses of episodic and semantic memory to patients with DAT. The performances of Alzheimer, HD, and AK patients were compared to those of young and elderly intact control subjects on memory for passages (i.e., episodic memory) and two (letter, category) verbal fluency tasks (i.e., semantic memory). Based on previous findings (12,13), it was anticipated that the quantitative and qualitative features of the AK and HD patients' responses would again reflect the role of an increased sensitivity to proactive interference (AK patients) and a general retrieval deficit (HD patients). Because patients with DAT also commit numerous perseveration and intrusion errors on episodic (7,23) and semantic (35) memory tasks, some similarities in the memory deficiencies of the AK and Alzheimer patients were anticipated. However, in view of Alzheimer patients' aphasic difficulties, they were expected to demonstrate a distinctive pattern of problems on the letter and category fluency tasks. If, as Martin and Fedio (28) have suggested, patients with DAT suffer an extensive reduction in the number of exemplars (e.g., dog, cat) comprising abstract categories (e.g., animals), they should be more impaired on category than on letter fluency tasks, especially in the very early stages of the disease.

The psychometric and demographic characteristics of the five subject groups participating in this study are shown in Table 1. The young normal controls were matched for age to the HD patients; and the old (i.e., elderly) normal controls were age-matched to the patients with DAT. It is important to stress that the three patient groups did *not* differ in terms of overall degree of dementia as assessed with the DRS. Such matching for general cognitive loss helps reduce the confounding of differences due to disease entity (e.g., HD versus DAT) with those due to severity of dementia (e.g., mild versus severe dementia). Because the three patient groups were equated in terms of the severity of their overall cognitive deficits, any differences among the groups' performances on the episodic and semantic memory tests are likely to reflect the pattern of memory decline associated with the particular neurologic diseases. As might be expected on the basis of Cummings and Benson's (18) proposed distinction between cortical (e.g., DAT) and subcortical (e.g., HD) dementias, only the Alzheimer patients showed a moderate degree of language dysfunction as assessed with the Boston Naming Test.

The episodic memory task involved the recall of four thematically neutral stories. Each story was composed of 23 arbitrarily designated phrases or units of information. All stories were similar in format and length to the Logical

TABLE 1. *Psychometric and demographic characteristics*

| Group | Age | Years of education | Dementia rating scale | Boston naming test |
|---|---|---|---|---|
| Young normal controls | 45.08 | 13.00 | 141.54 | 57.17 |
| (*n* = 13) | (9.56) | (1.47) | (2.18) | (1.75) |
| Old normal controls | 68.15 | 14.39 | 140.39 | 56.39 |
| (*n* = 13) | (4.54) | (2.93) | (2.40) | (2.66) |
| Huntington disease | 48.42 | 13.33 | 125.75 | 53.42 |
| patients (*n* = 12) | (13.60) | (2.31) | (7.57) | (5.92) |
| Alzheimer disease | 68.39 | 14.23 | 121.46 | 42.15 |
| patients (*n* = 13) | (7.32) | (2.62) | (10.55) | (14.18) |
| Alcoholic Korsakoff | 60.22 | 11.22 | 123.00 | 54.89 |
| patients (*n* = 9) | (4.52) | (3.23) | (5.45) | (4.34) |

Results are shown as the mean, with the SD in parentheses.

Memory Passages of the Wechsler Memory Scale, contained approximately the same amount of detail, and were written in the third person. The four stories were read aloud sequentially, and the subjects were instructed to listen closely and remember the story they were about to hear. Following the presentation of each story, the subjects were asked to count backward from 100 by 3s for 30 sec, and then were asked to recall as much of the story as they could remember. When the subjects indicated that they were unable to recall any additional material, they were allowed a 10-sec rest interval before the next story was presented. All stories were scored according to a verbatim scale that gave one point credit for each verbatim informational unit recalled by the subject. In addition to the items correctly recalled, the examiner recorded prior-story (i.e., a correctly recalled item from one story that is recalled as part of a subsequent story) and extra-story (i.e., ideas recalled by the subject that were never presented in any story) intrusion errors.

The evaluation of semantic memory was composed of two parts: a letter fluency task (FAS) developed by Benton and his colleagues (2,4) and a category fluency task. On the letter fluency task, the subjects were read the letters *F, A,* and *S* sequentially and asked to produce "as many *different* words as they could think of" that began with the given letter. They were instructed that proper nouns and the repetition of a word with a different suffix (e.g., *find, finding*) were not acceptable. For each of the three letters, the subjects were allowed 60 sec to orally generate words. On the category fluency task, the subjects were asked to produce "as many different *animals* as they could think of." The animal (i.e., category) fluency task was administered 60 sec after the end of the letter fluency test.

All of the subjects' responses (correct and incorrect) were recorded, and the examiner noted whether the responses were produced within the first, second, third, or fourth 15-sec quadrant of the given trial (i.e., whether they were produced between 0 and 15 sec, 16 to 30 sec, 31 to 45 sec, or 46 to 60 sec). Responses were categorized into four types: (a) correct responses, (b) perseveration errors, (c) intrusion errors, and (d) variation errors. Perseveration errors were defined as the repetition of a correct word within a given trial (e.g., generating *friend* as the first and eighth word to the letter *F*). Intrusion errors were responses that did not conform to the criteria established for the given letter or animal category (e.g., saying *house* on the *F* trial). Variation errors were words repeated within a given trial with a different or added suffix (e.g., saying *friend* and then *friendly* on the *F* trial).

The results for the episodic memory task (i.e., memory for passages) showed that all three patient groups were severely impaired compared to their age-matched controls in the number of phrases they correctly recalled (Fig. 1). The major differences among the three patient groups became apparent when the numbers of prior-story and extra-story intrusion errors were examined. Both the AK patients and the patients with DAT made more intrusion errors than did their age-matched controls and the HD patients. When the performances of the patient groups are evaluated in terms of proportions (percent) of total responses (Fig. 2), the differences among the three patient groups are even more striking. Although the HD patients did not recall many phrases from the four stories, what little they did recall was usually correct (78%). In contrast, less than 50% of the impaired recall of the AK and Alzheimer patients was correct; most of their recall represented some combination of prior- and extra-story intrusion errors.

The major results for the letter and category fluency tasks are shown in Fig. 3. On the left side of the figure, the total number of correct responses on the letter fluency test is displayed for each of the four 15-sec quadrants. On the right side of the figure, the total number of correct animal names generated in each 15-sec quadrant is shown. As anticipated on the basis of the literature (28,35,39), all subject groups displayed their greatest fluency during the first 15-sec quadrant, and their performances tended to decrease in a negatively decelerated fashion over the entire four quadrants.

Four major differences appeared among the five subject groups. (a) The HD patients were equally impaired on letter and category fluency tasks. Of the three patient groups, the HD patients were the most consistently and severely impaired in their attempts to retrieve information from semantic memory. (b) The AK patients showed mild to moderate impairment on both fluency tests, and like the HD patients the severity of their fluency problem was not related to the linguistic constraints (i.e., letter versus category fluency) of the semantic memory task. (c) The performance of the Alzheimer patients was directly related to the linguistic demands of the two fluency tasks. On the letter fluency test, the patients with DAT generated almost as many correct words as did their age-matched controls and actually produced more correct words than did the HD and AK patients. However, on the category fluency task, the performance of the patients with DAT was severely impaired. They generated significantly fewer correct animal names than did

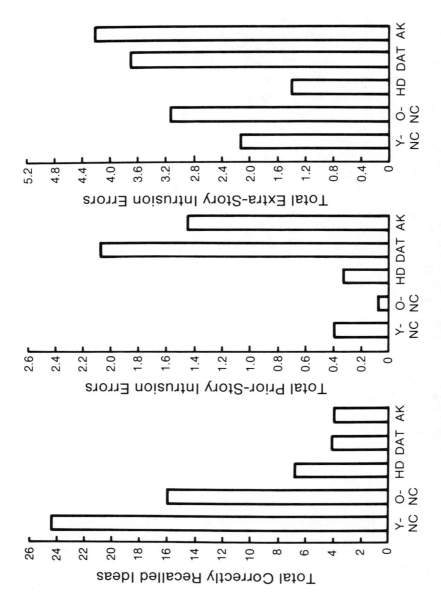

**FIG. 1.** Performance of young normal control (Y-NC) and old normal control (O-NC) subjects and patients with Huntington disease (HD), dementia of the Alzheimer type (DAT), and alcoholic Korsakoff (AK) syndrome on the story recall test. (Adapted from Butters et al., ref. 10.)

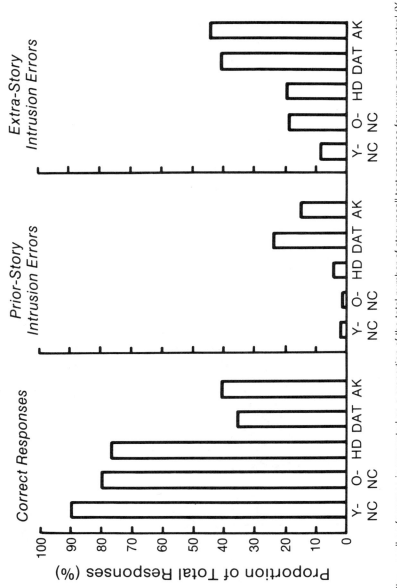

**FIG. 2.** Story recall performance is presented as a proportion of the total number of story recall test responses for young normal control (Y-NC) and old normal control (O-NC) subjects and for patients with Huntington disease (HD), dementia of the Alzheimer type (DAT), and alcoholic Korsakoff (AK) syndrome. (Adapted from Butters et al., ref. 10.)

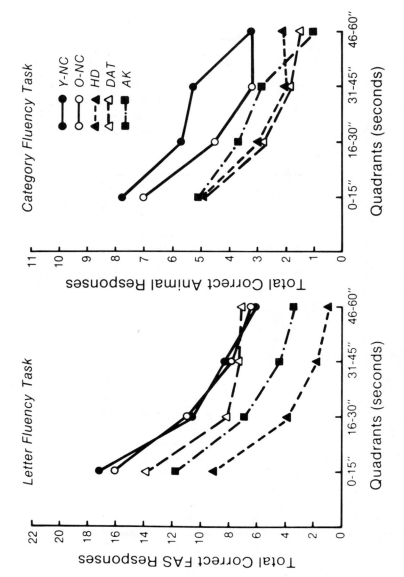

**FIG. 3.** Performance of young normal control (Y-NC) and old normal control (O-NC) subjects and patients with Huntington disease (HD), dementia of the Alzheimer type (DAT), and alcoholic Korsakoff (AK) syndrome on the letter (FAS) and category (animal) fluency tasks. (Adapted from Butters et al., ref. 10.)

their elderly age-matched controls, and their performance was indistinguishable from that of the severely impaired HD patients. (d) Although the young and elderly control subjects did not differ on the letter fluency task, the elderly controls generated significantly fewer animal names than did the young control subjects.

The total number of perseveration, intrusion, and variation errors on the letter fluency test is shown in Table 2. Although the HD patients and the young controls did not differ significantly in terms of perseveration errors, both the Alzheimer and Korsakoff patients committed more perseveration errors than did the elderly control subjects. Comparisons among the three patient groups indicated that the HD patients made significantly fewer perseveration errors than did the patients with DAT and the AK patients. For intrusion errors and variations, none of the differences among the subject groups approached statistical significance.

In order to correct for group differences in the total number of words produced on the letter fluency task, the proportion (percent) of each subject's total responses that were correct productions, perseveration errors, intrusion errors, and variations was calculated (Fig. 4). The HD patients did not differ from the young control subjects in terms of the percentage of correct responses, whereas the DAT and the AK patients had significantly lower percentages of correct responses than did the elderly control subjects. Group comparisons for perseveration errors showed that both the Alzheimer and AK patients repeated words significantly more often than did the elderly control subjects. The HD patients and the young control subjects did not differ in their tendency to commit perseveration errors. Analyses of intrusion errors and variations failed to yield any significant differences among the subject groups.

A similar comparison of perseveration and intrusion errors was conducted for the category fluency test. No significant group differences emerged from either of these two error types.

TABLE 2. *Total number of errors on the letter fluency task*

| Group | Perseverations | Intrusions | Variations |
|---|---|---|---|
| Young normal controls | 0.67 | 0.25 | 0.08 |
| | (0.99) | (0.45) | (0.29) |
| Old normal controls | 1.39 | 0.69 | 0.31 |
| | (1.71) | (0.86) | (0.63) |
| Huntington disease patients | 0.67 | 0.25 | 0.25 |
| | (1.16) | (0.62) | (0.45) |
| Alzheimer disease patients | 3.62 | 1.08 | 0.92 |
| | (3.57) | (1.66) | (1.32) |
| Alcoholic Korsakoff patients | 4.11 | 1.00 | 0.33 |
| | (2.03) | (1.00) | (0.50) |

Results are given as the mean, with the SD in parentheses.

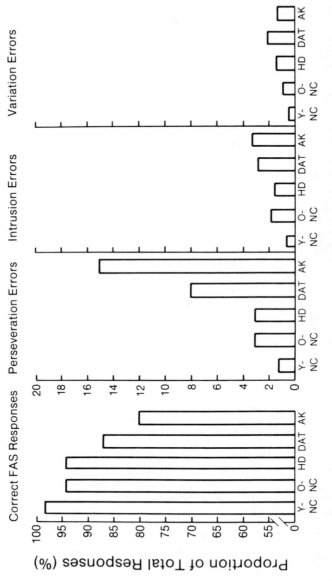

**FIG. 4.** Performance on the letter (FAS) fluency task is presented as a proportion of the total number of letter fluency task responses for young normal control (Y-NC) and old normal control (O-NC) subjects and for patients with Huntington disease (HD), dementia of the Alzheimer type (DAT), and alcoholic Korsakoff (AK) syndrome. (Adapted from Butters et al., ref. 10.)

These findings (10) indicate that patients with DAT have a pattern of deficits on episodic and semantic memory tasks that differentiates them from those with other dementing (e.g., HD) and amnesic (e.g., AK) disorders. When asked to recall short passages, the patients with DAT remembered few correct facts and made numerous prior-story and extra-story intrusion errors. The ubiquitousness of these intrusions exemplifies the Alzheimer patients' increased sensitivity to proactive interference and confirms other reports that intrusion errors are an important characteristic of these patients' episodic memory disorder (23,24).

On the two fluency tasks (i.e., semantic memory), the Alzheimer patients were adversely affected by their aphasic disorder (as evidenced by their severe impairment on the Boston Naming Test) as well as by their increased sensitivity to interference. Although the patients with DAT generated nearly as many correct responses as did the intact elderly controls on the letter fluency task, they emitted significantly more perseveration errors. Of even greater import for the Alzheimer patients' problems with semantic memory was the difference in their performances on the category and letter fluency tests. They were severely impaired in producing names of animals but encountered few problems on the letter fluency task. That is, their deficits in semantic memory were most apparent when they had to search for exemplars of an abstract category (i.e., animals). If, as Martin and Fedio (28) and Ober et al. (35) have suggested, the Alzheimer patients' language problems involve a reduction in the number of exemplars comprising an abstract category, scores on the category fluency task should be a highly sensitive measure of deficiencies in semantic memory. Because the letter fluency task can be performed using phonemic cues to search an extensive set of appropriate exemplars, impairments on this task may not be apparent until the disease has progressed beyond its earliest stages. It should also be noted that the significant difference between the elderly and young control subjects on the category fluency test suggests that some of the linguistic aberrations noted in Alzheimer patients may simply represent an acceleration of changes associated with "normal" aging.

These results (10) for the two fluency tests seem to conflict with some aspects of the findings of Rosen (39) and Ober et al. (35). They found that "mild" Alzheimer patients were impaired on both letter and category fluency tasks, and that their patients made numerous variation and intrusion as well as perseveration errors. A close scrutiny of these previous investigations suggests that the discrepancies between their findings and those just described (10) may be due to differences in the severity of the patients' dementia. Ober et al.'s (35) "mild" Alzheimer patients included patients with DRS scores as low as 95, whereas the lowest score of any patient with DAT in the present study (10) was 107. Although Alzheimer patients in the present study were selected on the basis of their DRS scores, their mean performance of 9.6 errors (SD 6.4) on Fuld's (22) 33-point mental status examination falls below the range of 11 to 19 errors compiled by Rosen's "mild" dementia patients on the same test. It appears then that the patients in the present study (10) represent an earlier stage of the disease than has been assessed in many other reports. If so, these early patients' performances on semantic memory tests seem dependent on the linguistic features of the to-be-retrieved memories. The more patients in the early stages of DAT must search for exemplars of an abstract, limited (i.e., relatively few exemplars) category the more obvious their deficiencies in semantic memory become. Impairments on the letter fluency task may require a more advanced stage of dementia in which paraphasic errors as well as dysnomia are apparent.

The HD patients' performances on the story recall and fluency tasks indicate that their episodic and semantic memory disorders involve processes different from those of Alzheimer patients. The HD patients were impaired on story recall and fluency measures, but their pattern of deficits and errors do not suggest a special role for proactive interference and general language dysfunctions. The HD patients displayed a relatively low proportion of intrusion and perseveration errors in comparison to Alzheimer patients and yet were severely impaired on both letter and category fluency tests. Although this study was not designed to evaluate the hypothesis that HD patients' episodic and semantic memory disorders reflect a general retrieval deficit (5,12,14), the findings are certainly consistent with this notion. Patients who encounter unusual difficulty in retrieving successfully stored information should be impaired on virtually all fluency tasks regardless of their linguistic demands. As has been noted previously (18), patients with subcortical dementias have difficulty initiating not only movement but also systematic problem-solving and retrieval strategies.

The alcoholics with Korsakoff's syndrome performed as anticipated on the episodic memory task. They recalled few verbatim items from the stories and made numerous prior- and extra-story intrusion errors. The prior-story intrusions serve as another indicator of the Korsakoff patients' well-known increased sensitivity to proactive interference (8), whereas the extra-story intrusions may be a remnant of these patients' tendency to confabulate during the acute phase of the disorder. The AK patients' propensity for perseverative intrusion errors was also evident on one of the semantic memory tasks (i.e., letter fluency), where they often repeated correct words (e.g., *field*, found, factory, *field*) during the 60-sec test period. Apparently, whether episodic or semantic memory is being assessed, those memories dominating a Korsakoff patient's response hierarchy at a given moment are repeatedly emitted and remain unmonitored by any inhibitory feedback.

Although the AK patients' poor story recall and error patterns were anticipated, their significant impairments on both fluency tasks are inconsistent with Weingartner et al.'s (51) report that such patients perform normally on letter fluency and other semantic memory tasks. A comparison of the psychometric (e.g., IQ, MQ) and demographic (e.g., age, education) characteristics of Weingartner et al.'s and the present population of Korsakoff patients does not yield any immediate clues as to the differences in the two studies, but a review of the available literature on the cognitive deficits of AK patients does suggest that these patients' semantic memories are not totally intact. For example, behavioral studies (43,47) have concluded that AK patients manifest at least moderate dysfunction of the prefrontal association cortex, a brain region shown to be vital for the maintenance of normal problem-solving (32) as well as verbal and nonverbal fluency (2,27,38). If Korsakoff patients are consistently impaired in initiating and shifting problem-solving strategies on numerous visuoperceptual sorting tasks (36,37,43,47), it should not be surprising that they also fail to adequately organize appropriate retrieval strategies on fluency tests.

Similarly, Butters and Cermak (9) have noted that AK patients may forget substantial amounts of semantic knowledge related to their professions. When patient P.Z., an eminent scientist who had acutely developed alcoholic Korsakoff's syndrome at 65 years of age, was queried about scientific terms he had defined and extensively discussed in numerous publications and textbooks, he was severely impaired in comparison to an age- and occupation-matched control subject. Butters and Cermak concluded that whereas semantic memories concerning the basic rules of grammar and arithmetic are preserved in Korsakoff's syndrome, complex and/or highly specialized semantic memories may not be accessible to the patient. From this viewpoint, AK patients (and perhaps all amnesics) have a relative, but not absolute, preservation of semantic memory.

The parallels in the performances of the Korsakoff and Alzheimer patients are deserving of some mention. As Butters (6) reported in a preliminary comparison of these patients' story recall and letter fluency, both Alzheimer and Korsakoff patients are prone to perseveration and intrusion errors. Although such error tendencies are not necessarily indicative of a specific brain dysfunction or etiology (42), one neuropathological report provided some basis for considering a common neurochemical factor in these two disorders. Arendt and his colleagues (1) have reported that the number of neurons in basal forebrain structures was reduced by 70% and 47% in the brains of Alzheimer and Korsakoff patients, respectively. Examination of the brains of HD patients revealed a significant loss of neurons in the globus pallidus but not in the basal forebrain. Given that the basal forebrain is the source of cholinergic input to the hippocampus and frontal association cortex, one might speculate that the common error patterns of Alzheimer and AK patients might reflect a similar underlying cholinergic deficiency. Although this suggestion is certainly worthy of further neurochemical and neuropathological investigation, the differences between Alzheimer and AK patients in terms of aphasic and dyspraxic symptoms must not be overlooked. The lack of aphasia and severe constructional apraxia in AK patients may be due to differences in the extent of basal forebrain damage or may be indications that the noted similarities in the two disorders are coincidental.

The possible involvement of the basal forebrain in alcoholic Korsakoff's syndrome may also help to explain why HD patients are not prone to perseverative tendencies and an increased sensitivity to proactive interference. Based on the major anatomical connections between the caudate nucleus and the frontal lobes (19,34,40), one might anticipate that HD patients would manifest the behavioral consequences (e.g., perseverative tendencies) of disruption of the corticostriatal system. The failure in the present study (10) to note these tendencies in the episodic and semantic memory performances of HD patients may reflect a number of possible factors. (a) In the early stages of HD a sufficient portion of the caudate nucleus and frontocaudal connections may remain to prevent the perseverative-type behavior so common in AK patients. (b) Korsakoff patients may endure more direct damage to the frontal cortex than do HD patients. In addition to the disturbance of fronto-diencephalic connections from lesions in the medial thalamus, AK patients, like all long-term alcoholics, may experience direct damage to the prefrontal cortex due to the neurotoxic effects of ethanol (6). (c) As indicated by Arendt et al. (1), the brains of AK, but not of HD, patients are characterized by a loss of neurons in various portions of the basal forebrain. Thus the maintenance of cholinergic input to the partially compromised frontal system of HD patients may be sufficient to ensure that perseverative tendencies and an increased sensitivity to proactive interference do not compound the patients' retrieval deficits.

Finally, the findings of our investigation (10) not only support the notion that episodic and semantic memory are disturbed in the dementias but also demonstrate that the processes underlying failures in episodic and semantic memory systems may vary from one patient population to another. Patients with HD perform poorly on both episodic and semantic memory tasks because of their inability to initiate suitable retrieval strategies, whereas the deficits of patients with DAT on these same memory tasks reflect at least some linguistic aberrations and an increased sensitivity to proactive interference. Based on these data, it seems reasonable to propose that future investigations should focus on the identification of additional factors that contribute to impairments in the episodic and semantic memory systems of an even broader range of dementing and amnesic disorders. Certainly, the notion that dementia represents a loss of both episodic and semantic memory seems too simplistic and likely blurs many important distinctions among various cortical and subcortical degenerative diseases.

## PROCEDURAL MEMORY

Based on Martone et al.'s (29) findings, Heindel et al. (26) examined the ability of HD and Alzheimer patients to acquire the motor skills underlying a pursuit rotor task. This classical test of skill learning had the advantage that it avoided some of the methodological problems encountered on the mirror reading task. For example, the HD patients' impairments in reading mirror-reflected words may have been more attributable to the eye movement problems associated with this disease than to a general impairment in skill learning. Also, the interpretation of Martone et al.'s results is further confounded by the failure of the HD patients to begin the mirror reading task at the same initial level of performance as the other subjects (i.e., they were slower than the Korsakoff patients and normal controls). Different levels of initial performance can often result in ceiling or floor effects that reduce the meaningfulness of the results. In Heindel et al.'s study, initial performance levels were equated by manipulating the difficulty (i.e., speed of rotation of the disk) of the pursuit rotor task. The use of this tracking task rather than a mirror reading test also reduced any effects attributable to the HD patients' abnormal eye movements.

A total of 45 patients participated in this study: 10 HD patients, 10 patients with DAT, 4 amnesic patients of mixed etiologies, and 20 intact control subjects. As in our fluency studies (10), the three patient groups were matched for overall degree of dementia with the DRS. The small group of amnesics (tested only on the pursuit rotor task) was included to confirm previous findings of spared motor learning in amnesia (15,17). The inclusion of Alzheimer as well as HD patients provided an opportunity to compare the performances of patients with cortical and subcortical dementias. Based on a report by Eslinger and Damasio (20) concerned with pursuit rotor learning in Alzheimer patients, it was anticipated that patients with DAT would demonstrate normal acquisition of this motor skill. Both the HD and Alzheimer groups were also administered a verbal recognition span test (33) to establish the severity of their deficits in learning new verbal information. Ten of the 20 normal control subjects were tested only on the pursuit rotor task; the remaining 10 control subjects were administered only the recognition span test.

On the pursuit rotor task subjects were told to try to maintain contact between a stylus held in their preferred hand and a small metallic disk (2 cm in diameter) on a rotating turntable (25 cm in diameter). The turntable could be adjusted to rotate at 15, 30, 45, or 60 rotations per minute (rpm) for a given 20-sec trial. All subjects were tested over three sessions of eight trials each, with each session separated by approximately 30 min of other psychometric testing. Within each test session, subjects were also allowed a 1-min rest interval between the fourth and fifth trials, thereby creating six blocks of four trials each. The total time on target was recorded for each 20-sec trial.

For each subject the first test session was preceded by a block of practice trials to determine the speed of rotation (i.e., 15, 30, 45, 60 rpm) of the turntable. On each successive practice trial the speed of the turntable was increased. The turntable was then set for the remainder of the subject's testing that speed associated with a score (i.e., time on target) closest to 5 sec (i.e., contact maintained 25% of time). In this manner the initial level of performance on the pursuit rotor task was equated for the four subject groups.

The verbal recognition span test has been described in detail elsewhere (33). It involves a delayed non-matching-to-sample procedure to estimate the longest span of words a subject can recognize before making an error and to assess immediate and delayed (2 min) recall of the words presented on the recognition test. Briefly, the subject and examiner were seated across from each other on opposite sides of a test board (61 × 46 cm) on which were mounted 30 yellow dots (12.5 mm in diameter) arranged in a 6 × 5 matrix. A black, opaque sliding door was mounted perpendicular to the front of the test board to ensure that placement of the stimuli could be shielded from the subject's view. The stimuli consisted in 14 brown plastic disks (5.08 cm in diameter), each with a unique five-letter word (low imagery nouns and verbs of moderate to high frequency in the English language).

Subjects were first shown the test board for 15 sec with only one disk (i.e., word) placed on it. The door was then closed, and a second disk was placed over one of the yellow dots on the test board. When the door was lifted again, the subject was asked to point to the *new* word. This procedure was repeated with yet another word until all 14 words (i.e., disks) had been presented to the subject. In order to eliminate spatial cues, the examiner moved the previously exposed disks to new positions at the same time he placed a new stimulus on the test board. All subjects were administered two consecutive series of 14 trials each. The subject's *recognition span* (i.e., the number of new words correctly identified before making an error) as well as the *total number of correct responses* (maximum 14) were recorded for both test series. In addition, *recall memory* was assessed by asking the subjects to recall, both immediately after the completion of recognition testing and again 2 min later, as many of the words as they could remember from the recognition test.

The results for the pursuit rotor task are shown in Fig. 5. It is evident that all four groups began at the same level of performance (approximately 25% time on target) and that three of the four groups evidenced systematic skill learning over the six blocks of testing. The Alzheimer and amnesic patients and the normal control subjects improved their performance to approximately 52% time on target on block 6, whereas the HD patients maintained contact between the stylus and the disk for only 36% of the time on this last test block. When difference scores (block 6 − block 1) were calculated to measure the amount of skill acquisition (Fig. 6), the HD patients showed significantly less learning than did the other three groups. As anticipated, the amnesic and Alzheimer patients did not differ from the intact control subjects on any measure of skill acquisition.

The results of the recognition span test are shown in Table 3. The Alzheimer and HD patients were both severely impaired in terms of length of verbal span and of immediate and delayed recall. However, although the HD

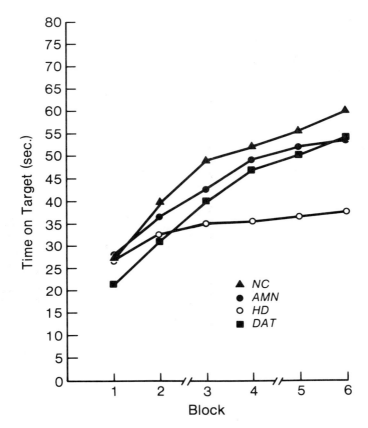

**FIG. 5.** Performance of normal control (NC) subjects, amnesic (AMN) and Huntington disease (HD) patients, and patients with dementia of the Alzheimer type (DAT) on the pursuit rotor task. (Adapted from Heindel et al., ref. 26.)

and Alzheimer patients did not differ on recognition span, the patients with DAT evidenced less recall and more rapid forgetting (i.e., immediate-delayed recall) than did the HD patients.

Like Martone et al.'s (29) findings, the results of Heindel et al.'s study (26) supported the notion that the basal ganglia (especially the neostriatum) are involved in the acquisition of motor skills. Because the four subject groups were matched for initial level of performance on the pursuit rotor task, the impairment of the HD patients cannot be attributed to ceiling or floor effects or to the motor limitations associated with the HD patients' choreiform movements. It should also be noted that the matching of the three patient groups in terms of overall level of dementia with the DRS reduces the

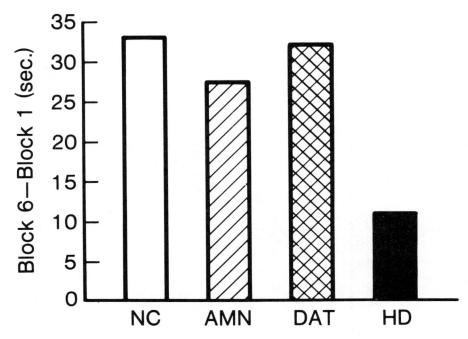

**FIG. 6.** Difference in performance between the last and first test blocks on the pursuit rotor task. NC = normal control subjects. AMN = amnesic patients. HD = patients with Huntington disease. DAT = patients with dementia of the Alzheimer type. (Adapted from Heindel et al., ref. 26.)

TABLE 3. *Verbal recognition span test: mean recognition performance, immediate and delayed recall, and savings scores*

| Group | Mean recognition span | Mean total correct responses (recognition) | Immediate recall | Delayed recall | Savings (%) |
|---|---|---|---|---|---|
| Huntington disease patients (*n* = 8) | 5.69 | 10.00 | 5.38 | 4.13 | 70 |
| Alzheimer disease patients (*n* = 9) | 5.89 | 9.39 | 2.44 | 0.89 | 32 |
| Normal controls (*n* = 10) | 11.90 | 13.00 | 6.80 | 6.50 | 98 |

possibility that the differences in the learning of the motor skill might reflect differences in degree of overall cognitive loss (i.e., dementia).

Despite their profound inability to learn a motor skill, the HD patients were not as impaired on the verbal memory test as were the Alzheimer patients. This pattern of results is similar to the double dissociation noted previously between HD and amnesic patients on a visuomotor skill (i.e., reading of mirror-reflected words) and a verbal recognition test (29). The ability of the HD patients to retain more information over a 2-min delay (i.e., savings scores for immediate and delayed recall) compared to the patients with DAT suggests that their respective memory impairments may be due to different processing deficits. Patients with degenerative diseases affecting the hippocampi (e.g., DAT) may be unable to store new factual information for more than a brief temporal period, whereas patients with dementias due to dysfunction of the basal ganglia (e.g., HD) may have a memory impairment characterized by deficient retrieval of relatively well stored information.

Although the linkage between the learning of factual data-based material and hippocampal-diencephalic structures appears firmly established (46), knowledge of the neuroanatomical substrate mediating the acquisition of motor skills and the learning of general procedures and rules is extremely limited. One possibility is that the different types of what Squire (44,46) has called *procedural memory* are mediated by distinct neural systems. The results of Heindel et al.'s investigation (26), in conjunction with those of a report concerning verbal priming in HD and Alzheimer patients (41) lend credence to this proposed dissociability of various forms of procedural memory (Fig. 7). Priming has been defined as the temporary facilitation of performance via prior exposure to stimuli and has been viewed as a form of procedural memory (45). For example, it has been shown that both amnesic patients and intact control subjects have a strong tendency (relative to chance) to complete three-letter word stems (e.g., *mot*) with previously presented words (e.g., *motel*) despite the failure of the amnesic patients to recall or recognize these words on standard memory tests (25). Although patients with DAT in Heindel et al.'s study showed intact learning of a motor skill, those in Shimamura et al.'s (41) study were severely impaired when compared to control and amnesic subjects on a stem-completion priming task. The reverse relation was found for HD patients who were severely impaired on Heindel et al.'s (26) pursuit rotor task yet exhibited normal levels of stem-completion priming (41).

This double dissociation between HD and Alzheimer patients on the stem-completion priming and pursuit rotor tasks suggests that various types of procedural memory do depend on different neuroanatomical substrates. The HD patients' impairments on pursuit rotor and mirror reading tests are certainly consistent with the proposed association between the acquisition of motor skills and the neostriatum, whereas the Alzheimer patients' deficiencies on verbal priming tasks may be attributable to the cortical neuropathology reported in DAT (3,48).

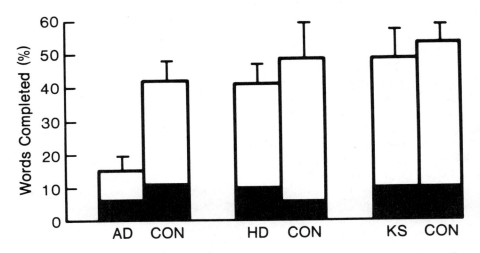

**FIG. 7.** Lexical priming ability as measured by the word completion test. Patients with Alzheimer disease (AD), Huntington disease (HD), and alcoholic Korsakoff disease (KS), as well as normal control (CON) subjects were shown words (e.g., motel) and later asked to complete three-letter word stems (e.g., mot) with the first words that came to mind. *Bars* represent the percentage of previously presented words that were used to complete word stems (total number of study words = 20). *Dark area* of each bar represents the baseline guessing performance, i.e., the tendency to complete the same words under conditions when they had not been presented. Performance of each patient group is shown next to its age-matched control group. (Adapted from Shimamura et al., ref. 41.)

The dissociation between the HD and Alzheimer patients has relevance for Cummings and Benson's (18) distinction between cortical and subcortical dementias. Patients with subcortical dementias (e.g., HD, Parkinson disease) usually have much less dysphasia and dyspraxia than do patients with cortical dementias (e.g., Alzheimer disease, Creutzfeldt-Jakob disease) but are also much slower to initiate and complete most cognitive, as well as motor, processes than are patients with cortical degenerative diseases. With regard to memory deficits, patients with cortical and subcortical dementias are supposed to have deficiencies in storage and retrieval, respectively. Our data are consistent with this storage-retrieval dichotomy, but they also point to another distinction between these two generic forms of dementia. Patients with cortical dementias have a preserved capacity to acquire and retain motor skills, although they may be severely impaired on other forms of procedural knowledge that depend on the intactness of the association cortex in the dominant hemisphere. In contrast, patients with subcortical dementias appear limited in their ability to learn motor skills despite their normal performance on procedural memory tasks mediated by verbal processes (e.g., stem-completion priming). Further investigations employing various types of cortical and subcortical dementias and larger batteries of procedural and rule learning tasks will determine the validity of this generalization.

## CONCLUSIONS

The neuropsychological studies reviewed in this chapter are consistent with the notion that patients with Alzheimer and Huntington diseases can be differentiated from each other and from patients with amnesic conditions. Although patients with DAT and HD patients are impaired on episodic and semantic memory tasks, they seen to fail for quite distinct reasons. The HD patients' capacity to store new verbal information seems relatively preserved, but these patients appear extremely deficient in initiating systemic retrieval strategies when asked to recall information from either episodic or semantic memory. In contrast, patients with DAT encounter unusual difficulty when consolidating new information, and their attempts to recall information from semantic memory are often hindered by their dysphasia. The deleterious effects of proactive interference are also more apparent in the episodic and semantic memory deficits of Alzheimer than of HD patients.

Investigations focusing on the learning of motor skills and other type of procedural memory usually preserved in amnesic patients suggest additional dissociations between cortical and subcortical dementias. Although HD patients appear severely impaired in their attempts to acquire motor skills, they perform normally on stem-completion priming tasks. The opposite relation is seen in patients with DAT. Alzheimer patients acquire and retain motor skills with the same facility as intact controls and amnesic patients, but they evidence little tendency to complete three-letter stems with words previously exposed to them. These findings suggest that the learning of motor skills and stem-completion priming depend on different neuroanatomical systems and also lend support to the previously proposed distinction between cortical and subcortical dementias.

From a clinical perspective, it is important to stress again that the present findings emanate from the application of concepts borrowed from cognitive psychology and from careful analyses of the processes underlying the patients' achievements and deficits. These demonstrations of the utility of experimental concepts with pathological populations also provide the constructs themselves with a form of validity and legitimacy unavailable through studies limited to normal subjects. In our view, the mutual benefits that have been described represent an ideal model for the interaction between experimental and clinical approaches to neuropsychology.

## ACKNOWLEDGMENTS

The research reported in this manuscript was supported by funds from the Medical Research Service of the Veterans Administration, by NIAAA grant AA-00187 to Boston University, and by NIA grant AG-05131 to the University of California at San Diego.

## REFERENCES

1. Arendt, T., Bigl, V., Arendt, A., and Tennstedt, A. (1983): Loss of neurons in the nucleus basalis of Meynert in Alzheimer's disease. *Acta Neuropathol. (Berl.)*, 61:101–108.
2. Benton, A. L. (1968): Differential behavioral effects in frontal lobe disease. *Neuropsychologia*, 6:53–60.
3. Blessed, G., Tomlinson, B. E., and Roth, M. (1968): The association between quantitative measures of dementia and of senile change in the cerebral grey matter of elderly subjects. *Br. J. Psychiatry*, 114:797–811.
4. Borkowski, J. G., Benton, A. L., and Spreen, O. (1967): Word fluency and brain damage. *Neuropsychologia*, 5:135–140.
5. Butters, N. (1984): The clinical aspects of memory disorders: contributions from experimental studies of amnesia and dementia. *J. Clin. Neuropsychol.*, 6:17–36.
6. Butters, N. (1985): Alcoholic Korsakoff's syndrome: some unresolved issues concerning etiology, neuropathology and cognitive deficits. *J. Clin. Exp. Neuropsychol.*, 7:181–210.
7. Butters, N., Albert, M. S., Sax, D. S., Miliotis, P., and Sterste, A. (1983): The effect of verbal elaborators on the pictorial memory of brain-damaged patients. *Neuropsychologia*, 21:307–323.
8. Butters, N., and Cermak, L. S. (1980): *Alcoholic Korsakoff's Syndrome: An Information-Processing Approach to Amnesia.* Academic Press, New York.
9. Butters, N., and Cermak, L. S. (1986): A case study of the forgetting of autobiographical knowledge: implications for the study of retrograde amnesia. In: *Autobiographical Memory*, edited by D. Rubin, pp. 253–272. Cambridge University Press, Cambridge.
10. Butters, N., Granholm, E., Salmon, D. P., Grant, I., and Wolfe, J. (1987): Episodic and semantic memory: a comparison of amnesic and demented patients. *J. Clin. Exp. Neuropsychol. (in press)*.
11. Butters, N., Sax, D. S., Montgomery, K., and Tarlow, S. (1978): Comparison of the neuropsychological deficits associated with early and advanced Huntington's disease. *Arch. Neurol.*, 35:585–589.
12. Butters, N., Wolfe, J., Granholm, E., and Martone, M. (1986): An assessment of verbal recall, recognition and fluency abilities in patients with Huntington's disease. *Cortex*, 22:11–32.
13. Butters, N., Wolfe, J., Martone, M., Granholm, E., and Cermak, L. S. (1985): Memory disorders associated with Huntington's disease: verbal recall, verbal recognition and procedural memory. *Neuropsychologia*, 6:729–744.
14. Caine, E., Hunt, R., Weingartner, H., and Ebert, M. (1978): Huntington's dementia: clinical and neuropsychological features. *Arch. Gen. Psychiatry*, 35:377–384.
15. Cermak, L. S., Lewis, R., Butters, N., and Goodglass, H. (1973): Role of verbal mediation in performance of motor tasks by Korsakoff patients. *Percept. Mot. Skills*, 37:259–262.
16. Cohen, N. J., and Squire, L. R. (1980): Preserved learning and retention of pattern analyzing skills in amnesia: dissociation of knowing how and knowing that. *Science*, 210:207–210.
17. Corkin, S. (1968): Acquisition of motor skill after bilateral medial temporal-lobe excision. *Neuropsychologia*, 6:255–265.
18. Cummings, J. L., and Benson, D. F. (1984): Subcortical dementia: review of an emerging concept. *Arch. Neurol.*, 41:874–879.
19. Divac, I. (1972): Neostriatum and functions of the frontal cortex. *Acta Neurobiol. Exp.*, 32:461–478.
20. Eslinger, P. J., and Damasio, A. R. (1986): Preserved motor learning in Alzheimer's disease: implications for anatomy and behavior. *J. Neurosci.*, 6:3006–3009.
21. Folstein, M. F., Folstein, S. E., and McHugh, P. R. (1975): "Mini-mental state": a practical method for grading the cognitive state of patients for the clinician. *J. Psychiatr. Res.*, 12:189–198.
22. Fuld, P. (1978): Psychological testing in the differential diagnosis of the dementias. In: *Alzheimer's Disease: Senile Dementia and Related Disorders*, edited by R. Katzman, R. D. Terry, and K. L. Bick, pp. 185–193. Raven Press, New York.
23. Fuld, P. A. (1983): Word intrusion as a diagnostic sign in Alzheimer's disease. *Geriatr. Med. Today*, 2:33–41.
24. Fuld, P. A., Katzman, R., Davies, P., and Terry, R. D. (1982): Intrusions as a sign of Alzheimer's dementia: chemical and pathological verification. *Ann. Neurol.*, 11:155–159.

25. Graf, P., Squire, L. R., and Mandler, G. (1984): The information that amnesic patients do not forget. *J. Exp. Psychol. [Hum. Learn. Mem.]*, 10:164–178.
26. Heindel, W. C., Butters, N., and Salmon, D. P. (1987): Impaired learning of a motor skill in patients with Huntington's disease. *Behav. Neurosci. (in press)*.
27. Jones-Gotman, M., and Milner, B. (1977): Design fluency: the invention of nonsense drawings after focal cortical lesions. *Neuropsychologia*, 15:653–674.
28. Martin, A., and Fedio, P. (1983): Word production and comprehension in Alzheimer's disease: the breakdown of semantic knowledge. *Brain Lang.*, 19:124–141.
29. Martone, M., Butters, N., Payne, M., Becker, J., and Sax, D. S. (1984): Dissociations between skill learning and verbal recognition in amnesia and dementia. *Arch. Neurol.*, 41:965–970.
30. Mattis, S. (1976): Mental status examination for organic mental syndrome in the elderly patient. In: *Geriatric Psychiatry*, edited by L. Bellack and T. B. Karasu, pp. 77–121. Grune & Stratton, New York.
31. McKann, G., Drachman, D., Folstein, M., Katzman, R., Price, D., and Stadlan, E. M. (1984): Clinical diagnosis of Alzheimer's disease: report of the NINCDS-ADRDA work group under the auspices of Department of Health and Human Services Task Force on Alzheimer's Disease. *Neurology*, 34: 939–944.
32. Milner, B. (1964): Some effects of frontal lobectomy in man. In: *The Frontal Granular Cortex and Behavior*, edited by J. M. Warren and K. Akert, pp. 313–334. McGraw-Hill, New York.
33. Moss, M. B., Albert, M. S., Butters, N., and Payne, M. (1986): Differential patterns of memory loss among patients with Alzheimer's disease, Huntington's disease and alcoholic Korsakoff's syndrome. *Arch. Neurol.*, 43:239–246.
34. Nauta, W. J. H. (1972): Neural associates of the frontal cortex. *Acta Neurobiol. Exp. (Warsz.)*, 32:125–140.
35. Ober, B. A., Dronkers, N. F., Koss, E., Delis, D. C., and Friedland, R. P. (1986): Retrieval from semantic memory in Alzheimer-type dementia. *J. Clin. Exp. Neuropsychol.*, 8:75–92.
36. Oscar-Berman, M. (1973): Hypothesis testing and focusing behavior during concept formation by amnesic Korsakoff patients. *Neuropsychologia*, 11:191–198.
37. Oscar-Berman, M., and Samuels, I. (1977): Stimulus preference and memory factors in Korsakoff's syndrome. *Neuropsychologia*, 15:99–106.
38. Peret, E. (1974): The left frontal lobe of man and the suppression of habitual responses in verbal categorical behavior. *Neuropsychologia*, 12:323–330.
39. Rosen, W. G. (1980): Verbal fluency in aging and dementia. *J. Clin. Neuropsychol.*, 2:135–146.
40. Rosvold, H. E. (1972): The frontal lobe system: cortical-subcortical interrelationships. *Acta Neurobiol. Exp. (Warsz.)*, 32:439–460.
41. Shimamura, A. P., Salmon, D. P., Squire, L. R., and Butters, N. (1987): Memory dysfunction and word priming in dementia and amnesia. *Behav. Neurosci.*, 101:347–351.
42. Shindler, A. G., Caplan, L. R., and Hier, D. B. (1984): Intrusions and perseverations. *Brain Lang.*, 23:148–158.
43. Squire, L. R. (1982): Comparisons between forms of amnesia: some deficits are unique to Korsakoff's syndrome. *J. Exp. Psychol. [Hum. Learn. Mem.]*, 8:560–571.
44. Squire, L. R. (1982): The neuropsychology of human memory. *Annu. Rev. Neurosci.*, 5:241–273.
45. Squire, L. R. (1984): The neuropsychology of memory. In: *The Biology of Learning*, edited by P. Marler and H. S. Terrace, pp. 667–685. Springer-Verlag, Berlin.
46. Squire, L. R. (1986): Mechanisms of memory. *Science*, 232:1612–1619.
47. Talland, G. A. (1965): *Deranged Memory*. Academic Press, New York.
48. Terry, R. D., and Katzman, R. (1983): Senile dementia of the Alzheimer type. *Ann. Neurol.*, 14:497–506.
49. Tulving, E. (1983): *Elements of Episodic Memory*. Oxford University Press, New York.
50. Victor, M., Adams, R. D., and Collins, G. H. (1971): *The Wernicke-Korsakoff Syndrome*. Davis, Philadelphia.
51. Weingartner, H., Grafman, J., Boutelle, W., Kaye, W., and Martin, P. (1983): Forms of memory failure. *Science*, 21:380–382.
52. Winocur, G., and Weiskrantz, L. (1976): An investigation of paired-associate learning in amnesic patients. *Neuropsychologia*, 14:97–110.

*Aging and the Brain*, edited by R. D. Terry.
Raven Press, New York © 1988.

# Cerebral Imaging and Function in the Dementias

## Richard S. J. Frackowiak

*MRC Cyclotron Unit, Hammersmith Hospital; and National Hospital for Nervous Diseases, London, W12 OHS, United Kingdom*

Computed tomographic (CT) reconstruction techniques have revolutionized diagnostic imaging. They permit visualization of deep structures within the body by noninvasive external detection of transmitted or emitted radiation or induced magnetic fields. The two most diagnostically useful techniques are x-ray CT and magnetic resonance imaging (MRI). Both give anatomical information. The former images structure as a function of density, i.e., the differential capacity of tissues to attenuate the transmission of x-rays directed through the body. The latter images proton density or functions dependent on proton–molecule or proton–proton interactions, which are determined largely by tissue water content and its physicochemical environment and to a lesser extent by fat content.

In contrast, positron emission tomography (PET) is a technique designed to measure regional tissue function. It is done by making use of a tomograph to measure tissue isotope concentrations regionally in the live, intact subject. The technique has exquisite sensitivity, being capable of the detection and quantification of picomolar concentrations of positron-labeled compounds in samples of tissue of 1 to 3 cm³. Measurements can be made in any region of the tissue of interest by using tomographic reconstruction techniques to register the distribution of the isotope in the plane of interest. The measurements of radioactivity derived from deep structures are accurate, despite the fact that they are made noninvasively with external detectors, because of the physical properties of positron annihilation and the method of coincidence detection of the resulting radiation.

Positron emission tomography uses tomographic data collection and reconstruction to make functional measurements from the distribution of the radiolabeled tracer, often as a function of time. As a result the data can be presented in the form of tomographic images. This presentation is advantageous because it allows the inspection and analysis of large amounts of data rapidly by eye. It has, however, led to the common erroneous view that PET scans can be readily interpreted visually, in the same way as CT or MRI scans. This view is in fact far from so.

The positron tomograph is therefore primarily an instrument for the measurement of local concentrations of radioactivity. These measurements must be made in absolute physical units (millicuries per milliliter) to be useful, so that results obtained in different laboratories can be compared and communicated with meaning. Measurement of radioactivity in absolute (rather than relative) physical units means that results obtained in one patient can be directly compared to those made at a different time in the same or any other patient.

Positron emission tomography measures function by using tracers. A tracer is a molecule that participates in a biological process of interest but is readily distinguished and hence measured, usually by being labeled with a radioisotope. It is normally introduced into the body in small quantities so that it does not disturb the kinetics of the process under study. In some cases the tracer is a labeled natural substrate for an enzyme or for a storage process. In these cases it is necessary to know the proportions of labeled to natural, unlabeled substrate delivered to the brain. In other cases analogs of substrates can be used as tracers. This approach may be useful because the analog has biochemical properties that distinguish it metabolically from the natural one. Such a feature serves to isolate a part of the biochemical process for study and measurement. To avoid significant competition by the tracer for natural substrate, transport mechanism, or receptor, the amounts given must be minute. PET is capable of detecting picomolar concentrations of the tracer if it can be synthesized with sufficiently high specific activity (i.e., amount of radioactivity per mole of tracer).

The use of a tracer with PET involves certain developmental steps. The identification of the process to be studied and a profound knowledge of the reactions and steps constituting that process *in vivo* are an essential prerequisite. The fate of the tracer must be understood from the moment of its introduction into the body through the various steps of transport, distribution, and metabolism that determine the distribution of the radioactive label at various times afterward.

The contribution of modern imaging to the study of the dementias may be considered under two broad headings. The first—essentially of practical clinical importance and of possible direct and immediate relevance to the management of the individual patient—is the need for a differential diagnostic test. It is suggested that modern imaging techniques should provide sensitive biological markers of disease with differential diagnostic specificity to permit early disease detection. The need for early diagnosis is dictated by the premise that therapeutic measures (preventive or curative) should be instigated as early as possible in the evolution of the disease to be effective. Thus the various diseases must be detected and distinguished early in their evolution. It is also relevant to ask if modern imaging techniques can be used to unravel the pathophysiological mechanisms leading to clinical dysfunction in the various disorders that result in dementia. The use of scanning for clinical research is of less obvious immediate relevance to the individual patient but potentially of much broader significance in the eventual understanding and rational management of the dementia. This chapter briefly reviews the information acquired as a result of the use of tomographic methods for the study of the dementias over the last few years.

## AGING

### Structural Studies

Are there changes intrinsic to normal aging that can be defined with CT and MRI? The quantitation of cortical and cerebral atrophy has been a difficult task, and often the terms have been used to convey a subjective interpretation of a CT image without objective measures and without reference to the range of "atrophic" changes encountered in normal people of the appropriately matched age cohort. Postmortem studies comparing brain volume with cranial capacity (which changes little with age) have shown a decrease in normal subjects with a loss of about 5% of brain volume into advanced old age (52). This finding compares with a mean loss of 13.4% in patients under 80 years of age with histologically proved Alzheimer disease. CT efforts at quantifying cerebral atrophy *in vivo* have centered on ventricular enlargement and widening of cerebral sulci and fissures (1,57,85). Methods have been hampered by partial volume artifacts. However, analyses of the reliability of linear, planimetric, and more recently volumetric measures have been published. None have been adopted for general clinical use (42).

Cortical, as opposed to generalized cerebral, atrophy is more difficult to assess quantitatively because of the proximity of cortex to bone and the lack of good gray white contrast (53). Methods such as measuring and summing the width of the four largest sulci have been proposed (60). These methods have obvious shortcomings when CT scanning is used but may become easier and more accurate with MRI. Other methods depend on computer analysis of the CT numbers in the scan that reflect tissue density. Cutoff points have been defined in an attempt to distinguish between cerebral tissue, bone, and CSF spaces (55). These techniques can give an approximation of volume if the physical size of the image voxels is known. There are also methods described that rely on the increase in surface area of the brain that accompanies the increased convolutions of the cortex consequent on atrophy. The increase can then be related to cranial capacity, again a measure that may be more precise with MRI (91). Such methods, though sometimes computerized, automated, and relatively easy to use, have gained little acceptance in clinical management largely because they are so machine-dependent. In terms of diagnostic sensitivity, patients with no cerebral atrophy and Alzheimer disease as well as normal subjects with marked atrophy have been regularly reported, so that atrophy does not constitute on its own a diagnostic criterion of much specificity. In this context there is an interesting report that compared apparently normal CT scan images of demented and nondemented subjects (80). The analysis involved measuring the mean CT number in a large region of interest in white matter of the centrum semiovale. A significantly lower CT number was observed in the demented patients with no overlap between demented and nondemented groups. This work has been extended to include cerebrospinal fluid (CSF) volume as an additional discriminatory variable giving added diagnostic sensitivity (2). No similar or parallel, systematic MRI studies that might pick up white matter change more readily have been reported. Of interest to research remains the observation by some workers of correlations between atrophy and neuropsychological tests of memory, orientation, and other cognitive functions (25,55,57).

## Function

Positron emission tomography studies of normal aging have concentrated on defining the normal regional changes in cerebral metabolism and hemodynamics, and describing the regional metabolic responses of the brain to physiological stimuli. In relation to energy metabolism the picture remains surprisingly confused, given the quantitative and spatial accuracy afforded by PET technology. A considerable part of the confusion may be ascribed to technical factors, as measurements have been made and reported concurrently with rapid advances in their technical precision. Such factors as appropriate measured corrections for the attenuation of radiation by the tissues of the body, the method of administering the tracer, blood sampling techniques necessary for quantification of the tracer distributions in terms of a biological variable, awareness of resolution effects on the sampling and size of regions of interest for making measurements, and an awareness of modeling assumptions and problems have all required careful solution.

The fractional extraction (OER) and consumption ($CMRO_2$) of oxygen have been measured using oxygen-15-labeled $O_2$ and $CO_2$ (35,83). This method also gives a measure of cerebral blood flow (CBF). The OER is in effect an expression of the relation between CBF (i.e., oxygen supply) and $CMRO_2$ (i.e., its utilization). The product of OER and the stable arterial oxygen content is the arteriovenous oxygen difference. The OER expresses the fractional extraction of oxygen, whereas the $AVO_2$ expresses the absolute oxygen extraction in milliliters of $O_2$ per milliliter of blood. The most commonly used and carefully validated technique is the steady-state method, and most of the studies of oxygen metabolism reported for aging and dementia have been done in this way (35,68).

Glucose metabolism has been measured for aging, and semiquantitative studies have been published of dementia using variations of Sokoloff's deoxyglucose technique (84,87,88). This technique is an analog method that depends on an adequate description of the relation between the handling of the analog and natural substrate (glucose) by the tissue. If this description is readily quantified, the use of the analog (e.g., [18]FDG) results in an accurate measure of the consumption of glucose.

Measurement of CBF in aging with PET suggests that in the gray matter a steady if small progressive decrease in perfusion occurs after the third decade of life (74,81). This conclusion was also drawn by Kety when he reviewed and summarized the findings in the literature up to 1965 that reported mean hemispheric measurements with the nitrous oxide technique (59). There appears to be no decrease of note in the white matter of the centrum semiovale. A significant criticism of these regional findings is that the human brain tends to lose weight (and volume) after the sixth decade of life. The measurements of CBF are made per volume (or weight) of brain tissue. If the volume of interest contains less gray matter, the corresponding flow value is underestimated. The main reason for thinking that this explanation of the finding is not sufficient is that measurements of $CMRO_2$ do not follow a similar pattern (see below).

Oxygen consumption shows a tendency to decrease with age between the third and eighth decades. However, it barely reaches significance, and there seems to be a definite difference between the rates of decrease of CBF and $CMRO_2$. This finding implies a gradual alteration of the relation between supply and demand and a tendency for the fractional oxygen extraction to increase. Kennedy and Sokoloff (58a) showed with the nitrous oxide technique that children had considerably higher CBF than adults during and beyond the third decade. Oxygen consumption was, however, much more comparable to adult values. The $AVO_2$ was 30% lower than in adults, as was the fractional oxygen extraction. There seems to be a trend throughout life for the fractional oxygen extraction to increase (37,38,69,74), which means that the range of normal OER varies from about 25% during childhood to 35 to 40% during adulthood, and 40 to 45% during old age. It is clear that there remains a considerable oxygen reserve in the perfusing blood, available to buffer any sudden changes in CBF or metabolism. For this reason, in no sense does this trend indicate cerebrovascular insufficiency. In an elderly person with an OER of 45%, the remaining 55% of unextracted oxygen should be capable of supporting a twofold increase in $CMRO_2$ even if no further increase in CBF were possible.

What is the physiological or morphological basis of this small but apparently definite trend toward a decrease in the hemodynamic reserve with age? The answer is not clear, but it is possible there is a decrease in the local capillary density with age. During normal aging the cerebral vessels are functionally normal and capable of appropriate cerebral vasoconstriction and dilatation. Cerebral autoregulation is maintained, as is $CO_2$ reactivity. There is therefore no evidence that the aging brain is chronically anoxic or somehow limited in its function by an inadequate nutrient supply.

The measurement of glucose consumption (CMRGlu) has provided less consistent results. Kuhl and his colleagues reported a decrease in CMRGlu (66) and compared this finding to the data on $CMRO_2$ published from Hammersmith Hospital (65). The decrease in CMRGlu was more pronounced than that in $CMRO_2$, suggesting that the brains of elderly subjects use energy substrates other than glucose (e.g., ketones). Some evidence for such a hypothesis had already been suggested by Gottstein et al. (46) using arteriovenous techniques. On the other hand, Rapoport and his colleagues at the National Institute of Aging (NIA) have reported no significant decrease in glucose consumption with age (21,22). Their study seems to be consistent with the 1960s National Institute of Health (NIH) study with arteriovenous difference techniques (16). The results of the latter study were at variance with those of most other workers at the time, and the discrepancy was attributed to the highly rigorous selection criteria for normality used. Similar criteria have been used in the subsequent PET study. Whether the "supernormal" or "normal" aged have different cerebral physiology is one question: its significance is another. Similarly, studies from Brookhaven suggest no decrease in CMRGlu with normal aging (19). It is important to realize that the coefficient of variation (COV) of the measurements in the studies from these two centers is of the order 20 to 25%, compared with an 8 to 10% COV in $CMRO_2$ in normal populations. This problem makes the demonstration of a small though significant negative correlation between CMRGlu and age difficult. There are still technical factors that require solution before definitive data concerning CMRGlu and normal aging are produced.

In terms of regional information, there is clarification of the distributions of CBF and energy metabolism in different cerebral structures. The hyperfrontal pattern described by Ingvar (54) in the awake, alert, normal individual is much less clearly seen than with the intracarotid [133]Xe technique. The reason is probably methodological and relates to siting of detectors and distribution of the [133]Xe after intracarotid injection. It appears that most cortical regions have similar perfusion, and the major difference lies between gray and white matter. The small differences registered by PET between different cortical areas may be partly explicable in terms of the resolution of the PET cameras. The cortical strip with a width averaging 3 to 4 mm has been examined to date by instruments with transaxial resolutions averaging 1 to 3 $cm^2$. Horwitz et al. reported that changes in the metabolic interrelations between different brain regions occur with aging (51). The physiological significance of these statistical correlations remains to be elucidated.

Mention should also be made of experiments relating alterations in the normal pattern of distribution of energy metabolism by specific physiological stimuli. Mazziotta and colleagues have demonstrated focal increases in cortical metabolism in response to visual, auditory, and alerting stimuli during the performance of memory and auditory discrimination tasks (75–78,82). This disturbance of the resting state pattern in the normal individual, when fully quantified, will provide the opportunity for working out intracerebral connections subserving complex functions in the brain. It is an exciting prospect for the fields of normal and abnormal neuropsychology. Of particular importance to the study of aging will be the comparison between the young and elderly of focal patterns and the capacity to augment cerebral metabolism locally in response to standard physiological stimuli. A disappointment until now has been the apparent inability to describe the effects of stimulation by absolute measures of energy metabolism in most cases. Many of the reports present results in terms of metabolic ratios: right/left, anterior/posterior, lobe/lobe, or local/global ratios. There are, however, studies that show a correlation between a graded physiological stimulus and increases in metabolism. Interestingly, the physiological response is not always linear (29,30,82).

## Structural/Functional Relations

The relation between structural and functional abnormalities in normal aging have been studied with combined CT and PET scan analysis by DeLeon and colleagues (18,19). Structural cortical changes were observed without change in CMRGlu, and the suggestion has been made that the normal brain undergoes structural change without metabolic correlate. This observation is opposite to that found in certain patients with Alzheimer disease. The problem with such correlative studies to date has been that the positron tomographs have had poor resolution compared to the CT scanners. There are also reservations about the interpretation of the metabolic data, as the CMRGlu values for young adults scatter widely between 3 and 5 mg/100 ml/ min. It is generally concluded that the addition of physiological data to structural data does not yet give information of sufficient sensitivity to allow discrimination of normal from pathological aging in individual cases, though group discrimination may be more precise.

## DEMENTIA

### Structure

Studies of cerebral structure with CT scanning in studies of aging and the dementias suggest a lack of sensitivity to disease (56,57). The pattern described as atrophy, comprising ventricular dilatation and sulcal widening, is commonplace in the clinically normal elderly population (53). So are changes in the white matter, with the occurrence of periventricular low attenuation lesions. Clearly these changes are representative of some form of structural alteration. Indeed pathological data presented by Brun (A. Brun, communicated at a meeting on dementia, Heidelberg, 1986) suggests the comparatively frequent occurrence of probably ischemic white matter change in apparently neurologically normal elderly subjects postmortem. However there is no clear relation between clinically detectable dysfunction and the presence or absence of atrophy detected by the radiologist from inspection of CT images. The common clinical experience is that normal elderly subjects may show atrophic scans with periventricular white matter change (which correlates better with late-onset epilepsy than dementia), and demented patients may have apparently normal scans (86). Attempts at quantitative analysis of CT images to define reliable criteria for the differentiation of dementia from normal aging have also been reported (6,14). Such methods have had limited clinical application because of inadequate specificity and sensitivity. It is worth remembering that cerebral "atrophy" on CT may be a reversible phenomenon. It is seen with severe dehydration and following alcohol ingestion, and it may even be iatrogenically produced (e.g., by corticosteroid therapy).

The differentiation of dementia due to multiple infarcts from that due to degenerative disease (especially Alzheimer disease) can in many cases be aided by CT scanning. However, the sensitivity of CT as a differential diagnostic test remains questionable. In the first place, ischemic change can occur without detectable changes on CT images. This finding may be due to the small size of strategically placed lacunes or because of healing and consequent secondary changes in x-ray attenuation with time, resulting in isodensity with brain. There may also be areas of brain where ischemia is mild and results in partial neuronal fallout rather than frank infarction, with little consequent change in structure visualized with CT. White matter changes occur that may correlate with hypertension, ischemic episodes, and dementia but that may equally well be associated with diabetes or normal aging with no clinically detectable cerebral dysfunction. Such white matter changes may rarely be confused with demyelination due to multiple sclerosis or with periventricular lucencies due to hydrocephalus. A final problem that is more fundamental relates to the not infrequent (20%) concurrence of ischemic cerebral change and Alzheimer pathology (90). At present one might take the pragmatic view that this matters little, given that effective therapy is available only in relation to preventing further ischemic disease, so that its detection, be it in isolation or in conjunction with Alzheimer changes, still constitutes an indication to appropriate management.

Only preliminary reports have appeared regarding MRI in degenerative dementia (5). However, MRI certainly appears to be more sensitive to structural change caused by ischemia than CT. A problem that may be theoretical rather than practical, if scans are interpreted in a clinical context, is that the method is relatively insensitive to the type of pathology. Thus similar signals can be obtained from lesions caused by edema, ischemia, or inflammation. A report of MRI in 20 consecutive elderly patients without structural disease evident on CT scans demonstrated changes in deep white matter in one-third (7). These patients showed a high incidence of hypertension, transient ischemic events, cardiac disease, and emotional lability. The sensitivity of MRI to ischemic, especially white matter, change is therefore high.

Changes have been described with CT scanning in the heads of the caudate nuclei in patients with established Huntington disease (67,89). In clinical practice this finding is rarely diagnostically useful. The changes frequently occur late, and patients with mild to moderate disease can have apparently normal caudate nuclei on CT.

Pick disease, characterized pathologically by severe frontal and temporal atrophy out of proportion to changes in the rest of the brain, may be difficult to distinguish clinically from Alzheimer disease in life. Structural scanning may provide clues to the true diagnosis because of localized frontotemporal atrophy on CT; however, such changes are not specific, and though indicative they cannot be considered diagnostic by themselves.

Similar problems of lack of specificity apply to the dementia associated with Creutzfeldt-Jakob disease (43) and acquired immunodeficiency disease (AIDS). In the latter condition, inflammatory changes or abscess formation may be readily detected and help in the differential diagnosis of some of the opportunistic infections associated with this syndrome and that can themselves cause a dementing clinical picture.

Detection of the syndrome of normal-pressure hydrocephalus is clinically less important now that the response to shunt therapy is seen to be less dramatic in most cases than initial reports may have suggested. The criteria differentiating chronic hydrocephalus from atrophy include dilation of the temporal horns, enlargement of the fourth ventricle, and obliterated or normal-sulci. In most cases of suspected normal-pressure hydrocephalus the structural changes observed by CT scanning constitute a relatively minor adjunct to the information obtained from a clinical history and examination.

In summary, changes of cerebral structure viewed by CT or MRI scanning provide important additional information to the clinical findings in the diagnosis and evaluation of dementing illnesses (24). The great strength of structural imaging lies in the exclusion of treatable structural disease (e.g., tumors, abscesses, diffuse inflammation) presenting with a dementing syndrome. The changes observed in the degenerative dementing diseases are not uniform or disease-specific and thus have little intrinsic diagnostic potential, especially if viewed out of clinical context. CT and MRI are, however, invaluable adjuncts to the overall evaluation of individual patients with dementia. They are also of major help in detecting ischemic changes and thus have a direct impact on patient management.

## Function

From the earliest studies of the dementias with PET, changes have been described in energy metabolism (36) that have subsequently been confirmed by all laboratories studying both oxygen and glucose consumption (17,22,26–28,40). The principal findings have been a progressive decrease in gray matter $CMRO_2$, CMRGlu, and CBF with increasing severity of dementia. This phenomenon is also seen in the white matter, whatever the pathology (i.e., Alzheimer or vascular) (36). This finding distinguishes the dementing process pathophysiologically from normal aging. White matter $CMRO_2$ does not correlate with the degree of atrophy seen on CT scanning. Patients with mild to moderate dementia exhibit an average 20% decrease in metabolic activity, and those with severe disease a 40% decrease compared to normal, age-matched subjects (36). No correlation has been demonstrated between gray matter CBF or $CMRO_2$ and clinicopathological type of dementia. This finding is at variance with the earlier (non-PET) CBF literature, which suggested that changes in CBF in early cases of dementia distinguished degenerative from multi-infarct disease (47). Patients with vascular dementia as a group have the same $CMRO_2$ as patients with degenerative disease of the same clinical functional severity (36). Therefore, in general, there is a correlation between global cortical metabolic hypofunction and severity but not type of disease.

Focal CBF and $CMRO_2$ abnormalities are seen in degenerative dementia of Alzheimer type. The most characteristic, seen in early to moderate disease, is a depression of metabolism in the posterior temporoparietal regions bilaterally (36). This region shows the smallest age-related decrease in $CMRO_2$ (9% decrease in normal aging with a further 29% fall in dementia). With increasing severity of disease the frontal regions also show striking depression of metabolism. There is relative sparing of occipital and primary motor-sensory cortices within the context of a generalized global decrease in cortical energy metabolism. The basis for this focal emphasis of pathology is not entirely clear.

Studies of glucose consumption show similar changes (22). The most commonly reported is the focalized posterior temporoparietal depression. Some reports suggest that the expression of cortical metabolic activity as a frontal/parietal ratio provides an index with high sensitivity to the presence of dementia (40). In patients with mild to moderate disease, it is claimed that the ratio distinguishes disease from normal aging with no overlap between the groups. The frontal decrease in energy metabolism seen with advanced disease has been confirmed in terms of CMRGlu (22).

Studies of glucose consumption have also addressed the question of the sensitivity of metabolic changes to dementia (13,48). There are reports that patients with mild but clinically evident dementia do not show a fall in cortical metabolism in comparison to normal volunteers. This finding is at variance with the reports measuring $CMRO_2$, in which a negative linear correlation has been demonstrated with disease severity. It is possible that small depressions in CMRGlu have not been recognized because of the large coefficient of variation in the normal CMRGlu data.

Focal abnormalities have been correlated with functional changes determined clinically (11,27,28). In particular, aphasia, apraxia, and visuospatial function have been correlated with changes in CMRGlu in the appropriate hemisphere. Such lobar changes have also been reported in terms of $CMRO_2$ but were demonstrated to be bilateral with some increased emphasis on the appropriate side (36). The resolution of earlier generation tomographs, with which many of these studies were performed, was poor, and it is likely that with newer cameras such focal structure–function relations may become more precisely defined.

Rare patients with apparent degenerative dementia of Alzheimer type have been described with remarkably asymmetrical abnormalities of parietal metabolism (CMRGlu) (11), and different hemispheric asymmetries have been reported in early- and late-onset Alzheimer disease (61). No specific reports of cases with atypical presentation of Alzheimer disease with focal disability (e.g., slowly progressive aphasia) have been reported. Members of a family with Alzheimer disease have been studied, and posterior temporoparietal changes indistinguishable from those seen in sporadic cases of the disease have been described in affected individuals (12). There has been insufficient length of follow-up to determine if at-risk individuals who develop disease show progressive metabolic changes and if they differ from at-risk subjects who do not develop dementia.

The interpretation of changes in cerebral metabolism of aging and dementia is made difficult because of the possible influence of atrophy on metabolic measurements. Metabolic measurements are made from regions (volumes) of interest defined by the axial resolution of the scanned tomographic plane and the transaxial area defined in analysis. Such volumes contain varying proportions of CSF, gray matter, white matter, and other intracranial contents. The choice of regions when making measurements must take cognizance of this fact. Atrophy of cortex, which significantly alters its volumetric dimensions, may result in regions of interest containing smaller or larger proportions of gray and white matter with a resultant apparent decrease in cortical metabolism. Herscovitch and colleagues (50) have described a method of attempted correction for atrophy based on CT scanning. They reported an expected 11% decrease in metabolism due to atrophic changes associated with normal aging. That it is not the whole story is demonstrated by the fact that CBF and $CMRO_2$ decrease at different rates with age, as already mentioned, and patients with dementia and without CT scan atrophy show metabolic changes that correlate better with severity of disease than CT abnormality. In any event, the argument is somewhat semantic in that the site of pathology, whether due to intrinsically decreased cellular metabolism or cell death, is clearly demonstrated. The resolution of the problem will come if a general tracer of living neurons can be developed and metabolic rates cited regionally in terms of neuronal density rather than volume. Correlations of structural and metabolic abnormalities have been attempted and reported in preliminary form. The different resolution of the two imaging modalities makes interpretation difficult, and too few patients have been reported to draw firm conclusions (20,39).

The question of the specificity of changes in energy metabolism in Alzheimer disease has been the subject of a number of studies. Kuhl et al. (63) have shown posterior temporoparietal hypometabolism in patients with parkinsonism and dementia. A striking case study in this report demonstrates a normal pattern of CMRGlu in a patient with normal mentation and parkinsonism that becomes abnormal 4 years later, coincidentally with the development of dementia. Whether the changes were due to a specific dementia of parkinsonism or represented the coincidence of two common diseases of the elderly is unclear.

Patients with dementia associated with progressive supranuclear palsy have shown a marked decrease in frontal CMRGlu without posterior changes (15). This pattern has also been demonstrated in terms of oxygen metabolism (70). A similar pattern has been described in patients with Pick disease (T. Chase, communicated at a meeting on dementia, Heidelberg, 1986). Patients with Huntington disease demonstrate global cortical hypometabolism without focal cortical emphasis but with marked metabolic depression in the caudate even when it appears structurally normal on CT (49,62). There are suggestions that the caudate metabolic changes may antedate the development of symptoms of the disease and therefore act as a marker of Huntington gene carrier status. More studies are needed to confirm whether this impression is true. Creutzfeldt-Jakob dementia has been reported to show changes similar to those of Alzheimer disease (41). Systematic studies of patients with pseudodementia (dementia of depression) are, however, lacking. Normal-pressure hydrocephalus has been differentiated from Alzheimer disease in metabolic terms as well (58).

Clearly, abnormalities of posterior temporoparietal energy metabolism are not specific for Alzheimer disease on their own, though in clinical context the changes assume greater significance.

## Degenerative and Vascular Dementia

Multi-infarct dementia constitutes a relatively small cause of mental deterioration in the elderly, though it may coexist with other degenerative diseases and particularly Alzheimer dementia (90). It assumes importance because therapeutic efforts can be made to attempt to halt its course. The study of vascular dementias cannot be considered in isolation from the pathophysiology of acute ischemic brain disease or from an appreciation of the homeostatic mechanisms that normally prevent ischemia in the face of acute or chronic decreases in cerebral perfusion. Reviews of insights into these normal and pathological mechanisms obtained with PET have appeared (32–34).

Studies of the ischemic pathogenesis of multi-infarct dementia have concentrated on establishing the relation between CBF and $CMRO_2$ in terms of oxygen extraction (36,44). In a comparison of patients with multi-infarct and degenerative dementia, no evidence has been found for a disturbance of the normal balance between CBF and $CMRO_2$ in either group of patients. All the patients with multi-infarct disease were examined during a stable phase of their disease, between acute ischemic events. The observation of a normal OER was true both regionally and globally. It was clear evidence for the absence of any pathogenic mechanism that might be termed "chronic ischemia." Ischemia is the pathological state in which energy metabolism, and hence function, is perfusion-limited. The blood supply to the brain is normally considerably in excess of metabolic requirements. Hence the extraction of oxygen is normally only 40% or so. The remainder constitutes a reserve that acts to buffer metabolism from normal moment-to-moment physiological fluctuations of blood flow. Before ischemia can occur, this reserve must be totally exhausted and oxygen extraction maximal, when oxygen delivery becomes limiting to metabolism.

We know from pathological studies that the substrate for vascular dementia is the accumulation of ischemic infarctions, usually beyond a threshold volume and sometimes with strategic placement (90). The pathophysiological sequence in these acute events is a fall in perfusion pressure and flow to levels that are less than half of normal. At this stage OER is maximal and ischemia is established. Depending on the depth and duration of the ischemia, cell death and or frank infarction occur. This phase is characterized by low $CMRO_2$ with high OER, which rapidly changes to low $CMRO_2$ and low OER with neuronal destruction. Eventually, tissue reparative processes lead to a recoupling of CBF and $CMRO_2$ and hence normalization of OER. If large infarctions occur, the OER may remain subnormal. It is of interest in this context that of the 23 patients with multi-infarct dementia studied in our laboratory during the stable interischemic phase of disease none exhibited global abnormalities of OER.

The pattern of metabolic decrease in multi-infarct dementia is different from that in Alzheimer disease, so some hope has been generated that PET can be of help in this important differential diagnosis. Certainly extreme dementias due to one or other pathology are readily distinguishable (4,36,64). In contrast to patients with Alzheimer disease, the pattern of dysfunction in vascular cases is characterized by punched-out, focal defects scattered throughout the brain in gray and white matter (79). Most such defects are found in the territory of the middle cerebral artery. Unfortunately, earlier-generation scanners are not capable of making the distinction reliably in the clinically less severe cases. The hope that new-generation scanners will be sensitive to such early change is, however, considerable.

In certain rare and specific cases, patients presenting primarily with dementia have been observed who have demonstrated a chronic focal elevation of OER in the territories of occluded cervical arteries (44). Such patients invariably have extensive neck vessel occlusions. The OER usually lies at submaximal levels of 50 to 70%. This situation is therefore a precarious preischemic one in which CBF is low and close to ischemic levels. The maintenance of cerebral oxygen delivery is entirely dependent on the small residual arterial oxygen reserve. The probability for further, frequent ischemic episodes seems *a priori* particularly great in such patients. This pathophysiological situation is rare, dangerous, but potentially amenable to revascularizing treatment.

### Neurochemistry *In Vivo*

Other functional aspects of cerebral metabolism have been examined with PET techniques in man. Studies of protein metabolism in Alzheimer dementia, though preliminary, show a distribution of defects of amino acid (methionine) incorporation into protein similar to that shown by the studies of energy metabolism (8–10). There is no change in the permeability of the blood–brain barrier to methionine, but the turnover of the free amino acid pool is greatly decreased, especially in frontal and temporoparietal areas.

The elaboration of methods to measure neurotransmitter function are in the early stages of development but constitute an important growth area in PET of potential significance to the study of aging and the pathogenesis of the degenerative dementias. [For example, changes in dopamine and serotonin receptors have been demonstrated to occur with normal aging (92).] There are also significant diagnostic implications, and preliminary studies are promising in this field. It has been shown that [76]Br-bromospiperone binding is decreased in the basal ganglia and in the frontal cortex of patients with progressive supranuclear palsy (3). This ligand is a potent dopamine D2 receptor antagonist with some serotonin S2 activity as well, probably explaining the cortical changes. On the other hand, studies of dopaminergic function with [18]F-DOPA show that there is also depressed uptake and retention of this ligand at presynaptic sites in the striatum (70). In parkinsonism patients a number of research groups have demonstrated decreased [18]F-DOPA associated uptake and retention in the striatum that correlates with disease severity (72). Normal [11]C-methylspiperone binding has been demonstrated in this disease (73). With Huntington disease [18]F-DOPA uptake is normal (71), but [11]C-methylspiperone binding is depressed (71). It is clear from these preliminary observations that there are different and characteristic patterns of pre- and postsynaptic dysfunction in these subcortical diseases associated with dementia. The combination of measures of energy metabolism and specific markers of neurotransmitter function seems to be a sensitive approach to the diagnosis of specific dementing diseases and may provide important information regarding pathogenesis in the future.

## REFERENCES

1. Albert, M., Naeser, M. A., Levine, H. L., and Garvey, A. J. (1984): Ventricular size in patients with presenile dementia of the Alzheimer type. *Arch. Neurol.*, 41:1258–1263.
2. Albert, M., Naeser, M. A., Levine, H. L., and Garvey, A. J. (1984): CT density numbers in patients with senile dementia of the Alzheimer type. *Arch. Neurol.*, 41:1264–1269.
3. Baron, J. C., Maziere, B., Loc'h, C., Cambon, H., Sgouropoulos, P., Bonnet, M., and Agid, Y. (1986): Loss of striatal ($^{76}$Br) bromospiperone binding sites demonstrated by positron tomography in progressive supranuclear palsy. *J. Cereb. Blood Flow Metab.*, 6: 131–136.
4. Benson, D. F., Kuhl, D. E., Hawkins, R. A., Phelps, M. E., Cummings, J. L. and Tsai, S. Y. (1983): The fluorodeoxyglucose $^{18}$F scan in Alzheimer's disease and multi infarct dementia. *Arch. Neurol.*, 40:711–714.
5. Besson, J. A. O., Corrigan, F. M., Iljon Foreman, E., Eastwood, L. M., Smith, F. W., and Ashcroft, G. W. (1985): Nuclear magnetic resonance (NMR). II. Imaging in dementia. *Br. J. Psychiatry*, 146:31–35.
6. Bondareff, W., Baldy, R., and Levy, R. (1981): Quantitative computed tomography in dementia. *Arch. Gen. Psychiatry*, 38:1365–1368.
7. Bradley, W. G., Waluch, V., Brant-Zawadzki, M., Yadley, R. A., and Wycoff, R. R. (1984): Patchy, periventricular white matter lesions in the elderly: a common observation during NMR imaging. *Noninvasive Med. Imaging*, 1:35–41.
8. Bustany, P., Henry, J. F., DeRotrou, J., Signoret, P., Cabanis E., Zarifian, E., Ziegler, M., Derlon, J. M., Crouzel, C., Soussaline, F., and Comar, D. (1985): Correlations between clinical state and positron emission tomography measurement of local brain protein synthesis in Alzheimer's disease, Parkinson's disease, schizophrenia and gliomas. In: *The Metabolism of the Human Brain Studied with Positron Emission Tomography,* edited by T. Greitz, D. Ingvar, and L. Widen, pp. 241–249. Raven Press, New York.
9. Bustany, P., Henry, J. F., Sargent, T., Zarifian, E., Cabanis, E., Colllard, P., and Comar, D. (1983): Local brain protein metabolism in dementia and schizophrenia: in vivo studies with $^{11}$C-L-methionine and positron emission tomography. In: *Positron Emission Tomography of the Brain,* edited by W-D. Heiss and M. E. Phelps, pp. 208–211. Springer-Verlag, New York.
10. Bustany, P., Henry, J. F., Soussaline, F., and Comar, D. (1983): Brain protein synthesis in normal and demented patients—a study by positron emission tomography with $^{11}$C-L-methionine. In: *Functional Radionuclide Imaging of the Brain,* edited by P. L. Magistretti, pp. 319–326. Raven Press, New York.
11. Chase, T. N., Foster, L. N., Fedio, P., Brooks, R, Mansi, L., and DiChiro, G. (1984): Regional cortical dysfunction in Alzheimer's disease as determined by positron emission tomography. *Ann. Neurol.*, 15 (Suppl.):S170–S174.
12. Cutler, N. R., Haxby, J. V., Duara, R., Grady, C. L., Moore, A. M., Parisi, J. E., White, J., Heston, L, Margolin, R. M., and Rapoport, S. I. (1985): Brain metabolism as measured with positron emission tomography: serial assessment in a patient with familial Alzheimer's disease. *Neurology*, 35:1556–1561.
13. Cutler, N. R., Haxby, J. V., Duara, R., et al. (1985): Clinical history, brain metabolism and neuropsychological function in Alzheimer's disease. *Ann. Neurol.*, 18:298–309.
14. Damasio, H., Eslinger, P., Damasio, A. R., Rizzo, M., Huang, H. K., and Demeter, S. (1983): Quantitative computed tomographic analysis in the diagnosis of dementia. *Arch. Neurol.*, 40:715–719.
15. D'Antona, R., Baron, J. C., Samson, Y., Serdaru, M., Viader, F., Agid, Y., and Cambier, J. (1985): Subcortical dementia: frontal cortex hypometabolism detected by positron tomography in patients with progressive supranuclear palsy. *Brain*, 108:785–800.
16. Dastur, D. K., Lane, M. H., Hansen, D. B., Kety, S. S., Butler, R. N., Perlin, S., and Sokoloff, L. (1963): Effects of aging on cerebral circulation and metabolism in man. In:

*Human Aging*, U.S. Public Health Service Publication 986, edited by J. E. Barren, R. N. Butler, S. W. Greenhouse, et al., pp. 59–76. U.S. Public Health Service, Washington, D.C.

17. DeLeon, M. J. Ferris, S. H., George, A. E., Christman, D. R., Fowler, J. S., Gentes, C., Reisberg, B., Gee, B., Emmerich, M., Yonekura, Y., Brodie, J., Kricheff, I. I., and Wolf, A. P. (1983): Positron emission tomographic studies of aging and Alzheimer's disease. *AJNR*, 4:568–571.

18. DeLeon, M. J., Ferris, S. H., George, A. E., Reisberg, B., Christman, D. R., Kricheff, I. I. and Wolf, A. P. (1983): Computed tomography and positron emission transaxial tomography evaluations of normal aging and Alzheimer's disease. *J. Cereb. Blood Flow Metab.*, 3:391–394.

19. DeLeon, M., George, A. E., Ferris, S. H., Christman, D. R., Fowler, J. S., Gentes, C. I., Brodie, J., Reisberg, B., and Wolf, A. P. (1984): Positron emission tomography and computed tomographic assessment of the human brain. *J. Comput. Assist. Tomogr.*, 8:88–94.

20. DeLeon, M. J., George, A. E., Ferris, S. H., Rosenbloom, S., Christman, D. R., Gentes, C. I., Reisberg, B., Kricheff, I. I., and Wolf, A. P. (1983): Regional correlation of PET and CT in senile dementia of Alzheimer type. *AJNR*, 4:553–556.

21. Duara, R., Grady, C., Haxby, J., Ingvar, D., Sokoloff, L., Margolin, R. A., Manning, R. G., Cutler, N. R., and Rapoport, S. I. (1984): Human brain glucose utilisation and cognitive function in relation to age. *Ann. Neurol.*, 16:702–713.

22. Duara, R., Grady, C., Haxby, J., Sundaram, M., Cutler, N. R., Heston, L., Moore, A., Schlageter, N., Larson, S., and Rapoport, S. I. (1986): Positron emission tomography in Alzheimer's disease. *Neurology*, 36:879—887.

23. Duara, R., Margolin, R. A., Robertson-Tschabo, E. A., London, E. D., Schwartz, M., Renfrew, J., Koziarz, B., Sundaram, M., Grady, C., Moore, A., Ingvar, D., Sokoloff, L., Weingartner, H., Kessler, R., Manning, R., Channing, M., Cutler, N., and Rapoport, S. (1983): Resting cerebral glucose utilisation as measured with positron emission tomography in 21 healthy men between the ages of 21 and 83 years. *Brain*, 106:761–775.

24. Erkinjuntti, T., Sipponen, J. T., Iivanainen, M., et al. (1984): Cerebral NMR and CT imaging in dementia. *J. Comput. Assist. Tomogr.*, 8:614–618.

25. Eslinger, P. J., Damasio, H., Graff-Radford, N., and Damasio, A. R. (1984): Examining the relationship between computed tomography and neuropsychological measures in normal and demented elderly. *J. Neurol. Neurosurg. Psychiatry*, 47:1319–1325.

26. Foster, N. L., Chase, T. N., Fedio, P., Patronas, N. J., Brooks, R. A., and DiChiro, G. (1983): Alzheimer's disease: focal cortical changes shown by positron emission tomography. *Neurology*, 33:961–965.

27. Foster, N. L. Chase, T. N., Mansi, L., Brooks, R., Fedio, P., Patronas, N. J. and DiChiro, G. (1984): Cortical abnormalities in Alzheimer's disease. *Ann. Neurol.*, 16:649–654.

28. Foster, N. L., Chase, T. N., Patronas, N. J., Gillespie, M. M., and Fedio, P. (1986): Cerebral mapping of apraxia in Alzheimer's disease by positron emission tomography. *Ann. Neurol.*, 19:139–143.

29. Fox, P. T., and Raichle, M. E. (1984): Stimulus rate dependence of regional cerebral blood flow in human striate cortex demonstrated by positron emission tomography. *J. Neurophysiol.*, 51:1109–1120.

30. Fox, P. T., and Raichle, M. E. (1985): Stimulus rate determines regional brain blood flow in striate cortex. *Ann. Neurol.*, 17:303–305.

31. Frackowiak, R. S. J. (1982): Human regional cerebral blood flow and oxygen metabolism studied with oxygen-15 and positron emission tomography. MD thesis, Cambridge University.

32. Frachowiak, R. S. J. (1985): Pathophysiology of human cerebral ischaemia: studies with positron tomography and oxygen-15. *Res. Publ. Assoc. Res. Nerv. Ment. Dis.*, 63:139–162.

33. Frackowiak, R. S. J. (1985): The pathophysiology of human cerebral ischaemia: a new perspective obtained with positron tomography. *Q. J. Med.*, 57:713–727.

34. Frackowiak, R. S. J. (1986): PET scanning: can it help resolve management issues in cerebral ischemic disease. *Stroke*, 17:803–807 (editorial).

35. Frackowiak, R. S. J., Lenzi, G. L., Jones, T., and Heather, J. D. (1980): Quantitative measurement of regional cerebral blood flow and oxygen metabolism in man using $^{15}0$ and positron emission tomography: theory, procedure and normal values. *J. Comput. Assist. Tomogr.*, 4:727–736.

36. Frackowiak, R. S. J., Pozzilli, C., Legg, N. J., DuBoulay, G. H., Marshall, J., Lenzi, G. L., and Jones, T. (1981): Regional cerebral oxygen supply and utilisation in dementia: a clinical and physiological study with oxygen-15 and positron tomography. *Brain,* 104:753–778.
37. Frackowiak, R. S. J., Wise, R. J. S., Gibbs, J. M., Jones, T., and Leenders, N. (1984): Oxygen extraction in the ageing brain. *Monogr. Neurol. Sci.,* 11:118–122.
38. Frackowiak, R. S. J., Wise, R. J. S., Gibbs, J. M., Jones, T., and Leenders, K. L. (1984): Oxygen extraction in the ageing brain. In: *Effects of Ageing on Regulation of Cerebral Blood Flow and Metabolism,* edited by C. Fieschi, G. L. Lenzi, and C. W. Loeb, pp. 180–186. Karger, Basel.
39. Friedland, R. P., Budinger, T. F., Brant-Zawadzki, M., and Jagust, W. J. (1984): The diagnosis of Alzheimer type dementia: a preliminary comparison of positron emission tomography and proton magnetic resonance. *JAMA,* 252:2750–2752.
40. Friedland, R. P., Budinger, T. F., Ganz, E., Yano, Y., Mathis, C. A., Koss, B., Ober, B. A., Huesman, R. H., and Derenzo, S. E. (1983): Regional cerebral metabolic alterations in dementia of the Alzheimer type: positron emission tomography with ($^{18}$F)-fluorodeoxyglucose. *J. Comput. Assist. Tomogr.,* 7:590–598.
41. Friedland, R. P., Prusiner, S. B., Jagust, W. J., Budinger, T. F., and Davis, R. L. (1984): Bitemporal hypometabolism in Creutzfeldt-Jacob disease measured by positron emission tomography with ($^{18}$F)-2-fluorodeoxyglucose. *J. Comput. Assist. Tomogr.,* 8:978–981.
42. Gado, M., Hughes, C. P., Danzinger, W., Chi, D., Jost, G., and Berg, L. (1984): Volumetric measurements of the cerebrospinal fluid spaces in demented subjects and controls. *Radiology,* 144:535–538.
43. Galvez, S., and Cartier, L. (1984): Computed tomography findings in 15 cases of Creutzfeldt-Jakob disease with histological verification. *J. Neurol. Neurosurg. Psychiatry,* 47:1244–1246.
44. Gibbs, J. M., Frackowiak, R. S. J., and Legg, N. J. (1986): Regional cerebral blood flow and oxygen metabolism in dementia due to vascular disease. *Gerontology,* 32 (Suppl. 1):84–88.
45. Goto, K., Ishii, N., and Fukasawa, H. (1981): Diffuse white matter disease in the geriatric population. *Radiology,* 141:687–695.
46. Gottstein, U., Muller, W., Berghoff, W., Gartner, H., and Held, K. (1971): Zur utilisation von nicht-veresterten Fettsauren und Ketonkorpen im Gehiren des Menschen. *Klin. Wochenschr.,* 49:406–411.
47. Harrison, M. J. G., Thomas, D. J., DuBoulay, G. H., and Marshall, J. (1979): Multi-infarct dementia. *J. Neurol. Sci.,* 40:97–103.
48. Haxby, J. V., Duara, R., Grady, C. L., Cutler, N. R., and Rapoport, S. I. (1985): Relations between neurophysiological and cerebral metabolic asymmetries in early Alzheimer's disease. *J. Cereb. Blood Flow Metab.,* 5:193–200.
49. Hayden, M. R., Martin, W. R. W., Stoessl, A. J., Clark, C., Hollenberg, S., Adam, M. J., Ammann, W., Harrop, R., Rogers J., Ruth, T., Sayre, C., and Pate, B. D. (1986): Positron emission tomography in the early diagnosis of Huntington's disease. *Neurology,* 36:888–894.
50. Herscovitch, P., Gado, M., Mintun, M. A., et al. (1984): The necessity for correcting for cerebral atrophy in global positron emission tomography measurements. *Monogr. Neural Sci.,* 11:93–97.
51. Horwitz, B., Duara, R., and Rapoport, S. I. (1986): Age differences in intercorrelations between regional cerebral metabolic rates for glucose. *Ann. Neurol.,* 19:60–67.
52. Hubbard, B. M., and Anderson, J. M. (1981): A quantitative study of cerebral atrophy in old age and senile dementia. *J. Neurol. Sci.,* 50:135–145.
53. Huckman, M. S., Fox, J., and Topel, J. (1975): The validity of criteria for the evaluation of cerebral atrophy by computed tomography. *Radiology,* 116:85–92.
54. Ingvar, D. H. (1979): Hyperfrontal distribution of the cerebral gray matter flow, in resting wakefulness: on the functional anatomy of the conscious state. *Acta Neurol. Scand.,* 60:12–25.
55. Ito, M., Hatazawa, J., Yamaura, H., and Matsuzawa, T. (1981): Age related brain atrophy and mental deterioration—a study with computed tomography. *Br. J. Radiol.,* 54:384–390.
56. Jacoby, R. J., and Levy, R. (1980): Computed tomography in the elderly. 2. Senile dementia: diagnosis and functional impairment. *Br. J. Psychiatry,* 136:256–269.
57. Jacoby, R. J., Levy, R., and Dawson, J. M. (1980): Computed tomography in the elderly. 1. The normal population. *Br. J. Psychiatry,* 136:249–255.

58. Jagust, W. J., Friedland, R. P., and Budinger, T. F. (1985): Positron emission tomography with ($^{18}$F)fluorodeoxyglucose differentiates normal pressure hydrocephalus from Alzheimer type dementia. *J. Neurol. Neurosurg. Psychiatry*, 48:1091–1096.

58a. Kennedy, C., and Sokoloff, L. (1957): The adaptation of the nitrous oxide technique to the study of the cerebral circulation in children: normal values for cerebral blood flow and cerebral metabolic rate in childhood. *J. Clin. Invest.*, 36:1130–1137.

59. Kety, S. S. (1956): Human cerebral blood flow and oxygen consumption as related to ageing. *Res. Publ. Assoc. Res. Nerv. Ment. Dis.*, 35:31–45.

60. Kohlmeyer, K., and Shamena, A. R. (1981): The size of the lateral ventricles and cortical sulci in old age subjects with and without dementia. *Neuroradiology*, 138:89–92.

61. Koss, E., Friedland, R. P., Ober, B. A., and Jagust, W. J. (1985): Differences in lateral hemispheric asymmetries of glucose utilisation between early and late onset Alzheimer-type dementia. *Am. J. Psychiatry*, 142:638–640.

62. Kuhl, D. E., Markham, C. H., Metter, E. J., Reige, W. H., Phelps, M. E., and Mazziotta, J. C. (1985): Local cerebral glucose utilisation in symptomatic and pre-symptomatic Huntington's disease. *Res. Publ. Assoc. Res. Nerv. Ment. Dis.*, 63:199–209.

63. Kuhl, D. E., Metter, E. J., Benson, D. F., Ashford, J. W., Riege, W. H., Fujikawa, D. G., Markham, C. H., Mazziotta, J. C., Maltese, A., and Dorsey, D. A. (1985): Similarities of cerebral glucose metabolism in Alzheimer's and parkinsonian dementia. *J. Cereb. Blood Flow Metab.*, 5(Suppl. 1):S169–S170.

64. Kuhl, D. E., Metter, E. J., and Riege, W. H. (1985): Patterns of cerebral glucose utilisation in depression, multiple infarct dementia and Alzheimer's disease. *Res. Publ. Assoc. Res. Nerv. Ment. Dis.*, 63:211–225.

65. Kuhl, D. E., Metter, E. J., Riege, W. H., and Hawkins, R. A. (1984): The effect of normal ageing on patterns of local cerebral glucose utilisation. *Ann. Neurol.*, 15(Suppl.):S133–S137.

66. Kuhl, D. E., Metter, E. J., Riege, W. H., and Phelps, M. E. (1982): Effects of human ageing on patterns of local cerebral glucose utilisation determined by the $^{18}$F-fluorodeoxyglucose method. *J. Cereb. Blood Flow Metab.*, 2:163–171.

67. Kuhl, D. E., Phelps, M. E., Markham, C. H., Metter, E. J., Riege, W. H., and Winter, E. J. (1982): Cerebral metabolism and atrophy in Huntington's disease determined by $^{18}$FDG and computed tomographic scans. *Ann. Neurol.*, 12:425–434.

68. Lammertsma, A. A., Wise, R. J. S., Heather, J. D., Gibbs, J. M, Leenders, K. L., Frackowiak, R. S. J., Rhodes, C. G., and Jones, T. (1983): The correction for the presence of intravascular oxygen-15 in the steady state technique for measuring regional oxygen extraction ratio in the brain. 2. Results in normal subjects, brain tumour and stroke patients. *J. Cereb. Blood Flow Metab.*, 3:425–431.

69. Lebrun-Grandie, P., Baron, J. C., Soussaline, F., Loc'h, C., Sastre, J., and Bousser, M. G. (1983): Coupling between regional blood flow and oxygen utilisation in the normal human brain. *Arch. Neurol.*, 40:230–236.

70. Leenders, K. L., Frackowiak, R. S. J., and Lees, A. J. (1987): Steele-Richardson-Olszewski syndrome: brain energy metabolism, blood flow and fluorodopa uptake measured by positron emission tomography. *Brain (in press)*.

71. Leenders, K. L., Frackowiak, R. S. J., Quinn, N., and Marsden, C. D. (1986): Brain energy metabolism and dopaminergic function in Huntington's disease measured in vivo using positron emission tomography. *Movement Disord.*, 1:69–77.

72. Leenders, K. L, Palmer, A. J., Quinn, N., Clark, J. C., Firnau, G., Garnett, E. S., Nahmias, C., Jones, T., and Marsden, C. D. (1986): Brain dopamine metabolism in patients with Parkinson's disease measured with positron emission tomography. *J. Neurol. Neurosurg. Psychiatry*, 49:853–860.

73. Leenders, K. L., Palmer, A., Turton, D., Quinn, N., Firnau, G., Garnett, S., Nahmias, C., Jones, T., and Marsden, C. D. (1986): DOPA uptake and dopamine receptor binding visualised in the human brain in vivo. In: *Recent Developments in Parkinson's Disease*, edited by S. Fahn, C. D. Marsden, P. Jenner, and P. Teychenne, pp. 103–113. Raven Press, New York.

74. Lenzi, G. L., Gibbs, J. M., Frackowiak, R. S. J., and Jones, T. (1983): Measurement of cerebral blood flow and oxygen metabolism by positron emission tomography and the 150 steady-state technique: aspects of methodology, reproducibility and clinical application. In:

*Functional Radionuclide Imaging of the Brain,* edited by P. L. Magistretti, pp. 291–304. Raven Press, New York.

75. Mazziotta, J. C., Phelps, M. E., and Carson, R. E. (1984): Tomographic mapping of human cerebral metabolism: subcortical responses to auditory and visual stimulation. *Neurology,* 34:825–828.

76. Mazziotta, J. C., Phelps, M. E., Carson, R. E., and Kuhl, D. E. (1982): Tomographic mapping of human cerebral metabolism: auditory stimulation. *Neurology,* 32:921–937.

77. Mazziotta, J. C., Phelps, M. E., Carson, R. E., and Kuhl, D. E. (1982): Tomographic mapping of human cerebral metabolism: sensory deprivation. *Ann. Neurol.,* 12:435–444.

78. Mazziotta, J. C., Phelps, M. E., Miller, J., and Kuhl, D. E. (1981): Tomographic mapping of human cerebral metabolism: normal unstimulated state. *Neurology,* 31:503–516.

79. Metter, E. J., Mazziotta, J. C., Itabashi, H. H., Mankovich, N. J., Phelps, M. E. and Kuhl, D. E. (1985): Comparison of glucose metabolism, x-ray CT and post-mortem data in a patient with multiple cerebral infarcts. *Neurology,* 35:1695–1701.

80. Naeser, M. A., Gebhardt, C., and Levine, H. L. (1980): Decreased computerised tomography numbers in patients with presenile dementia: detection in patients with otherwise normal scans. *Arch. Neurol.,* 37:401–409.

81. Pantano, P., Baron, J. C., Lebrun-Grandie, P., Duquesnoy, N., Bousser, M. G., and Comar, D. (1984): Regional cerebral blood flow and oxygen consumption in human ageing. *Stroke,* 15:635–641.

82. Phelps, M. E., Mazziotta, J. C., Kuhl, D. E., Nuwer, M., Packwood, J., Metter, J., and Engel, J. R. (1981): Tomographic mapping of human cerebral metabolism: visual stimulation and deprivation. *Neurology,* 31:517–529.

83. Raichle, M. E. (1985): Measurement of local brain blood flow and oxygen utilisation using oxygen-15 radiopharmaceuticals: a rapid dynamic imaging approach. In: *Positron Emission Tomography,* edited by M. Reivich and A. Alavi, pp. 241–247. Alan R. Liss, New York.

84. Reivich, M., Kuhl, D., Wolf, A., Greenberg, J., Phelps, M. E., Ido, T., Casella, V., Fowler, J., Hoffman, E., Alavi, A., and Sokoloff, L. (1979): The [18]F-fluorodeoxyglucose method for the measurement of local cerebral glucose utilisation in man. *Circ. Res.,* 44:127–137.

85. Schwartz, M., Creasey, H., Grady, C. L., Deleo, J. M., Frederickson, H. A., Cutler, R. N., and Rapoport, S. I. (1985): Computed tomographic analysis of brain morphometrics in 30 healthy men, aged 21 to 81 years. *Ann. Neurol.,* 17:146–157.

86. Soininen, H., Puranen, J., and Riekkinen, P. J. (1982): Computed tomography findings in senile dementia and normal ageing. *J. Neurol. Neurosurg. Psychiatry,* 45:50–54.

87. Sokoloff, L. (1981): Localisation of functional activity in the central nervous system by measurement of glucose utilisation with radioactive deoxyglucose. *J. Cereb. Blood Flow Metab.,* 1:7–36.

88. Sokoloff, L., Reivich, M., Kennedy, C., DesRosiers, M. H., Patlak, C. S., Pettigrew, K. D., Sakurada, O., and Shinohara, M. (1977): The (C-14)-deoxyglucose method for the measurement of local glucose utilisation: theory, procedure and normal values in the conscious, anaesthetised albino rat. *J. Neurochem.,* 28:897–916.

89. Stober, T., Wussow, W., and Schimrigk, K. (1984): Bicaudate diameter—the most specific and simple CT parameter in the diagnosis of Huntington's disease. *Neuroradiology,* 26:25–28.

90. Tomlinson, B. E., Blessed, G., and Roth, M. (1970): Observations on the brains of demented old people. *J. Neurol. Sci.,* 11:205–242.

91. Turkheimer, E., Cullum, C. M., Hubler, D. W., Paver, S. W., Yeo, R. A., and Bigler, E. D. (1984): Quantifying cortical atrophy. *J. Neurol. Neurosurg. Psychiatry,* 47:1314–1318.

92. Wong, D. F., Wagner, H. N., Dannals, R. F., Links, J. M., Frost, J. J., Ravert, H. T., Wilson, A. A., Rosenbaum, A. E., Gjedde, A., Douglass, K. H., Petronis, J. D., Folstein, M. F., Toung, J. K. T., Bruns, H. D., and Kuhar, M. J. (1984): Effects of age on dopamine and serotonin receptors measured by positron tomography in the living human brain. *Science,* 226:1393–1396.

*Aging and the Brain,* edited by R. D. Terry.
Raven Press, New York © 1988.

# Some Morphometric Aspects of Alzheimer Disease and of Normal Aging

## Robert D. Terry and Lawrence A. Hansen

*Department of Neurosciences, School of Medicine, University of California,
San Diego, La Jolla, California 92093*

For many years it has been the belief of most workers in the field and even of the public that normal human aging is necessarily associated with a massive loss of neocortical neurons. This widespread opinion was based largely on the data of Brody (2), whose cell counts were done on 13 specimens from patients between the ages of 16 and 95. His conclusions were reinforced by others' observations concerning, on the one hand, psychological (4) and motor (7) changes in the elderly and, on the other, clear autoptic and radiologic evidence of cerebral shrinkage. Nevertheless, our own morphometric study on about 50 cases indicates far less neuronal loss than has been previously believed to occur (9).

This semiautomated morphometric work began not on normal aging but, rather, on senile dementia of the Alzheimer type (SDAT) (10). The latter involved patients aged between 70 and 90 years, and more recently a group of patients aged 50 to 65, all with the classic Alzheimer clinical picture. Necessarily, both groups were compared with age-matched normals. Subsequently, a sizable group of normal subjects aged 20 to 100 have been assembled for examination.

The purposes of this chapter are therefore threefold: (a) to enumerate the relatively mild regressive changes of the neocortex of normal aging; (b) to compare neocortical morphometry of young Alzheimer patients with that of the senile age group; and (c) to compare neocortical populations in normals with those in Alzheimer specimens.

## METHODS

Most of the Alzheimer patients had been studied clinically by my colleagues in the Department of Neurology at the Albert Einstein College of Medicine and more recently in the Department of Neurosciences at the University of California in San Diego. The patients displayed dementia in the form of memory loss and a multiplicity of other cognitive deficits including the functions of orientation, work finding, judgment, praxia, etc. Most of the normal subjects came by a similar route, having been judged to have normal mentation on neurologic and psychological bases. Other normals were sent by colleagues at outside institutions and had come from life situations incompatible with dementia.

Histologic proof of normality was gained by careful gross examination and screening of many microscopic sections from each case. Any evidence of anoxia other than terminal, Parkinson's disease, or ischemic changes caused us to rule out the subject from this normal series. More than three plaques or any tangles per neocortical ×125 field brought similar exclusion. Alzheimer disease (AD) and SDAT were diagnosed histologically on finding numerous plaques in the neocortex—at least as many as prescribed by Khachaturian (5). Neocortical tangles were invariably present in those below age 75 but were lacking in about 30% of those who were older (11). The entorhinal cortex was always intensely involved, and the hippocampus pyramidal layer usually showed many lesions in the AD/SDAT specimens.

Cell counting was performed with a semiautomatic image analysis apparatus: the Quantimet 720 and more recently the Quantimet 920. Formalin-fixed tissue blocks from midfrontal, superior temporal, and inferior parietal areas were dehydrated in alcohol, cleared in xylene or Histoclear, embedded in paraffin, sectioned at 20 $\mu$m, and stained with cresyl violet. Care was taken so that the cortex along the side of the sulcus was perpendicular to the pial surface. The apparatus recognizes cells on the basis of the stained density of the glial or neuronal perikaryon, the area of which was measured in 10 size classes. Video editing separated contiguous cells, eliminated vessels and artifacts, and filled imcompletely stained cell bodies. This sort of editing is essential for accuracy (8). Previous work had shown that perikarya smaller than 40 $\mu$m² were almost always glial, whereas neurons were almost always larger than 40 $\mu$m². The eight size classes of neurons were divided for purposes of presentation into two size groups: small, between 40 and 90 $\mu$m² in cross-sectional area; and large, more than 90 $\mu$m².

Neuritic plaques and neurofibrillary tangles were counted on paraffin sections 10$\mu$m thick stained with thioflavin S and taken serially from the same blocks as were the cresyl violet sections. These counts were done manually with a fluorescence microscope using filtration identical to that designed for work with fluorescein (FITC). Plaques were enumerated in three fields along the side of the gyrus at a total magnification of ×125. Tangles were enumerated similarly at a magnification of ×500. The thioflavin stain was chosen rather than a silver impregnation stain because of the former's high resolution and because of the rapidity, facility, and consistency of the technique as well as its low cost in labor and material. Its sensitivity is at least as great as that of the best silver impregnations, and its resolution is better as there are no aggregates of silver particles to obscure the cytologic detail. Furthermore, the stain demonstrates vascular amyloid as well as plaques and tangles. Silver reactions do not have this capacity.

## RESULTS

### Normal Aging

Fifty-one normal specimens were available for analysis of brain weight. The weight of both male and female specimens decreased equally and significantly at about 6 g/year. Pearson's coefficient of correlation ($r$) was $-0.67$. This weight loss remains significant even if one subtracts the secular change. Cortical thickness lessened slightly but significantly in midfrontal and superior temporal areas but not significantly in the inferior parietal region.

The thickness of the midfrontal cortical laminae was measured with an eyepiece reticule in more than 30 cases, and it was found that only layer 3 showed a significant absolute as well as a relative decrease.

The number of glia increased in midfrontal and superior temporal areas but not significantly in the inferior parietal lobe. By utilizing antiserum against glial fibrous acidic protein with the peroxidase antiperoxidase technique of Sternberger (6), it was shown that the number of fibrous astrocytes also increased significantly as a function of normal aging in layers 2 to 6 of the frontal region (3). This cell type was not counted in other areas.

We found that the number of large neurons (those with a cross-sectional perikaryon area greater than 90 $\mu m^2$) decreased significantly ($r = -0.64$) in all three cerebral areas as a function of normal aging. The decrease was seen particularly in the largest cell subclasses. There was additional positive correlation ($r = 0.64$, $p < 0.001$) between the number of large neurons and the total brain weight. Whereas the number of large neurons decreased in normal aging, there was an actual increase in the number of cells falling into the 40 to 90 $\mu m^2$ classes, i.e., small neurons. When we averaged the number of small neurons in the specimens up to age 49 and compared them to the average of the specimens from patients aged 70 and above, it was found that in the older group the mean increase in small neurons equaled the average decrease of large neurons. Thus the total number of neurons did not change as a function of normal aging. We concluded that the large neurons shrank into these smaller neuron classes. In general, the changes in midfrontal and superior temporal regions were more marked than those in the inferior parietal area. Dividing the patients into a younger group (aged 20–49) for comparison with the group aged 70 and above revealed differences similar to those found by the regression analyses. Large neurons decreased about 40%, small neurons increased about 22%, and glia increased by about 50%.

An unexpected finding was that in normal specimens within an age group the cell populations did not vary significantly by analysis of variance among midfrontal, superior temporal, and inferior parietal areas; that is, in groups of normal specimens aged 20 to 50, 51 to 69, or 70 and up, there were approximately the same numbers of large neurons, small neurons, and glia in the three areas within each age group.

## Comparing Presenile with Senile Alzheimer Disease

Both patients and normal controls were split into two groups according to age: (a) 50 to 65, and (b) above 69. The 5-year interval was left between the groups because patients dying at the intermediate age might well have had the onset of disease during the presenile period. The most important difference between the two groups of patients was that in about 30% of the older group neocortical tangles were absent, whereas they were always found in the younger patients. Noting that fact, we redivided the older patients into two groups: one with cortical plaques and tangles, the other with plaques only. We found that there were no differences between these two groups using the Blessed et al. psychological score (1), the rate of change of the Blessed et al. score, the brain weight, neuron and glial counts, plaque counts, and concentrations of choline acetyltransferase. We therefore concluded that the disease with neocortical plaques and tangles is not different from the one with neocortical plaques so far as the SDAT population is concerned (11).

Other than the tangle counts, major differences between presenile and senile Alzheimer disease were not found in comparisons of brain weights, numbers of glia and neurons, or concentration of plaques. For each parameter the younger group showed slightly, but not significantly, more disease.

## Alzheimer Disease Compared with Normal Aging

The changes in the older group have been superimposed on those of normal aging, so that the differences between SDAT and aged normals are less than those between presenile Alzheimer disease and the 50- to 65-year-old normals. Those differences between SDAT and the normal elderly remain statistically significant. Even after age 80, significant differences remain between SDAT and normals as to large neurons, plaques, tangles, and choline acetyltransferase (ChAT) concentrations (Table 1). The tangle concentration decreases because 30% of the SDAT cases in this age group do not have any.

The 50- to 65-year-old Alzheimer group has lost about 50% of the large neocortical neurons, whereas the 70- to 100-year-old patients have lost only 28% of these cells compared with age-matched groups. The younger AD specimens displayed a 13% loss of brain weight, whereas the older ones are down only 7%. All these figures are statistically significant. By definition, the differences as to plaques and tangles are total. In a large group of Alzheimer patients both plaques and tangles decrease significantly with age (Tables 2 and 3).

TABLE 1. *Old SDAT (80–100 years) vs. normals (80–100 years): differences of means*

| Measurement | Midfrontal | | Superior temporal | | Inferior parietal | |
|---|---|---|---|---|---|---|
| | % | p < | % | p < | % | p < |
| Cortical thickness | −6 | NS | −5 | NS | −15 | 0.02 |
| Total neurons | −18 | 0.05 | −6 | NS | −6 | NS |
| Large neurons | −24 | 0.05 | −15 | NS | −26 | 0.05 |
| Small neurons | −15 | NS | −3 | NS | 0 | NS |
| Glia | −16 | NS | −10 | NS | +4 | NS |
| Neuron/glia ratio | 0 | NS | −5 | NS | −4 | NS |
| Plaques | +96 | 0.001 | +100 | 0.001 | +100 | 0.001 |
| Tangles | +100 | 0.05 | +100 | 0.05 | +100 | NS |
| ChAT | −47 | 0.05 | −51 | 0.02 | −54 | 0.02 |
| Brain weight | +2 | NS | | | | |

TABLE 2. *Young AD (50–65 years) vs. normals (50–65 years): differences of means*

| Measurement | Midfrontal | | Superior temporal | | Inferior parietal | |
|---|---|---|---|---|---|---|
| | % | p < | % | p < | % | p < |
| Cortical thickness | −15 | 0.05 | −14 | NS | −26 | 0.02 |
| Total neurons | −23 | 0.02 | −26 | 0.02 | −36 | 0.01 |
| Large neurons | −50 | 0.001 | −44 | 0.01 | −58 | 0.001 |
| Small neurons | −9 | NS | −17 | NS | −25 | 0.05 |
| Glia | +35 | NS | −12 | NS | 0 | NS |
| Brain weight | −13 | 0.01 | | | | |

TABLE 3. *Young AD (50–65 years) vs. old SDAT (70–100 years): midfrontal*

| Measurement | % | p < |
|---|---|---|
| Cortical thickness | +5 | NS |
| Total neurons | +2 | NS |
| Large neurons | +17 | NS |
| Small neurons | −2 | NS |
| Glia | +5 | NS |
| Brain weight | −2 | NS |

## CONCLUSIONS

The messsages here are as follows: (a) the findings in patients with Alzheimer disease at any age are clearly different from those of age-matched normal controls; (b) the "younger" disease is more severe than the "older"; and (c) neuron loss per unit volume in normally aging neocortex is much less marked than previously thought.

## REFERENCES

1. Blessed, G., Tomlinson, B. E., and Roth, M. (1968): The association between quantitative measures of dementia and of senile changes in the cerebral gray matter of elderly subjects. *Br. J. Psychiatry,* 114:797–811.
2. Brody, H. (1955): Organization of the cerebral cortex, part three, a study of aging in the human cerebral cortex. *J. Comp. Neurol.,* 102:551–556.
3. Hansen, L. A., Armstrong, D. M., and Terry, R. D. (1987): An immunohistochemical quantification of fibrous astroctyes in the aging human cerebral cortex. *Neurobiol. Aging,* 8:1–6.
4. Katzman, R., and Terry, R. D. (1983): Normal aging of the nervous system. In: *The Neurology of Aging,* edited by R. Katzman and R. D. Terry, pp. 15–50. Davis, Philadelphia.
5. Khachaturian, Z. S. (1985): Diagnosis of Alzheimer's disease. *Arch. Neurol.,* 42:1097–1105.
6. Sternberger, L. A. (1979): *Immunocytochemistry,* 2nd ed. Wiley, New York.
7. Teravainen, H., and Calne, D. B. (1983): Motor system in normal aging and Parkinson's disease. In: *The Neurology of Aging,* edited by R. Katzman and R. D. Terry, pp. 85–109. Davis, Philadelphia.
8. Terry, R. D., and DeTeresa, R. (1982): The importance of video editing in automated image analysis in studies of the cerebral cortex. *J. Neurol. Sci.,* 53:413–421.
9. Terry, R. D., DeTeresa, R., and Hansen, L. A. (1987): Neocortical cell counts in normal human adult aging. *Ann. Neurol.,* 21:530–539.
10. Terry, R. D., DeTeresa, R., Schechter, R., and Horoupian, D. S. (1981): Some morphometric aspects of the brain in senile dementia of the Alzheimer type. *Ann. Neurol.,* 10:184–192.
11. Terry, R. D., Hansen, L. A., DeTeresa, R., Davies, P., Tobias, H., and Katzman, R. (1987): Senile dementia of the Alzheimer type without neocortical neurofibrillary tangles. *J. Neuropathol. Exp. Neurol.,* 46:262–268.

Aging and the Brain, edited by R. D. Terry.
Raven Press, New York © 1988.

# "Classical" Neurotransmitters in Alzheimer Disease

## D. M. Bowen, A. M. Palmer, P. T. Francis, A. W. Procter, and S. L. Lowe

*Miriam Marks Department of Neurochemistry, Institute of Neurology, University of London, London, WC1N 1PJ, United Kingdom*

Reductions in the activity of acetylocholinesterase in Alzheimer disease (AD) brain reported in 1964 by Pope and colleagues provided an indication that the cholinergic system may be affected in this condition. The large reductions in choline acetyltransferase (ChAT) activity that were reported more than a decade later indicated that specific neurotransmitter deficits may underlie the symptoms of the disease and suggested the possibility that these symptoms could be ameliorated by pharmacological manipulation (reviewed in ref. 12). It is argued here that cognitive and noncognitive symptoms are likely to involve cholinergic and serotonergic cells and their action on cortical pyramidal neurons.

### CHOLINERGIC NEURONS

Choline acetyltransferase is apparently present in large excess over normal requirements for acetylcholine synthesis and is generally considered not to be the rate-limiting step in this process. Thus the effects of the reductions in this enzyme activity on acetylcholine synthesis in intact tissue were not readily predictable. To resolve this issue the synthesis of [$^{14}$C]acetylcholine from [U-$^{14}$C]glucose was measured by Sims et al. (50–52) in tissue prisms (minislices) prepared from fresh neocortical tissue samples from patients with dementia. In this study as in subsequent investigations of biopsied brain, control values were obtained using apparently normal neocortex removed as a necessary part of surgery (usually to gain access to deep-seated tumors). Samples from demented patients, in which diagnosis of AD was confirmed histologically, showed markedly lower synthesis of acetylcholine under both resting (5 mM K$^+$) and depolarized (31 mM K$^+$) conditions. The reductions were similar in both frontal and temporal lobes.

Measurement of high-affinity choline uptake into the prisms was similarly reduced in the biopsy samples from patients with AD (51). Comparable reductions in high-affinity choline uptake were also found by Rylett et al. (49) in synaptosomes prepared from frontal cortex of fresh autopsy brains from AD cases. Synaptosomes prepared from hippocampus showed even less preservation of activity, suggesting an even greater loss of cholinergic function within this region.

Several years ago Whitehouse and colleagues reported that in AD patients there was a significant loss of large acetylcholinesterase-positive neuronal cell bodies in the nucleus basalis of Meynert, which provide the major cholinergic projection to the neocortex. This observation has been confirmed in a number of studies (reviewed in ref. 43). The identification of reductions in ChAT activity led rapidly to attempts to ameliorate the defects using cholinergic agonists or acetylcholinesterase inhibitors (reviewed in refs. 12,21,55). Such trials were encouraged by early reports that the numbers of muscarinic receptors were similar in AD and control brains, suggesting that suitable targets for the agonists were available or there was an increased acetylcholine signal.

The findings that there may be two or more subclasses of muscarinic receptors (distinguished at present largely from their antagonist binding properties) has led to a reexamination of the status of these receptors in AD. Nicotinic receptors are also present in human brain, albeit representing only a small proportion of total cholinergic binding sites. Studies indicate that binding at these sites, as well as at the lower-affinity muscarinic sites, is reduced in AD patients (30,57). The function of both sites is poorly defined, and the biological significance of the observed disease-induced alterations cannot at present be predicted.

The available evidence from the effects of drugs and lesions in humans and animals suggests a role for the cholinergic system in memory and cognitive function, but the specific functions of cholinergic inputs in the limbic system and particularly the diffuse projection to the neocortex remain poorly defined. A correlation between ChAT activity in autopsy brain and an overall measure of cognitive function determined within 6 months prior to death was found for a group of patients presenting with either AD or depression (40). In patients with AD who were biopsied, there was also a significant correlation between an overall clinical assessment of the degree of dementia and [$^{14}$C]-acetylcholine synthesis [although not ChAT activity (33)]. Among specific psychometric tests [Wechsler Adult Intelligence Scales (WAIS), token test, and visual reaction time], only the reaction time showed a significant correlation with the rate of acetylcholine synthesis. The observed significant correlations do not allow any conclusions to be drawn as to a cause-and-effect relation but do indicate that cholinergic deficits and the degree of dementia advance in parallel and are at least consistent with there being a cholinergic contribution to the development of the symptoms of AD.

Other "classical" neurotransmitters as well as neuropeptides have been examined in AD patients, but none has been identified that relates to the clinical course of dementia in AD.

## NEOCORTICAL NEURONS

### Interneurons

Glutamic acid decarboxylase (GAD) activity is affected by the way patients die. For this reason the concentration of $\gamma$-aminobutyric acid (GABA) in autopsy samples has been used to estimate this major (23) inhibitory cortical interneuron. No widespread loss was found in AD patients (48).

Examination of biopsy samples of frontal cortex from AD patients at approximately the midpoint of the disease does not show altered GAD activity, whereas cholinergic markers are reduced (2). Fresh tissue from the temporal cortex of AD patients has been mechanically chopped in two planes to provide preparations for the determination of the $K^+$-induced release of endogenous neurotransmitter. Electron microscopy of such tissue prisms has shown that, as previously reported for adult rat brain, these samples are primarily preparations of intact synaptic endings (reviewed in ref. 16). The release of GABA is not altered in AD (Table 1).

Neuropeptides (somatostatin, cholecystokinin, neuropeptide Y, vasoactive intestinal peptide, substance P, neurotensin) are quite stable postmortem, so they have been extensively investigated in AD, although as a group they are found in only a few ($<10\%$) cortical interneurons (23). Somatostatin-like immunoreactivity (SLIR) is the only peptide measurement found to be consistently reduced. Francis et al. (15) have related this change to the results of positron emission tomographic and histopathologic investigations, which indicate that in AD patients there is not a uniformly diffuse degenerative process in the neocortex. The temporal lobe is always severely degenerated (i.e., always contains numerous senile plaque and tangles) and has consistently shown a reduction in the concentration of SLIR. There is evidence of reduced SLIR content in the parietal cortex, and this lobe often shows pronounced degeneration. In frequently less degenerated areas (frontal lobe and anterior cingulate cortex) the content is often unaffected. Some inconsistency does seem to exist as the concentration of SLIR is reduced in the motor cortex, which is only slightly degenerated, and not all studies report a reduced SLIR content in the parietal lobe.

The concentrations of SLIR in both frontal and temporal cortex from AD biopsy samples were not significantly different from those of control cortex (15), and $K^+$-induced release was not significantly altered (Table 1).

Antibody to the peptide stains some tangle-bearing neurons, but in the biopsy tissue there was no correlation between tangle count and SLIR concentration (15). Perry (42) pointed out that the neuronal types affected by tangles is an underresearched area but there is a tendency in elderly or moderately advanced cases for supragranular pyramidal neurons to be more susceptible.

TABLE 1. *Neurosurgical specimens: 50 mM K+-induced release of endogenous neurotransmitters and somatostatin from tissue prisms of neocortex*

| Neurotransmitter | Control (pmol/mg protein) | Alzheimer disease (pmol/mg protein) |
|---|---|---|
| Serotonin | 0.34 ± 0.05 (6) | 0.17 ± 0.05 (6)[a] |
| Acetylcholine[b] | 6.33 ± 1.23 (6) | 3.21 ± 0.66 (7)[a] |
| GABA | 1,810 ± 570 (6) | 1,690 ± 240 (7) |
| SLIR | 0.052 ± 0.038 (7) | 0.067 ± 0.038 (6) |
| Glutamate | 7,020 ± 2,330 (6) | 9,870 ± 2,550 (7) |
| Aspartate | 1,850 ± 550 (6) | 2,160 ± 550 (7) |
| Dopamine | 0.24 ± 0.09 (5) | 0.46 ± 0.35 (6) |
| Norepinephrine | 0.55 ± 0.44 (5) | 0.41 ± 0.25 (6) |

Tissue is from the temporal lobe except for SLIR, dopamine, norepinephrine, and 5-HT, which are from the frontal lobe (cholinergic markers are reduced by about the same extent in both lobes). Values are means and standard deviations. Sample numbers are in parentheses.

[a]The only values significantly different from control.

[b]Acetylcholine release (dpm/mg protein/min) is based on the determination of [14C]acetylcholine synthesis in medium containing 31 mM K+. Other experiments (53) indicate that the medium contains more than 80% of the total [14C]acetylcholine.

Data are from refs. 15,35,54.

## Pyramidal Neurons

Many would argue that the excitatory amino acids glutamic acid and perhaps aspartate are the major neurotransmitters for cortical pyramidal neurons (especially of the hippocampus and corticostriatal pathway) but not corticopetal cells. The biochemical investigation of these neurotransmitters in conventional autopsy samples is at present unreliable. Phosphate-activated glutaminase activity is subject to unexplained variability (56; A. W. Procter et al., *unpublished results*) and membranes used for Na+-dependent binding of $^3$H-D-aspartic acid (36,45) may be contaminated by saccules containing neurotransmitter (10).

An indirect method for assessing the integrity of these neurons in autopsy material may be to measure recognition sites for neurotransmitters that act directly on the cell. The serotonin (5-hydroxytryptamine, 5-HT)$_{1A}$ receptor is one such site based on neurophysiological studies of the action of 8-hydroxy-2-(di-*n*-propylamino)tetralin (8-OH-DPAT) (5). Further support observed in two independent studies (35,38) for such a close association of corticopetal serotonergic fibers and pyramidal cells is provided by the correlation between the density of tangle-bearing (pyramidal) cells and the concentration of 5-hydroxyindoleacetic acid (5-HIAA). [$^3$H]8-OH-DPAT binding is not reduced in the temporal cortex in AD (32). Lacking knowledge about the proportion of 5-HT$_{1A}$ recognition sites on pyramidal neurons, it is impossible to confidently use the above information for establishing whether either shrinkage or loss of pyramidal cells occurs. A marker of 5-HT$_2$ recognition sites, $^3$Hketanserin binding is reduced in both temporal cortex and the entire temporal lobe (6; A. W. Procter et al., *unpublished results*) which has been equated with loss of interneurons (6). Loss of nerve cell membrane from the entire lobe occurs based on reduced ganglioside content (2), but data obtained by cell counting techniques (reviewed in ref. 11) suggests that loss of large or pyramidal neurons (rather than interneurons) is a feature of AD particularly in severe or presenile AD patients (42). Other morphological data (33,39) indicate that the neocortical cytoarchitecture and regional interconnections are disrupted in AD patients, with the degree of disruption being correlated with severity of dementia. However, this correlation neither allows conclusions to be drawn as to a cause-and-effect relation nor allows for the known changes in the hippocampus and amygdala (17,36), which almost certainly contribute to cognitive decline.

$Na^+$-dependent uptake of $[^3H]$-D-aspartic acid, a metabolically stable false neurotransmitter, has been used by Procter et al. (44) to assess the number or functional state of excitatory dicarboxylic amino acid (glutamic and aspartic acid)-releasing nerve endings. Brains obtained promptly after death were processed into tissue prisms (4) as for the neurosurgical samples. Other samples were obtained from patients undergoing surgical treatment for intracerebral tumor where the removal of apparently normal tissue was a necessary part of the procedure. Three patients had causes of cognitive impairment other than AD, and three patients had AD with widespread senile plaque and neurofibrillary tangle formation. The latter also had the lowest uptake values in almost all regions examined. Both groups included subjects with a short (<1 hour) and a long (3 days) terminal coma, but there appeared to be no effect of a magnitude comparable to that of AD. Another patient was found to have few neocortical tangles but abundant plaques. This patient had an uptake value in the temporal lobe within the range of the neurosurgical specimens, and elsewhere intermediate between the florid AD cases and the patients with other dementias.

On $K^+$ stimulation, tissue prisms of neocortex obtained at diagnostic craniotomy from AD patients responded in a manner similar to that of controls, with an enhanced and preferental efflux of only 3 of the 13 amino acids measured. These three were the putative transmitters: aspartate, glutamate, and GABA. The absolute amounts released by AD samples were not significantly altered from the age-matched control values, for either unstimulated or $K^+$-stimulated prisms, although acetylcholine release was greatly reduced (Table 1).

## NONCHOLINERGIC CORTICOPETAL NEURONS

### Serotonergic Cells

Like cholinergic cells, serotonergic neurons also innervate large areas of cerebral cortex from discrete subcortical nuclei. However, the integrity of serotonergic neurons has been less thoroughly investigated in AD, largely because of the difficulty of measuring the activity of tryptophan hydroxylase in postmortem brain. With the exception of studies of the 5-HT carrier, all other estimates of serotonergic neurons in postmortem samples have relied on determination of the concentrations of 5-HT and 5-HIAA. The 5-HT concentration in the neocortex from AD subjects has in general been found to be reduced, whereas 5-HIAA was unaltered except according to one report of reduced concentration. This discrepancy may be related to postmortem delay, which was shorter in the latter study than in other investigations. Postmortem changes are known to affect the indoleamines, particularly in the cortex. Moreover, as oxygen is a cofactor for tryptophan hydroxylase, the terminal hypoxia usually associated with AD may be partly responsible for some of the observed changes (reviewed in refs. 34,38).

Problems associated with postmortem material have been circumvented by assessing the integrity of serotonergic varicosities in AD biopsy samples. Uptake of [3H]5-HT has been shown to be reduced in such material (3). Three additional indices of serotonergic neurons have now been studied: (a) uptake of [3H]5-HT dependent on a specific 5-HT uptake inhibitor; (b) K+-evoked release of endogenous 5-HT; and (c) concentrations of 5-HT and 5-HIAA (34). All these indices were substantially reduced in AD biopsy samples, which is a selective change as markers of dopaminergic neurons were not reduced in the same samples. Serotonergic dysfunction was shown to occur in patients who probably had had the disease for 2 years or less. The biopsy specimens were typically taken 3.5 years after onset of symptoms, which is approximately at the midpoint of the disease. At this stage the temporal cortex of the average patient has lost some 60% of each of the markers for serotonergic and cholinergic neurons. The serotonergic lesion was more severe in the temporal cortex, as was found postmortem (38). These findings presumably reflect the spread of the disease process and are consistent with serotonergic denervation occurring in AD as a result of changes in the neocortex. Neurofibrillary degeneration and neuronal loss from the raphe nucleus have been reported (9,26), but it is not known if the affected cells relate topographically to areas of pronounced neocortical damage.

In contrast to presynaptic cholinergic dysfunction, serotonergic denervation does not correlate with the dementia rating. It may be because, unlike in the case of the cholinergic system, the neuropsychological consequences of impaired serotonergic neurotransmission can also involve marked loss of 5-HT receptors, in particular the 5-HT$_2$ type (reviewed in refs 6,31). Alternatively, serotonergic denervation could predispose patients to amnesia, with the increasing severity of dementia being due to other overriding changes within the cortex such as pyramidal neuron loss or cholinergic denervation, both of which correlate with dementia rating (33). A compensatory increase in the rate of 5-HT turnover in the remaining neurons may account for the reported (34) increase observed in the concentration of 5-HIAA in cerebrospinal fluid

(CSF) as the disease intensifies (based on dementia rating). There is other evidence for increased 5-HT turnover in AD (38) and for similar changes in dopamine and norepinephrine metabolism in neurodegenerative disease, including AD (46).

Indices of serotonergic cells did not significantly correlate with indices of cholinergic neurons, pyramidal cell number, or plaque formation. However, in agreement with data from postmortem tissue (38), 5-HIAA concentration significantly correlated (negatively) with tangle counts, suggesting that intrinsic cortical change may be a determinant of serotonergic denervation.

The selective loss of serotonergic receptors (2,6,31) has been equated with degeneration of cortical neurons containing 5-HT receptors (possibly glutamergic pyramidal or somatostatin neurons), which may then lead to denervation of the ascending 5-HT projection by retrograde degeneration (3,36,39). The observed correlation between tangle formation (which occurs predominantly in pyramidal cells) and 5-HIAA is consistent with such a mechanism involving the pyramidal neuron. Moreover, increased glucose oxidation [which occurs *in vitro* in AD and correlates with 5-HIAA concentration (34)] is also likely to be due to alterations in pyramidal neurons [as these are the largest and most abundant type of cortical nerve cell, and many have terminal fields within their own and other cortical areas, whereas serotonergic and cholinergic varicosities and somatostatin cells are only minor components of neurophils (3,34)]. As loss of cortical pyramidal neurons correlates with dementia rating (33), investigation of the action of serotonergic drugs on pyramidal neurons may provide a novel therapeutic approach for AD.

## Catecholaminergic Cells

Cell loss from the noradrenergic locus cerulus is a well-documented feature of AD, and evidence is emerging of the loss of corticopetal dopaminergic nerve cells (28). Catecholaminergic varicosities have not been thoroughly investigated in AD, as the enzymes responsible for the synthesis of dopamine (DA) and norepinephrine (NE) are unstable postmortem. Apart from two studies of dopamine-β-hydroxylase activity postmortem—one indicating reduced activity and the other finding no change—neurochemical studies of the cerebral cortex have focused on determination of the concentrations of DA and NE and their principal metabolites (homovanillic acid, HVA; and 3-methoxy-4-hydroxyphenylglycol, MHPG). DA concentrations have consistently been found not to be reduced, as have the concentrations of a minor DA metabolite dihydroxyphenylacetic acid (DOPAC). HVA concentrations were also unaltered in some regions but elevated in others. Reduced concentrations of NE have generally been found, whereas concentrations of MHPG have been reduced, unaltered, or even elevated. These discrepancies may be a reflection of the postmortem accumulation of MHPG, which together with the high turnover rate and low concentrations of DA and NE in the cortex, question the validity of determining tissue concentrations postmortem (reviewed in refs. 35,38). As oxygen is a cofactor of both tyrosine hydroxylase and dopamine-$\beta$-hydroxylase, the terminal hypoxia usually associated with AD may also be partly responsible for some of the observed changes.

Problems associated with postmortem tissue have again been circumvented by Palmer et al. (35) using neocortical tissue from presenile AD patients obtained antemortem at diagnostic craniotomy. Several markers have been measured: (a) uptake of [³H]NE; (b) K⁺-evoked release of endogenous DA and NE; and (c) concentrations of DA, NE, DOPAC, HVA, and MHPG. The present study confirms postmortem indications of a presynaptic noradrenergic deficit in the temporal cortex, as two indices were substantially reduced (Table 2). Marked cell loss hase been reported from the locus ceruleus, so the simplest explanation for the present deficits is that they reflect a loss of noradrenergic neurons. These deficits suggest that noradrenergic denervation, like cholinergic and serotonergic denervation, occurs at a relatively early stage of the disease.

Cerebrospinal fluid data show evidence of selective changes in AD as the concentrations of HVA and the principal 5-HT metabolite (5-HIAA) are reduced whereas the concentration of MHPG is unaltered (37). The lesion in the cortex itself also displays some specificity as neurochemical dopaminergic markers are spared (Table 2), in agreement with postmortem studies (1,7,20,22,38). The selectivity of the cortical lesion is further illustrated in the frontal cortex, where the release of 5-HT from tissue prisms is reduced whereas the release of DA and NE was spared (Table 1).

Morphological studies implicate catecholaminergic varicosities in the formation of senile plaques (24,27,29), but, as in postmortem neurochemical studies (7,38,41), catecholaminergic markers were not found here to correlate with plaque density. Indices of dopaminergic cells correlated with densities of tangles and pyramidal cells in antemortem AD tissue, which provides evidence that disease-related changes occur in dopaminergic neurons, possibly secondary to the "cortical perikaryal disorder" of AD (Table 3). Other data for a similar group of samples show that presynaptic cholinergic markers correlate with densities of both pyramidal cells and plaques, and the 5-HIAA concentration correlates with tangle density (33,34). Thus only cholinergic and serotonergic varicosities show evidence of large losses in AD that advance in parallel with the degree of histological damage (Table 3).

Studies of humans and experimental animals are said to suggest a role for noradrenergic neurons in the physiological process underlying mood and affect (20) as well as learning and memory (25,47). However, the noradrenergic markers in the cortex of AD patients were not influenced by the presence or absence of mood disturbance, nor did they significantly correlate with dementia rating or other psychometric test scores (35). It may be because noradrenergic denervation is effectively complete at a very early stage of the disease so that progressive clinical deterioration is not accompanied by any further reduction

TABLE 2. *Catecholamine neurotransmitters and metabolite concentrations, NE uptake, and ChAT activity of neocortex obtained at diagnostic craniotomy of Alzheimer patients and controls*

| Measurement | Controls | Alzheimer disease (AD) | AD as % of control |
|---|---|---|---|
| *DA neurons* | | | |
| DA | | | |
| Temporal cortex | 1.55 ± 0.36 (17) | 0.83 ± 0.20 (11) | 54 |
| Frontal cortex | 0.98 ± 0.31 (20) | 0.63 ± 0.07 (4) | 64 |
| HVA | | | |
| Temporal cortex | 62 ± 6 (22) | 56 ± 4 (15) | 90 |
| Frontal cortex | 35 ± 6 (26) | 32 ± 7 (9) | 91 |
| DOPAC | | | |
| Temporal cortex | 3.03 ± 0.67 (17) | 1.04 ± 0.16 (10) | 34 |
| Frontal cortex | 1.54 ± 0.47 (17) | 0.61 ± 0.09 (4) | 40 |
| HVA/DA | | | |
| Temporal cortex | 7.8 ± 2.2 (14) | 40.9 ± 29.1 (11) | 524 |
| *NE neurons (temporal cortex)* | | | |
| NE | 1.77 ± 0.36 (17) | 0.57 ± 0.21 (11) | 32[a] |
| MHPG | 0.54 ± 0.10 (11) | 0.53 ± 0.08 (8) | 102 |
| MHPG/NE | 0.6 ± 0.3 (9) | 10.2 ± 0.67 (8) | 1,700[a] |
| [$^3$H]Ne uptake (per minute) | | | |
| Total | 0.55 ± 0.07 (10) | 0.26 ± 0.08 (12) | 47[a] |
| DMI-dependent | 0.28 ± 0.08 (7) | 0.13 ± 0.04 (9) | 46[b] |
| *Cholinergic neurons* | | | |
| ChAT activity (per minute) | | | |
| Temporal cortex | 91 ± 8 (12) | 32 ± 3 (12) | 35[c] |
| Frontal cortex | 103 ± 11 (20) | 37 ± 4 (17) | 36[a] |

Values are the mean ± SEM. Numbers of subjects are in parentheses. Results are expressed in picomole per milligram of homogenate or prism protein.
[a]$p < 0.01$.
[b]$p < 0.06$ (trend).
[c]$p < 0.001$ compared with controls.
After Palmer et al. (35).

in noradrenergic function. (Similar threshold effects could also account for the lack of any relation between the histopathological measures of cortical damage and the loss of noradrenergic markers.) The alternative explanation is that noradrenergic denervation is not a clinically critical change in AD, possibly because of compensatory mechanisms. For example, the sprouting of new noradrenergic varicosities in response to denervation has been demonstrated in the adult rat (8), and there is evidence for similar neuronal plasticity of hippocampal cholinergic circuits in AD (18). Alterations in monoamine metabolite/transmitter ratios have previously been used to index changes in transmitter turnover in Parkinson disease, so the elevation in the MHPG/NE

TABLE 3. *Summary of neurochemical findings for corticopetal and somatostatinergic neurons assessed antemortem in Alzheimer disease*

| | | | Correlations of neuron type with | | |
| Neuron type | Evidence of severe loss | Increased transmitter turnover | "Cortical perikaryal disorder" | Plaque formation | Dementia score |
| --- | --- | --- | --- | --- | --- |
| Cholinergic | + | − | + | + | + |
| Dopaminergic | − | − | + | − | − |
| Noradrenergic | + | + | − | − | − |
| Serotonergic | + | + | + | − | − |
| Somatostatinergic | − | − | − | − | − |

Tangle formation and reduced pyramidal neuron density are measures that Neary et al. (33) considered reflect a "cortical perikaryal disorder" in AD.

( + ) presence. ( − ) absence.

After refs. 15, 33–35.

ratio in AD (Table 2, which confirms postmortem data) (38) may reflect increased activity of remaining neurons. Moreover, Raskind et al. (46) found that the concentration of MHPG is CSF from severely affected AD patients was higher than that of controls, suggesting that NE turnover may increase as the disease progresses. Such a change, which probably also occurs in serotonergic neurons (38), could obscure the functional consequences of the loss of some corticopetal innervation.

## CONCLUSIONS

In AD, markers of excitatory dicarboxylic amino acid-releasing nerve endings are reduced in only our autopsy series. Glutamic acid concentration of the florid AD patients in the region examined (temporal cortex) is low in comparison with most other specimens (A. W. Procter et al., *unpublished results*). Similar samples show no gross loss of $5\text{-HT}_{1A}$ recognition sites, and glutamate release from neurosurgical samples is not altered. Perhaps the simplest interpretation is that the autopsy marker of these nerve endings is particularly sensitive to postmortem changes in Alzheimer tissue (e.g., uptake may be altered secondary to a spuriously low glutamate content). Glutamate release and glucose oxidation by the tissue prisms of the AD patients correlates, so it has been argued (2) that glutamate release reflects altered energy metabolism rather than the density of nerve endings.

SLIR and GABA concentrations are consistently reduced only in severely affected regions (e.g., temporal cortex) at the end of the disease. When these and other markers are assayed in tissue obtained by cerebral biopsy of patients at an earlier stage of the disease no such loss is observed. Thus cholinergic and serotonergic cells (Table 1), but not these two types of cortical interneuron, seem to degenerate early in the disease. By analogy, the data for excitatory dicarboxylic amino acid-releasing nerve endings in prompt autopsies may indicate a loss of these structures only in the late stage of the disease.

A preliminary estimate made of the synapses in the neurosurgical specimens suggests that the density is reduced by some 30% (11) in the samples assayed for release. The overall density of the nerve endings of the major corticopetal fibers affected in AD probably account for no more than 10% of all cortical nerve endings (3). Thus if excitatory dicarboxylic amino acid-releasing nerve endings are intact, the neurotransmitter associated with the remaining lost terminals is still to be identified. Glutaminase immunoreactivity seems to mark all neurons considered to use excitatory dicarboxylic amino acids as neurotransmitter, with the exception of some supragranular pyramidal neurons (14). Neurotransmitter candidates for these cells and excitatory cortical interneurons (23) are unknown, but 2-amino-4-sulfobutanoic acid is one of a group of compounds (13) that have some characteristics of such neurotransmitters.

Our neurochemical studies of AD show evidence for denervation of noradrenergic tracks (as well as loss of cholinergic and serotonergic fibers) with sparing of GABAergic, somatostatinergic, and dopaminergic markers. From postmortem data it was concluded that, of the changes in corticopetal neurons, cholinergic denervation was most closely related to the clinical course of AD. The summary of results in Table 3 is in agreement with this conclusion, as markers of only cholinergic denervation significantly correlated with the overall degree of cognitive impairment and reduced cortical cholinergic activity may even precede cortical damage (17). Only a small proportion of demented patients are nursed in hospital. The need for institutional care itself appears to be determined not by cognitive impairment but, rather, by other symptoms such as aggression (19) and depression (J. E. B. Lindesay, *unpublished results*). The amelioration of such symptoms will thus have important social and economic consequences. There is experimental evidence that some of these behaviors are mediated by alterations in 5-HT metabolism (reviewed in ref. 31).

## REFERENCES

1. Arai, H., Kosaka, K., and Iizuka, R. (1984): Changes of biogenic amines and their metabolites in postmortem brains from patients with Alzheimer-type dementia. *J. Neurochem.*, 43:388–393.
2. Bowen, D. M., and Davison, A. N. (1986): Biochemical studies of nerve cells and energy metabolism in Alzheimer's disease. *Br. Med. Bull.*, 42:75–80.
3. Bowen, D. M., Allen, S. J., Benton, J. S., Goodhardt, M. J., Haan, E. A., Palmer, A. M., Sims, N. R., Smith, C. C. T., Spillane, J. A., Esiri, M. M., Snowden, J. S., Wilcock, G. K., and Davison, A. N. (1983): Biochemical assessment of serotonergic and cholinergic dysfunction and cerebral atrophy in Alzheimer's disease. *J. Neurochem.*, 41:266–272.
4. Bowen, D. M., Sims, N. R., Lee, K. A. D., and Marek, K. L. (1982): Acetylcholine synthesis and glucose oxidation are preserved in human brain obtained shortly after death. *Neurosci. Lett.*, 31:195–199.

5. Colino, A., and Halliwell, J. V. (1986): 8-OH-DPAT is a strong antagonist of 5-HT action in rat hippocampus. *Eur. J. Pharmacol.*, 130:151–153.
6. Cross, A. J., Crow, T. J., Ferrier, I. N., and Johnson, J. A. (1986): The selectivity of the reduction of serotonin S2 receptors in Alzheimer-type dementia. *Neurobiol. Aging*, 7:3–8.
7. Cross, A. J., Crow, T. J., Johnson, J. A., Joseph, M. H., Perry, E. K., Perry, R. H., Blessed, G., and Tomlinson, B. E. (1983): Monoamine metabolism in senile dementia of Alzheimer type. *J. Neurol. Sci.*, 60:383–392.
8. Crutcher, K. A., Brothers, L., and Davis, J. N. (1981): Sympathetic noradrenegric sprouting in response to central cholinergic denervation: a histochemical study of neuronal sprouting in the rat hippocampal formation. *Brain Res.*, 210:115–128.
9. Curcio, C. A., and Kemper, T. (1984): Nucleus raphe dorsalis in dementia of the Alzheimer type: neurofibrillary changes and neuronal packing density. *J. Neuropathol. Exp. Neurol.*, 43:359–368.
10. Danbolt, N. C., and Storm-Mathisen, J. (1986): Na⁺-dependent binding of D-aspartate in brain membranes is largely due to uptake into membrane-bounded saccules. *J. Neurochem.*, 47:819–824.
11. Davies, C. A., Mann, D. M. A., Sumpter, P. Q., and Yates, P. O. (1986): A quantitative morphometric analysis of the neuronal and synaptic content of the frontal and temporal cortex in patients with Alzheimer's disease. *J. Neurol. Sci. (in press).*
12. DeKosky. S., and Bass, N. H. (1985): Biochemistry of senile dementia. In: *Handbook of Neurochemistry*, edited by A. Lajtha, pp. 617–649. Plenum Press, New York.
13. Do, K. Q., Herrling, P. L., Streit, P., Turski, W. A., and Cuenod, M. (1986): In vitro release and electrophysiological effects in situ of homocysteic acid, an endogenous N-methyl-(D-aspartic acid agonist, in the mammalian striatum. *J. Neurosci.*, 6:2226–2234.
14. Donoghue, J. P., Wenthold, R. J., and Altschuler, R. A. (1985): Localization of glutaminase-like and aspartate aminotransferase-like immunoreactivity in neurons of cerebral neocortex. *J. Neurosci.*, 5:2597–2608.
15. Francis, P. T., Bowen, D. M., Lowe, S. L., Neary, D., Mann, D. M. A., and Snowden, J. S. (1986): Somatostatin content and release measured in cerebral biopsies from demented patients. *J. Neurol. Sci. (in press).*
16. Francis, P. T., Palmer, A. M., Sims, N. R., Bowen, D. M., Davison, A. N., Esiri, M. M., Neary, D., Snowden, J. S., and Wilcock, G. K. (1985): Neurochemical studies of early-onset Alzheimer's disease: possible influence on treatment. *N. Engl. J. Med.*, 313:7–11.
17. Francis, P. T., Pearson, R. C. A., Lowe, S. L., Neal, J. W., Stephens, P. H., Powell, T. P. S., and Bowen, D. M. (1986): The dementia of Alzheimer's disease: an update. *J. Neurol. Neurosurg. Psychiatry (in press).*
18. Geddes, J. W., Monaghan, D. T., Cotman, C. W., Lott, T., Kim. R. C., and Chui, H. C. (1985): Plasticity of hippocampal circuiting in Alzheimer's disease. *Science*, 230:1179–1181.
19. Gilchrist, P. N., Rozenbilds, U. T., Martin, E., and Connolly, M. (1985): A study of 100 consecutive admissions to a psychogenetic unit. *Med. J. Aust.*, 143:236–240.
20. Gottfries, C. G., Adolfsson, R., Aquilonius, S. M., Carlsson, A., Eckernas, S-A., Nordberg, L., Oreland, L., Svennerholm, L., Wilberg, A., and Winblad, B. (1983): Biochemical changes in dementia disorders of Alzheimer type (AD/SDAT). *Neurobiol. Aging*, 4:261–271.
21. Hollander, E., Mohs, R. C., and Davis, K. L. (1986): Cholinergic approaches to the treatment of Alzheimer's disease. *Br. Med. Bull.*, 42:97–100.
22. Iversen, L. L., Rosser, M. N., Reynolds, G. P., Hills, R., Roth, M., Mountjoy, C. Q., Foote, J. H., Morrison, J. H., and Bloom, F. E. (1984): Loss of pigmented dopamine-beta-hydroxlase positive cells from locus coeruleus in senile dementia of Alzheimer's type. *Neurosci. Lett.*, 39:95–100.
23. Jones, E. G. (1986): Neurotransmitters in the cerebral cortex. *J. Neurosurg.*, 65:135–153.
24. Kitt, C. A., Struble, R. G., Cork, L. C., Mobley, W. C., Walker, L. C., Joh, T., and Price, D. C. (1986): Catecholaminergic neurites in senile plaques in pre-frontal cortex of aged nonhuman primates. *Neuroscience*, 16:691–699.
25. Mair, R. G., McEntee, W. J., and Zatorre, R. J. (1985): Monoamine activity correlates with psychometric deficits in Korsakoff's disease. *Behav. Brain Res.*, 15:247–254.
26. Mann, D. M. A., and Yates, P. O. (1983): Serotonergic nerve cells in Alzheimer's disease. *J. Neurol. Neurosurg. Psychiatry*, 46:96.
27. Mann, D. M. A., Yates, P. O., and Marcyniuk, B. (1984): Alzheimer's presenile dementia,

senile dementia of Alzheimer's type and Down's syndrome in middle age have an age related continuum of pathological changes. *Neuropathol. Appl. Neurobiol.,* 10:185–207.

28. Mann, D. M. A., Yates, P. O., and Marcyniuk, B. (1986): Dopaminergic neurotransmitter systems in Alzheimer's disease and in Down's syndrome at middle age. *J. Neurol. Neurosurg. Psychiatry (in press).*

29. Marcyniuk, B., Mann, D. M. A., and Yates, P. O. (1986): Loss of nerve cells from the locus coeruleus in Alzheimer's disease is topographically arranged. *Neurosci. Lett.,* 64:247–252.

30. Mash, D. C., Flynn, D. D., and Porter, L. T. (1985): Loss of M2 muscarine receptors in the cerebral cortex in Alzheimer's disease and experimental cholinergic denervation. *Science,* 228:1115–1117.

31. Middlemiss, D. N., Bowen, D. M., and Palmer, A. M. (1986): Serotonin neurones and receptors in Alzheimer's disease. In: *New Concepts in Alzheimer's Disease,* edited by M. Briley, A. Kato, and M. Weber. Macmillan, London *(in press).*

32. Middlemiss, D. N., Palmer, A. M., Edel, N., and Bowen, D. M. (1986): Binding of the novel serotonin agonist 8-hydroxy-2-(di-n-propylamino) tetralin in normal and Alzheimer brain. *J. Neurochem.,* 46:993–996.

33. Neary, D., Snowden, J. S., Mann, D. M. A., Bowen, D. M., Sims, N. R., Northern, B., Yates, P. O., and Davison, A. N. (1986): Alzheimer's disease: a correlative study. *J. Neurol. Neurosurg. Psychiatry,* 49:229–237.

34. Palmer, A. M., Francis, P. T., Benton, J. S., Sims, N. R., Mann, D. M. A., Neary, D., Snowden, J. S., and Bowen, D. M. (1986): Presynaptic serotonergic dysfunction in patients with Alzheimer's disease. *J. Neurochem. (in press).*

35. Palmer, A. M., Francis, P. T., Bowen, D. M., Benton, J. S., Neary, D., Mann, D. M. A., and Snowden, J. S. (1986): Catecholaminergic neurones assessed ante-mortem in Alzheimer's disease. *Brain Res. (in press).*

36. Palmer, A. M., Procter, A. W., Stratmann, G., and Bowen, D. M. (1986): Excitatory amino acid-releasing and cholinergic neurons in Alzheimer's disease. *Neurosci. Lett.,* 66:199–204.

37. Palmer, A. M., Sims, N. R., Bowen, D. M., Neary, D., Palo, J., Wikstrom, J., and Davison, A. N. (1984): Monoamine metabolite concentrations in lumbar cerebrospinal fluid of patients with histologically verified Alzheimer's dementia. *J. Neurol. Neurosurg. Psychiatry,* 47:481–484.

38. Palmer, A. M., Wilcock, G. K., Esiri, M. M. Francis, P. T., and Bowen, D. M. (1986): Monoaminergic innervation of the frontal and temporal lobe in Alzheimer's disease. *Brain Res. (in press).*

39. Pearson, R. C. A., Esiri, M. M., Hiorns, R. W., Wilcock, G. K., and Powell, T. P. S. (1985): Anatomical correlates of the distribution of the pathological changes in the neocortex in Alzheimer's disease. *Proc. Natl. Acad. Sci. USA,* 82:4531–4534.

40. Perry, E. K., Tomlinson, B. E., Blessed, Y., Bergmann, K., Gibson, P. H., and Perry, R. H. (1978): Correlation of cholinergic abnormalities with senile plaques and mental test scores in senile dementia. *Br. Med. J.,* 2:1457–1459.

41. Perry, E. K., Tomlinson, B. E., Blessed, G., Perry, R. H., Cross, A. J., and Crow, T. J. (1981): Neuropathological and biochemical observations on the noradrenergic system in Alzheimer's disease. *J. Neurol. Sci.,* 51:279–287.

42. Perry, R. H. (1986): Recent advances in neuropathology. *Br. Med. Bull.,* 42:34–41.

43. Price, D. L. (1986): New perspectives on Alzheimer's disease. *Annu. Rev. Neurosci.,* 9:489–512.

44. Procter, A. W., Palmer, A. M., Bowen, D. M., Murphy, E., and Neary, D. (1987): Glutamatergic denervation in Alzheimer's disease—a cautionary note. *J. Neurol. Neurosurg. Psychiatry (in press).*

45. Procter, A. W., Palmer, A. M., Stratmann, G. C., and Bowen, D. M. (1986): Glutamate/aspartate-releasing neurons in Alzheimer's disease. *N. Engl. J. Med.,* 314:1711.

46. Raskind, M. A., Peskind, E. R., Halter, J. B., and Jimerson, D. C. (1984): Norepinephrine and MHPG levels in CSF and plasma in Alzheimer's disease. *Arch. Gen. Psychiatry,* 41:343–346.

47. Robbins, T. W., Everitt, B. J., Cole, B. J., Archer, T., and Mohammed, A. (1985): Functional hypotheses of the coeruleocortical noradrenergic projection: a review of recent experimentation and theory. *Physiol. Psychol.,* 13:127–150.

48. Rossor, M. N., Garrett, N. J., Johnson, A. L., Mountjoy, C. Q., Roth, M., and Iversen,

L. L. (1982): A post-mortem study of the cholinergic and GABA systems in senile dementia. *Brain*, 105:313–330.

49. Rylett, R. J., Ball, M. J., and Colhoun, E. H. (1983): Evidence of high affinity choline transport in synaptosomes prepared from hippocampus of patients with Alzheimer's disease. *Brain Res.*, 289:169–175.

50. Sims, N. R., Bowen, D. M., and Davison, A. N. (1981): [$^{14}$C]Acetylcholine synthesis and [$^{14}$C]carbon dioxide production from [U-$^{14}$C]glucose by tissue prisms from human neocortex. *Biochem. J.*, 196:867–876.

51. Sims, N. R., Bowen, D. M., Allen, S. J., Smith, C. C. T., Neary, D., Thomas, D. J., and Davison, A. N. (1983): Presynaptic cholinergic dysfunction in patients with dementia. *J. Neurochem.*, 40:503–509.

52. Sims, N. R., Bowen, D. M., Smith, C. C. T., Flack, R. H., Davison, A. N., Snowden, J. S., and Neary, D. (1980): Glucose metabolism acetylcholine synthesis in relation to neuronal activity in Alzheimer's disease. *Lancet*, 1:333–336.

53. Sims, N. R., Marek, K. L., Bowen, D. M., and Davison, A. N. (1982): Production of [$^{14}$C]carbon dioxide from [U-$^{14}$C]glucose in tissue prisms from ageing rat brain. *J. Neurochem.*, 38:488–492.

54. Smith, C. C. T., Bowen, D. M., Sims, N. R., Neary, D., and Davison, A. N. (1983): Amino acid release from biopsy samples of temporal neocortex from patients with Alzheimer's disease. *Brain Res.*, 264:138–141.

55. Summers, W. K., Lawrence, V. M., Marsh, G. M., Tachiki, K., and Kling, A. (1986): Oral tetrahydroaminoacridine in long-term treatment of senile dementia, Alzheimer type. *N. Engl. J. Med.*, 315:1241–1245.

56. Svenneby, G., Roberg, B., Hogstad, S., Torgner, I. A., and Kvamme, E. (1986): Phosphate-activated glutaminase in the crude mitochondrial fraction (P2 fraction) from human brain cortex. *J. Neurochem.*, 47:1351–1356.

57. Whitehouse, P. J., Martino, A. M., Antuono, P. G., Lowestein, P. R., Coyle, J. T., Price, D. L., and Kellar, K. J. (1986): Nicotinic acetylcholine binding sites in Alzheimer's disease. *Brain Res.*, 371:146–151.

*Aging and the Brain*, edited by R. D. Terry.
Raven Press, New York © 1988.

# Some Observations on the Significance of Neurotransmitter Changes in Alzheimer Disease

Joseph B. Martin, M. Flint Beal, Michael Mazurek, Neil W. Kowall, and John H. Growdon

*Neurology Service and Department of Neurology, Massachusetts General Hospital and Harvard Medical School, Boston, Massachusetts 02114*

Among the variety of experimental approaches directed toward understanding Alzheimer disease (AD), the search for abnormalities in neurotransmitter content or function has received considerable attention. The rationale behind these studies has been threefold. First, it is hoped that delineation of neurotransmitter changes in AD might lead, as it did in Parkinson disease, to the development of an effective treatment. Second, the changes might identify the selectivity or specificity of the cytopathologic events occurring in nerve cells or neuropil. Third, the events themselves might provide clues to the nature of the neurodegenerative process. To date, none of these expectations has been fulfilled. Nevertheless, the data accumulated have provided a basis for speculation about the distribution and possibly the neuronal systems involved in AD.

Radioimmunoassays and immunohistochemistry have been applied to human brain tissue obtained at either surgery or autopsy. The results have shown that neuropeptides in postmortem tissue are remarkably stable, allowing detailed anatomic study and analysis of changes in tissue concentration associated with disease. A degree of variation in tissue levels does occur so that studies must include sufficient numbers of cases to detect significant differences and to control for antemortem factors, e.g., age, sex, drug treatment, other coincident illness, and cause of death.

Studies of peptide stability in postmortem tissue have shown little correlation of peptide concentration with delay to autopsy. Substance P (19,23,24,39), somatostatin (19,23,28,39,42), cholecystokinin (CCK) (39,41,80,93) met-enkephalin (43), thyrotropin-releasing hormone (TRH) (16,79), gonadotropin-releasing hormone (GnRH) (79), neurotensin (16,19,23,67), vasoactive intestinal polypeptide (VIP) (80), and neuropeptide Y (NPY) (2,12) have all been shown to be stable in human brain by this criterion. Even more convincing evidence of postmortem stability of neuropeptides has come from animal experiments where rodent brains are cooled at a rate simulating human autopsy conditions (104). Substance P (35), somatostatin (27,37,42,64), CCK (93), VIP (36), met-enkephalin (35), and NPY (15) have all been shown to be stable in animal brains for at least 24 hr and in some studies for as long as 72 hr postmortem. Prolonged agonal status also has no effect on postmortem concentrations of VIP, somatostatin, CCK, and neurotensin (81).

Biochemical separation methods to define peptide degradation products have generally also given evidence for stability. Immunoreactive substance P (8,35,68), CCK (80,93), VIP (36), NPY (2,12), met-enkephalin (35), and neurotensin (67) in extracts of human brain have all been shown to migrate as single chromatographic peaks. In the case of somatostatin, where higher-molecular-weight forms of immunoreactive material can generally be found in extracts of postmortem brain, the substances separated closely resemble precursor forms known to be present in extracts from animal brains.

Immunocytochemical techniques applied to human postmortem brain tissue and use of multiple labeling techniques, i.e., antibodies to anti-peroxidase or to fluorescence-labeled probes, has permitted double labeling experiments to examine for co-localization of two or more peptides or of peptides with other neurotransmitters or cellular markers (49,54,56,60,96). With use of such techniques it has been possible to examine the relation of neuropeptides to pathologic processes such as senile plaques (6,7,29,105,106) and cells with neurofibrillary tangles.

## NEUROCHEMICAL ANATOMY OF THE CEREBRAL CORTEX

Neurons of the cerebral cortex can be divided into two general categories: *intrinsic* (local circuit) *neurons* and *projection neurons*. Intrinsic neurons are characterized by their multipolar, bipolar, or stellate shape and have axons that arborize within a local region of cortex. It has been suggested that up to 40% of these intrinsic neurons utilize γ-aminobutyric acid (GABA) as a transmitter (82), whereas others use a variety of neuropeptides. Projection neurons have a pyramidal-shaped cell body with an apical dendrite projecting toward the cortical surface. The pyramidal neurons in the outer cortical layers (II–III) are thought to be involved in corticocortical connections, and those in deeper layers project to the striatum, thalamus, brainstem, and spinal cord. On the basis of lesion and uptake experiments it has been proposed that pyramidal neurons utilize glutamate or aspartate as their neurotransmitters (31). Many of the currently known neuropeptides are found in intrinsic neurons of the cerebral cortex in higher primates and man (21,60,74,102). VIP, somatostatin, CCK, NPY, corticotropin-releasing factor (CRF), substance P, and dynorphin have each been demonstrated in intrinsic cortical neurons and fiber plexuses (34,48,50,54).

## NEUROTRANSMITTER ALTERATIONS IN AD

### Acetylcholine, Norepinephrine, Serotonin

Most of the acetylcholine in cortex is present in the synaptic terminals of neurons originating in the basal nucleus of Meynert. Similarly, virtually all of the norepinephrine and serotonin found in cortex appears to derive from cell bodies in the locus ceruleus and dorsal raphe nuclei, respectively. Each of these subcortical neurotransmitter systems is pathologically affected in AD. Cholinergic efferents originating in the basal nucleus of Meynert are severely depleted in AD (18,32). Abnormalities of cortical norepinephrine and serotonin, reflecting neuronal degeneration in locus ceruleus and the dorsal raphe nucleus, respectively, have also been described (1,18,25,112,116).

### Neuropeptides

In contrast to the cholinergic, noradrenergic, and serotonergic systems, which project to cortex form subcortical cell bodies, virtually all of the neuropeptides present in cerebral cortex are found in intrinsic neurons with small (8–10 μm) diameter perikarya concentrated in layers II/III and VI and subjacent white matter (54) (Fig. 1). These peptidergic neurons give rise to vertically oriented processes that form distinct plexuses in layers I/II and layer VI. All peptidergic neurons found in cortex appear to be morphologically similar (54). No peptide immunoreactivity has been detected in other neuronal populations, e.g., pyramidal cells, basket cells, or chandelier cells. Of the peptides thus far identified in cortex, somatostatin, NPY, CCK, and VIP have the highest concentrations, each being observed in roughly 2 to 3% of the neurons present. Somatostatin and NPY appear to be co-localized in almost all cells examined. Furthermore, most of these somatostatin/NPY cells, as well as all CCK neurons, also contain GABA. Somatostatin/NPY cells terminate on the small peripheral dendrites of pyramidal neurons, and CCK- and VIP-immunoreactive terminals synapse on pyramidal cell somata. Neurons staining for substance P, dynorphin, met-enkephalin, or CRF are also found in cortex but are considerably fewer in number than those containing somatostatin/NPY, CCK, or VIP. Neither vasopressin nor oxytocin has been detected in intrinsic cortical neurons.

Because GABA is found in a high percentage of cortical neurons, it is interesting to consider whether all GABA-containing neurons also contain neuropeptides. Evidence suggests that most of the eight or nine morphologic types of cortical intrinsic neurons are GABAergic, *but that only one class, described above, contains neuropeptides* (46,47,51). The GABA-containing basket cells, which are much larger than the peptidergic neurons, have not, to

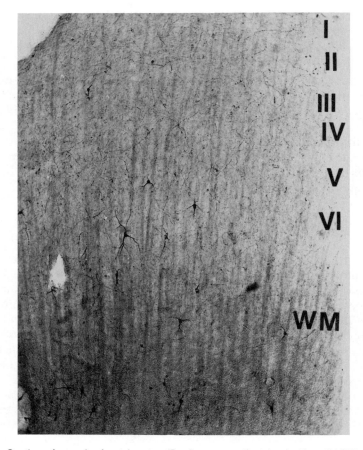

**FIG. 1.** Section of superior frontal cortex (Brodman area 8) stained with anti-NPY antiserum using an avidin-bioten immunoperoxidase procedure. A few immunoreactive neurons are seen in layers II/III. Most are found in layers V/VI and the subcortical plate region. *WM* = white matter. Original magnification ×40.

date, shown any immunoreactivity to the known neuropeptides found in cortex (46,51). Certain of the same peptidergic cell types also contain acetylcholine (33). It can be concluded that data obtained to date suggest that all neuropeptides in primate cortex co-localize with either GABA or acetylcholine. On the other hand, morphologic evidence suggests that neuropeptides do not co-localize with the excitatory neurotransmitters glutamate and aspartate, as these neurotransmitters are thought to be localized in pyramidal neurons of layers II, III, V, and VI (31).

## Neuropeptide Alterations in Cerebral Cortex in AD

### Somatostatin and neuropeptide Y

The most consistent peptidergic abnormality described in AD is a loss of somatostatin in cerebral cortex. Davies et al. (28) first reported reduced cortical somatostatin in AD in 1980. They subsequently demonstrated significant reductions of somatostatin in all cortical areas examined except the anterior cingulate cortex (26). The decreases in somatostatin were much greater in younger (age 66 or less) than older patients. Several other laboratories have confirmed the somatostatin loss in AD, with differing degrees of peptide reduction being found. Rossor et al. first reported a reduction in somatostatin only in the temporal cortex, but subsequent observations demonstrated that younger patients (under age 79) had more widespread decreases of greater magnitude (89,92). Nemeroff et al. (76) found reductions in both cortical and subcortical somatostatin in AD. Ferrier et al. (39) found reduced somatostatin levels in temporal, frontal, and parietal cortex as well as septum, but other subcortical regions including both nucleus accumbens and amygdala were not affected. Interestingly, they reported significantly *increased* concentrations in the substantia innominata. This finding, however, was not confirmed in the study of Arai et al. (5), where significant reductions of somatostatin were found in orbital cortex, hippocampus, and putamen with no change in substantia innominata. We have found a widespread reduction of somatostatin in virtually all cortical regions examined (11) (Fig. 2). The most profound changes are found in the temporal lobe, but there are also major reductions in

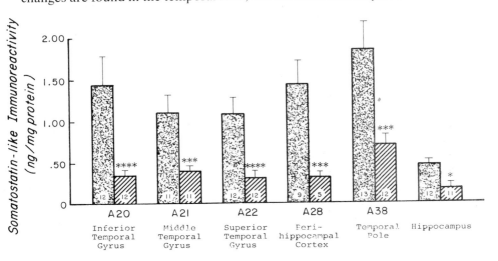

**FIG. 2.** Somatostatin concentrations in control (*left column*) and AD (*right column*) samples from temporal lobe and hippocampus. *$p < 0.05$. ***$p < 0.005$. ****$p < 0.001$.

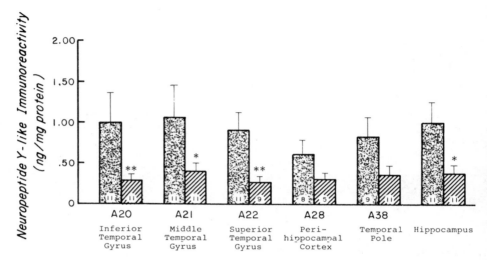

**FIG. 3.** Neuropeptide Y concentrations in control (*left column*) and AD (*right column*) samples from temporal lobe and hippocampus. $*p < 0.05$. $**p < 0.025$.

both frontal and occipital cortex and in hippocampus. We find no changes in somatostatin in subcortical regions, including the amygdala and substantia innominata.

Because somatostatin and NPY are at least 80% co-localized in both monkey and human cortical neurons, it would be expected that parallel losses of both somatostatin and NPY would occur if these neurons or their terminals degenerate in AD. We measured concentrations of NPY in AD cerebral cortex and found widespread reductions that correlate closely with reductions of somatostatin (12) (Fig. 3). The discrepancy with the earlier report (2) may reflect differences in the ages of the patients, the patients studied previously being older than those in our study.

Several possibilities may account for changes in concentrations of these neuropeptides. Altered degradation or processing, increased release with insufficient synthesis, transsynaptic effects due to alteration of other neurotransmitters, or selective neuronal degeneration could account for the observations. The finding of reduced levels of somatostatin in cerebrospinal fluid (CSF) argues against increased release, as CSF somatostatin concentrations are remarkably stable (14). The acetylcholine deficit in AD probably does not account for the somatostatin reductions, as lesions in rats that reduce hippocampal choline acetyltransferase activity have no effect on hippocampal somatostatin (72). Nor do reductions in somatostatin appear to be a consequence of altered degradation or processing, as chromatographic profiles in AD and control frontal cortex are identical (11). In addition, we have measured concentrations of somatostatin 28 (1–12) in AD and have found reductions that are highly correlated with those of somatostatin (9). The similar reductions in two molecular weight species of somatostatin argues against altered degradation or processing as an etiology.

The most parsimonious explanation of the findings is that there is extensive degeneration of somatostatin/NPY neurons in AD cerebral cortex. Several immunocytochemical studies have provided evidence to corroborate this concept. One study showed somatostatin-staining neurons to be shrunken and irregularly shaped in AD cortex compared with age-matched controls (57). In another, cortical somatostatin perikarya exhibited morphologic changes that were interpreted as being consistent with neuronal degeneration, and some were shown to contain tangles (86). In a third study, swollen bulbous profiles and beaded processes were interpreted as representing degenerating somatostatin neurons (73). Similar dystrophic changes have been reported for NPY neurons (20), and we have observed similar changes in our own material (62).

We have found that somatostatin receptors are also reduced in AD cerebral cortex (13) (Fig. 4). The loss of receptors correlates with reductions of somatostatin. The localization of these receptors is unknown, but it is possible that the loss of receptors results from transneuronal degenerative changes in somatostatin neurons or terminals.

*CRF, VIP, CCK*

Corticotropin-releasing factor is also localized in a smaller number of cortical neurons, and concentrations of this neuropeptide have been found to be reduced in AD cerebral cortex (17). In contrast to our findings with

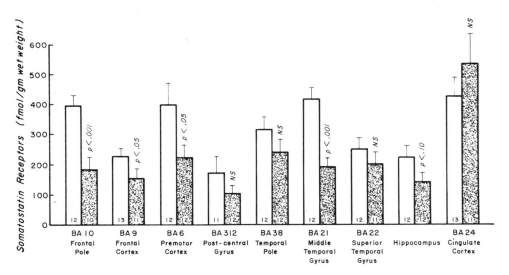

**FIG. 4.** Somatostatin receptor concentrations in control (*left column*) and AD (*right column*) samples. The levels of significance using the Mann-Whitney U test are shown.

somatostatin, receptors for CRF were increased in AD cerebral cortex (17). The authors suggested that loss of CRF and synaptic sites may result in "up-regulation" of CRF receptors. Why this difference occurs between somatostatin and CRF receptors remains unexplained. In contrast, neither VIP nor CCK concentrations are altered in AD cerebral cortex (39,82,93), although in one study aqueous extracted CCK was decreased in severe cases (82). CCK receptors are also normal in AD cortex (45). Because VIP and CCK are contained in cortical neurons showing morphologic features similar to those of somatostatin, NPY, and CRF, their preservation indicates a degree of selectivity of the degenerative process. Met-enkephalin concentrations are also unaltered in AD cerebral cortex (88). Three studies have found no alterations in neurotensin concentrations in AD (39,76,117). Neurotensin had been thought to be present in nerve terminals in cerebral cortex, but immunohistochemical studies have shown its presence in small numbers of cortical neurons as well. There is a large number of neurotensin neurons in the subiculum of the hippocampus (95). Because prominent pathologic findings are frequently found in the subiculum in AD, it would be useful to examine neurotensin concentrations in this region.

### Hypothalamic hypophysiotropic peptides

The hypothalamic hypophysiotropic neuropeptides are localized for the most part within neuronal perikarya confined in the hypothalamus with terminals projecting to other regions. Concentrations of both TRH (16,76,118) and GnRH (118) are unaltered in AD. Vasopressin is of particular interest in AD because of its putative role in memory functions (30). In an initial study reduced concentrations were found in the globus pallidus and locus ceruleus; however, many brain regions could not be measured owing to inadequate assay sensitivity (91). We have examined concentrations of vasopressin in AD and have found reduced concentrations in the globus pallidus, nucleus accumbens, and hippocampus (70). Concentrations were increased in cerebral cortex, presumably reflecting tissue atrophy with preserved vasopressin terminals. In contrast to the reduced vasopressin concentrations in hippocampus, concentrations of oxytocin were significantly increased in the hippocampus (70). Because oxytocin has been hypothesized to inhibit memory consolidation and vasopressin to enhance memory, it is conceivable that the above-mentioned alterations might play a role in the memory deficits of AD. Morphometric studies have shown a loss of vasopressin neurons in the suprachiasmatic nucleus in AD but no change in supraoptic and paraventricular oxytocin and vasopressin neurons (40,109).

### Relation of Neuropeptides to Amino Acid Neurotransmitters

Another issue with regard to neuropeptide deficits in AD is their relation to those of amino acid neurotransmitters. It has been estimated that GABA accounts for as many as 40% of all cortical synapses (52), and GABA is co-localized with somatostatin, NPY, and CCK in cortical neurons (50,96,101). GABA content was found to be reduced in AD cerebral cortex by Rossor et al. particularly in younger patients (90,92). We have confirmed this finding and have documented a widespread 30 to 40% reduction in cortical GABA content, with the most marked reductions being found in temporal cortex (33a). It is possible therefore that reduced somatostatin and NPY in AD reflect loss of a subpopulation of GABAergic neurons.

## HISTOCHEMICAL STUDIES OF PEPTIDERGIC NEURONS IN AD

Histochemical methods can be used to study the relation of biochemical changes to the classic neuropathologic alterations associated with AD: the senile plaque and neurofibrillary tangle (NFT). Typically well-defined senile plaques contain aggregates of distorted neuronal processes, termed neurites, that surround a core of amyloid. Both local circuit neurons and subcortical input fibers contribute to senile plaque formation. A number of neurotransmitters have been localized to individual neurites within senile plaques in cortex. Among the peptidergic fibers identified in senile plaques are somatostatin (63,73), NPY (20,63), substance P (6,29), VIP, CCK, neurotensin, bombesin, leu-enkephalin (106), melanoctye-stimulating hormone (MSH), ACTH (85), and CRF (83). Every neurotransmitter histochemically identified within neuronal processes in human brain to date has been found in senile plaque neurites irrespective of their quantitative depletion in AD cortex. For example, somatostatin (11,26,28) and CRF (17) are greatly depleted in AD cortex, whereas neurotensin (16,117,118) and CCK (93) peptides are mildly depleted if at all; yet both are found in senile plaques. This fact suggests that senile plaques indiscriminately incorporate fibers surrounding them as they develop. Before this conclusion can be reached, however, further quantitative studies of neurotransmitter-specific plaque distribution must be performed. In one study (7) somatostatin neurites were identified in up to 50% of plaques, depending on the region of cortex studied. It is not known what proportion of senile plaques contain other peptidergic fibers. If other peptides are rarely found in plaques, their concentrations in cortex may not be reduced. Thus it may be premature to assume that senile plaque formation is necessarily accompanied by depletion of peptide concentrations. At present no single neurotransmitter specific fiber type has been found in individual senile plaques. It is not known if senile plaques are sometimes associated with a particular subset of neurons.

Cortical NFTs are mainly found in layers III and V projection neurons, which are thought to use glutamate or aspartate as a neurotransmitter. Roberts et al. (86) examined human hippocampal cortex using silver staining to detect NFTs followed by immunoperoxidase staining for somatostatin and found that somatostatin neurons contain NFTs. We have examined sections of temporal neocortex with double immunofluorescence methods to detect tangles and somatostatin or NPY simultaneously (62). Despite the widespread occurrence of morphologic abnormalities in somatostatin/NPY neurons, tangles were not found in any of these neurons (62). This finding suggests that not all neurons affected by AD form NFTs as they degenerate. Further studies delineating the neurotransmitter content of NFT-bearing neurons are required to clarify these conflicting findings.

Several groups have discovered that the microtubule-associated protein tau is an important component of the paired helical filaments (58a,111) found in NFTs (44,59,114,115). We have found that the normal axonal distribution of tau in human brain is dramatically altered in AD (61). Aside from its localization in NFTs and the neuritic portion of senile plaques, myriad tau immunoreactive short curly fibers are found coursing randomly throughout the cortex. This finding suggests that the cytoskeletal disruption found in AD is more widespread than previously thought. Attempts to correlate behavioral and quantitative neurochemical changes with senile plaques or NFTs may therefore be overly simplistic because these phenomena represent only the most severe pathologic alteration.

## NEUROPEPTIDES IN CSF

Measurement of neuropeptide concentrations in Alzheimer CSF offers a number of potential advantages over the study of tissue levels in postmortem brain. First, the serial measurement of CSF transmitters may permit the biochemical charting of disease progression. A second, potential advantage is the opportunity to correlate neurochemical data with clinical and radiologic information and with specific drug regimens. Third, the investigation of CSF chemistry has the potential of providing a diagnostic marker, or at least a diagnostic profile, of AD. It would not only assist in the selection of patients for experimental protocols but might also enable AD patients to be reliably distinguished from those who have other forms of dementia, in which the treatment program would perhaps be quite different.

These potential advantages notwithstanding, there are limitations to CSF studies. The usefulness of CSF neuropeptide concentrations in AD depends on the assumption that these levels reflect the functional release of those peptides from brain. A reasonable case can be made that CSF peptides largely derive from the CNS, as they appear stable in CSF (10,53) and the blood–brain barrier insulates CSF peptide concentrations from all but the largest fluctuations in plasma levels (4,22,55). There is less evidence concerning exactly which regions of the central nervous system contribute to CSF peptide levels. Even when information is available concerning rostral-caudal gradients, it is not always clear what proportion of the material measured in lumbar CSF originates in brain, as opposed to spinal cord. Furthermore, CSF levels

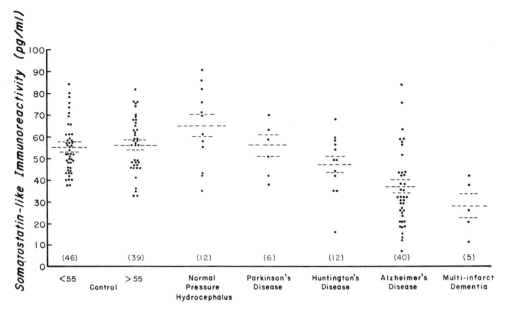

**FIG. 5.** Somatostatin concentrations in CSF for a variety of dementing neurologic illnesses. Mean concentrations in both AD and multi-infarct dementia are significantly reduced from those of controls ($p < 0.05$).

of some peptides may undergo diurnal variations (3,22). These caveats should be kept in mind when interpreting studies of neurotransmitter concentrations in CSF.

## CSF Peptides in AD

The most clearly established peptide abnormalities in Alzheimer CSF are decreased levels of somatostatin (13,100,115) (Fig. 5) and vasopressin (71,84,103,108) (Fig. 6). There is evidence that the CSF concentrations of somatostatin reflect, at least to some extent, release of the peptide in neocortex (10). It is therefore not particularly surprising, given the marked reductions of somatostatin found in AD cortex, that somatostatin levels should be decreased in the CSF in AD. The origin of vasopressin in CSF, by contrast, is unlikely to be neocortex, as levels there are very low. Rather, studies indicate that CSF vasopressin derives at least partially from the suprachiasmatic nuclei of the hypothalamus (97). In light of the reduced CSF vasopressin levels found in AD, it is of interest that 50% decreases in the volume and number of vasopressin cell bodies in the suprachiasmatic nucleus, but not the supraoptic or paraventricular nuclei, have been observed in AD brain (40,109).

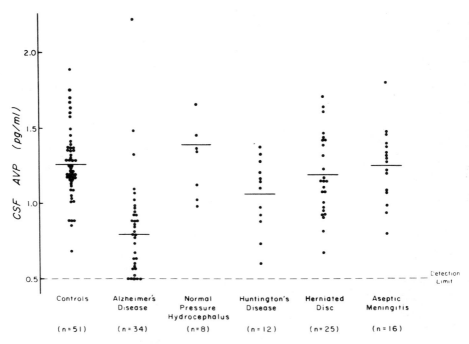

**FIG. 6.** Vasopressin concentrations in CSF in controls, AD, and other neurologic illness. Concentrations for AD patients were significantly ($p < 0.05$) reduced from those of controls.

The findings of reduced somatostatin and vasopressin levels in Alzheimer CSF should not be taken to mean the measurement of these peptides provides a reliable guide to diagnosing the disease in individual cases. As shown in Figs. 5 and 6, there is overlap between values in the AD group and those of controls. Furthermore, the CSF changes are not specific to AD, somatostatin being reportedly decreased in multi-infarct dementia (14) and depression (94) and vasopressin being reduced in Korsakoff psychosis (65). A more promising approach to diagnosing individual cases of AD may be to use CSF somatostatin and vasopressin determinations in conjunction with other neurotransmitter markers, with the aim of developing a comprehensive neurochemical profile of the disease. VIP and β-lipotropin appear to be normal in Alzheimer CSF (98,107,113) and concentrations of β-endorphin and CRF are reported to be either normal or decreased (38,58,69,77,84,107).

One of the most important potential applications of CSF neuropeptide measurement may be in the differentiation of normal-pressure hydrocephalus from AD; the former often responds to ventricular shunting whereas AD does not. The data from several studies indicate that, unlike AD, normal-pressure hydrocephalus is associated with normal levels of CSF somatostatin and vasopressin (13,71,103) (Figs. 5 and 6). These findings raise the possibility that very low CSF somatostatin and vasopressin levels might serve as a means of identifying patients who are unlikely to benefit from ventricular shunting.

## IMPLICATIONS OF NEUROPEPTIDE ALTERATIONS IN AD

Several questions remain unresolved concerning neuropeptides and their role in the pathophysiology of neurologic illness. It is as yet unclear what relation alterations in neuropeptides have to clinical symptoms in AD and if they are associated with alterations in the functional activity of neurons. Several approaches to further clarification of these issues are possible. If specific pure peptide receptor agonists or antagonists can be developed that can cross the blood-brain barrier, these drugs can be used to investigate a causal relation between a given symptom or behavior and neuropeptide alterations. Currently, pure antagonists are available only for the opioid peptides.

Another approach to studying the dynamics of peptide alterations is to use molecular biology techniques. Concentrations and localization of messenger RNA can be detected in postmortem tissue either by analysis of extracted message or by *in situ* hybridization to message in tissue sections. Messenger RNA concentrations have been shown to correlate with functional activity of neurons in a variety of paradigms, and cDNA probes are available for most neuropeptides (32,66,87,99,110). Improved knowledge of the significance of neuropeptide alterations may arise from such observations in AD. Quantitative correlations with immunocytochemical findings may provide useful information.

A crucial question is whether alterations in neuropeptides give any clues to fundamental disease processes. Several hypotheses have been advanced to explain neuronal death in the degenerative neurologic diseases. They include genetically programmed cell death, loss of neuronal growth factors, the excitotoxin hypothesis, slow-virus-mediated cell death, and immunologically mediated cell death. The best characterized neuropeptide abnormality in AD disease is the apparent vulnerability of somatostatin and NPY neurons in AD cerebral cortex. If selective neuronal growth factors can be found for somatostatinergic neurons, it is possible that they might be found to be deficient in AD. Because the somatostatin gene has been localized to chromosome 3 (75), further studies of its linkage in AD could provide clues to genetic factors. In addition, detailed knowledge of neuropeptide alterations in neurologic disease can provide a background on which one may test the validity of experimental models of neurologic illness. For instance, one can examine whether scrapie infections or aluminum intoxication can reproduce the neurochemical characteristics of AD. If specific subsets of neurons are selectively spared or vulnerable in an illness, an examination of their biochemistry may provide clues to the nature of the disease process. It might then be possible to develop therapies to retard or halt the underlying degenerative process.

## SUMMARY AND CONCLUSIONS

1. There are many neurotransmitter abnormalities in AD, as documented by alterations in tissue levels, contributions of neuronal processes to senile plaques, and altered levels in the CSF. It may be most useful in future studies to define the degree of their involvement in the disease process rather than to attempt to show selective vulnerability or selective sparing. It appears likely that in the severest form of the disease all categories of cortical neurons may be affected, either by NFTs or by participating in the formation of senile plaques. Further quantitation and correlation with the stage of the disease may permit delineation of neuronal subtypes that are affected early from those that are affected late in the course of the disease.

2. It seems probable that neuronal processes of all cellular types may participate in senile plaque formation. Furthermore, individual plaques appear to contain neurites contributed from multiple neuronal types. An extension of this conclusion is that senile plaques represent a reaction to a cellular degenerative process, with random incorporation of neuronal elements into their formation.

3. Neurons that contain NFTs are predominantly, if not exclusively, of the projection type—either to other cortical regions or to subcortical nuclear structures (thalamus, basal ganglia, brainstem). To date, neuropeptides have not been conclusively found in any of these neurons, and peptide-containing neurons do not appear to be subject to formation of NFTs.

4. It seems probable that all of the characteristic cellular changes in AD, including alterations in tissue levels of neuropeptides, are secondary phenomena caused by the underlying disease process.

5. Because of the widespread extent of the cortical lesions in AD and the variety of neurotransmitter changes associated with them, it seems unlikely that a successful therapeutic strategy will evolve from the studies of these changes.

## ACKNOWLEDGMENTS

This work was supported by the Massachusetts Alzheimer's Disease Center, NIH 1P50AG05134. The authors acknowledge the valuable technical assistance of Geetinder K. Chatta, Kenton Swartz, Samantha Knowlton, and Linda Lorenz. Patricia Clougherty typed the manuscript.

## REFERENCES

1. Adolfsson, R., Gottfries, G. C., Roos, B. E., and Winblad, B. (1979): Changes in brain catecholamines in patients with dementia of Alzheimer-type. *Br. J. Psychiatry*, 135:216–223.
2. Allen, J. M., Ferrier, I. N., Roberts, G. W., et al. (1984): Elevation of neuropeptide Y (NPY) in substantia innominata in Alzheimer's type dementia. *J. Neurol. Sci.*, 64:325–331.
3. Amico, J. A., Tenicela, R., Johnston J., and Robinson, A. G. (1983): A time-dependent peak of oxytocin exists in cerebrospinal fluid but not in plasma of humans. *J. Clin. Endocrinol. Metab.*, 57:947–951.
4. Ang, V. T. Y., and Jenkins, J. S. (1982): Blood-cerebrospinal fluid barrier to arginine-vasopressin in the dog. *J. Endocrinol.*, 93:319–325.
5. Arai, H., Moroii, T., and Kosaka, K. (1984): Somatostatin and vasoactive intestinal polypeptide in postmortem brains from patients with Alzheimer-type dementia. *Neurosci. Lett.*, 52:73–78.
6. Armstrong, D. M., and Terry, R. D. (1985): Substance P immunoreactivity within neuritic plaques. *Neurosci. Lett.*, 58:139–144.
7. Armstrong, D. M., Leroy, S., Shields, D., and Terry R. D. (1985): Somatostatin-like immunoreactivity with neuritic plaques. *Brain Res.*, 338:71–79.
8. Aronin, N., Cooper, P. E., Lorenz, L. J., et al. (1983): Somatostatin is increased in the basal ganglia in Huntington's disease. *Ann. Neurol.*, 13:519–526.
9. Beal, M. F., Benoit, R., Mazurek, M. F., Bird, E. D., and Martin, J. B. (1986): Somatostatin-28 (1-12)-like immunoreactivity is reduced in Alzheimer's disease cerebral cortex. *Brain Res.*, 368:380–383.
10. Beal, M. F., Mazurek, M. F., Black, P. B., and Martin, J. B. (1985): CSF somatostatin in neurological disease. *J. Neurol. Sci.*, 71:91–104.
11. Beal, M. F., Mazurek, M. F., Chattha, G., and Martin, J. B. (1985): Somatostatin-like immunoreactivity in Alzheimer's disease. *Ann. Neurol.*, 18:144.
12. Beal, M. F., Mazurek, M. F., Chattha, G., Bird, E. D., and Martin, J. B. (1985): Neuropeptide Y immunoreactivity is reduced in Alzheimer's disease cerebral cortex. *Neurosci. Abstr.*, 11:1119.
13. Beal, M. F., Mazurek, M. F., Tran, V. T., et al. (1985): Somatostatin receptors are reduced in cerebral cortex in Alzheimer's disease. *Science*, 229:289–291.
14. Beal, M. F., Mazurek, M. F., Black, P. B., and Martin, J. B. (1985): CSF somatostatin in neurological diseases. *J. Neurol. Sci.*, 71:91–104.
15. Beal, M. F., Mazurek, M. F., Lorenz, L. J., et al. (1986): An examination of neuropeptide Y post-mortem stability in an animal model simulating human autopsy conditions. *Neurosci. Lett.*, 64:69–74.
16. Biggins, J. A., Perry, E. K., McDermott, J. R., et al. (1983): Post mortem levels of thyrotropin-releasing hormone and neurotensin in the amygdala in Alzheimer's disease, schizophrenia and depression. *J. Neurol. Sci.*, 58:117–122.
17. Bissette, G., Reynolds, G. P., Kilts, C. D., Widerlov, E., and Nemeroff, C. B. (1985): Corticotropin-releasing factor-like immunoreactivity in senile dementia of the Alzheimer type. *JAMA*, 254:3067–3069.
18. Bondareff, W., Mountjoy, C. Q., and Roth M. (1981): Selective loss of neurones of origin of adrenergic projection to cerebral cortex (nucleus locus coeruleus) in senile dementia. *Lancet*, 1:783–784.
19. Buck, S. H., Deshmukh, P., Burks, T. F., and Yamamura, H. I. (1981): A survey of substance P, somatostatin, and neurotensin levels in aging in the rat and human central nervous system. *Neurobiol. Aging*, 2:257–264.
20. Chan-Palay, V., Lang, W., Allen, Y. S., Haesler, U., and Polak, J. M. (1985): Cortical neurons immunoreactive with antisera against neuropeptide Y are altered in Alzheimer's-type dementia. *J. Comp. Neurol.*, 238:390–400.
21. Chronwall, B. M., Chase, T. N., and O'Donohue, T. L. (1984): Coexistence of neuropeptide Y and somatostatin in rat and human cortical and rat hypothalamic neurons. *Neurosci. Lett.*, 52:213–217.

22. Coleman, R. J., and Reppert, S. M. (1985): CSF vasopressin rhythm is effectively insulated from osmotic regulation of plasma vasopressin. *Am. J. Physiol.*, 248:E346–E352.
23. Cooper, P. E., Fernstrom, M. H., Rorstad, O. P., Leeman, S. E., and Martin, J. B. (1981): The regional distribution of somatostatin, substance P and neurotensin in human brain. *Brain Res.*, 218:219–232.
24. Crystal, H. A., and Davies, P. (1982): Cortical substance P-like immunoreactivity in cases of Alzheimer's disease and senile dementia of the Alzheimer type. *J. Neurochem.*, 38:1781–1784.
25. Curcio, C. A., and Kemper, T. (1984): Nucleus raphe dorsalis in dementia of the Alzheimer type: neurofibrillary changes and neuronal packing density. *J. Neuropathol. Exp. Neurol.*, 143:359–368.
26. Davies, P., and Terry, R. D. (1981): Cortical somatostatin-like immunoreactivity in cases of Alzheimer's disease and senile dementia of the Alzheimer type. *Neurobiol. Aging*, 2:9–14.
27. Davies, P., and Thompson, A. (1981): Postmortem stability of somatostatin-like immuno-reactivity in mouse brain under conditions simulating handling of human autopsy material. *Neurochem. Res.*, 6:787–791.
28. Davies, P., Katzman, R., and Terry, R. D. (1980): Reduced somatostatin-like immuno-reactivity in cerebral cortex from cases of Alzheimer disease and Alzheimer senile dementia. *Nature*, 288:279–280.
29. Dawbarn, D., and Emson, P. C. (1985): Neuropeptide Y-like immunoreactivity in neuritic plaques of Alzheimer's disease. *Biochem. Biophys. Res. Commun.*, 126:289–294.
30. Dewied, D. (1976): Behavioral effects of intraventricularly administered vasopressin and vasopressin fragments. *Life Sci.*, 19:685–690.
31. Donoghue, J. P., Wenthold, R. J., and Altschuler, R. A. (1985): Localization of glutaminase-like and aspartate aminotransferase-like immunoreactivity in neurons of cere-bral cortex. *J. Neurosci.*, 5:2597–2608.
32. Ebewine, J., and Roberts, J. (1984): Glucocorticoid regulation of pro-opoimelanocortin gene transcription in the rat pituitary. *J. Biol. Chem.*, 259:2166–2170.
33. Eckenstein, F., and Baughman, R. (1984): Two types of cholinergic innervation in cortex, one co-localized with vasoactive intestinal polypeptide. *Nature*, 309:153–155.
33a. Ellison, D. N., Beal, M. F., Mazurek, M. F., Bind, E. D., and Martin, J. B. (1986): A post mortem study of amino acid neurotransmitters in Alzheimer's disease. *Ann. Neurol.*, 20:616–621.
34. Emson, P. C., and Hunt, S. P. (1981): Anatomical chemistry of the cerebral cortex. In: *The Organization of the Cerebral Cortex*, edited by F. O. Schmitt, F. G. Worden, G. Adelman, and S. G. Dennis, pp. 325–345. MIT Press, Cambridge.
35. Emson, P. C., Arregui, A., Clement-Jones, V., et al. (1980): Regional distribution of methionine-enkephalin and substance P-like immunoreactivity in normal human brain and in Huntington's disease. *Brain Res.*, 199:147–160.
36. Emson, P. C., Fahrenkrug, J., and Spokes, E. G. S. (1979): Vasoactive intestinal poly-peptide (VIP): distribution in normal human and in Huntington's disease. *Brain Res.*, 173:174–178.
37. Emson, P. C., Rossor, M., and Lee, C. M. (1981): The regional distribution and chromato-graphic behavior of somatostatin in human brain. *Neurosci. Lett.*, 22:319–324.
38. Facchinetti, F., Nappi, G., Petraglia, F., Martignoni, E., Sinforiani, I. E., and Genazzani, A. R. (1984): Central ACTH deficit in degenerative and vascular dementia. *Life Sci.*, 35:1691–1697.
39. Ferrier, I. N., Cross, A. J., Johnson, J. A., et al. (1983): Neuropeptides in Alzheimer type dementia. *J. Neurol. Sci.*, 62:159–170.
40. Fliers, E., Swaab, D. F., Pool, C. W., and Vermer, R. W. H. (1985): The vasopressin and oxytocin neurons in the human supraoptic and paraventricular nucleus: changes with aging and senile dementia. *Brain Res.*, 342:45–53.
41. Geola, F. L., Hershman, J. M., Warwick, R., et al. (1981): Regional distribution of cholecystokinin-like immunoreactivity in the human brain. *J. Clin. Endocrinol. Metab.*, 53:270–275.
42. Geola, F. L., Yamada, T., Warwick, R. J., Tourtellotte, W. W., and Hershman, J. M. (1981): Regional distribution of somatostatin-like immunoreactivity in the human brain. *Brain Res.*, 299:35–42.

43. Gramsch, C., Hollt, V., Mehraein, P., et al. (1979): Regional distribution of methionine-, enkephalin- and beta-endorphin-like immunoreactivity in human brain and pituitary. *Brain Res.*, 171:261–270.
44. Grunke-Igbel, I., Igbal, K., Quinlan, M., et al. (1982): MAP tau, a component of Alzheimer paired helical filament. *J. Biol. Chem.*, 261:6084–6089.
45. Hayes, S. E., and Paul, S. M. (1982): CCK receptors and human neurological disease. *Life Sci.*, 31:319–322.
46. Hendry, S. H. C., and Jones, E. G. (1981): Sizes and distributions of intrinsic neurons incorporating tritiated GABA in monkey sensory-motor cortex. *J. Neurosci.*, 1:390–408.
47. Hendry, S. H. C., Houser, C. R., Jones, E. G., and Vaughn, J. E. (1983): Synaptic organization of immunocytochemically identified GABA neurons in the monkey sensory-motor cortex. *J. Neurocytol.*, 12:639–660.
48. Hendry, S. H. C., Jones, E. G., and Beinfeld, M. C. (1983): CCK immunoreactive neurons in rat and monkey cerebral cortex make symmetric synapses and have intimate associations with blood vessels. *Proc. Natl. Acad. Sci. USA*, 80:2400–2404.
49. Hendry, S. H. C., Jones, E. G., and Emson, P. C. (1984): Morphology, distribution, and synaptic relations of somatostatin- and neuropeptide Y-immunoreactive neurons in rat and monkey neocortex. *J. Neurosci.*, 4:2497–2517.
50. Hendry, S. H. C., Jones, E. G., Defelipe, J., et al. (1984): Neuropeptide-containing neurons of the cerebral cortex are also GABAergic. *Proc. Natl. Acad. Sci. USA*, 81:6526–6530.
51. Houser, C. R., Hendry, S. H. C., Jones, E. G., and Vaughn, J. E. (1983): Morphological diversity of immunocytochemically identified GABA neurons in monkey sensory-motor cortex. *J. Neurocytol.*, 12:617–638.
52. Iversen, L. L., and Bloom, F. E. (1979): Studies of the uptake of $^3$H-GABA and $^3$H-glycine in slices and homogenates of rat brain and spinal cord by electron microscopic autoradiography. *Brain Res.*, 41:131–143.
53. Jackson, I. M. D. (1980): Significance and function of neuropeptides in cerebrospinal fluid. In: *Neurobiology of Cerebrospinal Fluid*, edited by J. H. Wood, pp. 625–650. Plenum Press, New York.
54. Jones, E. G., and Hendry, S. H. C. (1986): The peptide containing neurons of the primate cerebral cortex. In: *Neuropeptides in Neurologic and Psychiatric Disease*, edited by J. B. Martin and J. D. Barchas, pp. 163–178. Raven Press, New York.
55. Jones, P. M., and Robinson, I. C. A. F. (1982): Differential clearance of neurophysin and neurohypophyseal peptides from the cerebrospinal fluid in conscious guinea pigs. *Neuroendocrinology*, 34:297–302.
56. Jones, E. G., Hendry, S. H. C. (1985): GABAergic, substance P-immunoreactive neurons in monkey cerebral cortex. *Neurosci. Abstr.*, 11:145.
57. Joynt, R. J., and McNeill, T. H. (1984): Neuropeptides in aging and dementia. *Peptides*, 5(Suppl. 1):269–274.
58. Kaiya, H., Tanaka, T., Takeuchi, K., et al. (1983): Decreased levels of beta-endorphin like immunoreactivity in cerebrospinal fluid of patients with senile dementia of Alzheimer type. *Life Sci.*, 33:1039–1043.
58a. Kidd, M. (1963): Paired helical filaments in electron microscopy of Alzheimer's disease. *Nature*, 197:192–193.
59. Kosik, K. S., Joachim, C. L., and Selkoe, D. J. (1986): MAP tau is a major actigenic component of paired helical filaments in Alzheimer's disease. *Proc. Natl. Acad. Sci. USA*, 83:4044–4048.
60. Kowall, N., Ferrante, R. J., Beal, M. F., and Martin, J. B. (1985): Characteristics, distribution and interrelationships of somatostatin, neuropeptide Y, and NADPH-diaphorase in human caudate nucleus. *Neurosci. Abstr.*, 11:209.
61. Kowall, N. W., and Kosik, K. S. (1986): Tau histochemistry reveals widespread cytoskeletal disorganization in Alzheimer's disease. *Soc. Neurosci. Abstr.*, 12:943.
62. Kowall, N. W., Beal, M. F., and Martin, J. B. (1986): Somatostatin, neuropeptide Y and NADPH diaphorase neurons do not contain neurofibrillary tangles in Alzheimer's disease cortex. *Ann. Neurol.*, 20:124.
63. Kowall, N. W., Beal, M. F., and Martin, J. B. (1986): Somatostatin neuropeptide Y and NADPH diaphorase reactive fibers contribute to senile plaque formation in Alzheimer's disease. *Neurology*, 36(Suppl. 1):224.

64. Lee, C. M., Emson, P. C., and Iversen, L. L. (1981): Chromatographic behavior and post-mortem stability of somatostatin in the rat and mouse brain. *Brain Res.*, 220:159–166.
65. Mair, R. G., Langlais, P. J., Mazurek, M. F., Beal, M. F., Martin, J. B., and McEntee, W. J. (1986): Reduced concentrations of arginine vasopressin and MHPG in lumbar CSF of patients with Korsakoff's amnesia. *Life Sci.*, 38:2301–2306.
66. Majoub, J., Rich, A., Von Boon, J., and Habener, J, (1983): Vasopressin oxytocin mRNA regulation in the rat assessed by hybridization with synthetic oligonucleotides. *J. Biol. Chem.*, 258:14061–14064.
67. Manberg, P. J., Youngblood, W. W., Nemeroff, C. B., et al. (1982): Regional distribution of neurotensin in human brain. *J. Neurochem.*, 38:1777–1780.
68. Mauborgne, A., Javoy-agid, F., LeGrand, J. C., et al. (1983): Decrease of substance P-like immunoreactivity in the substantia nigra and pallidum of parkinsonian brains. *Brain Res.*, 268:167–170.
69. May, C., Kay, A., Hill, B., et al. (1985): Cerebrospinal fluid corticotropin releasing factor is reduced in Alzheimer's disease. *Neurology*, 35(Suppl. 1):91.
70. Mazurek, M. F., Beal, M. F., and Martin, J. B. (1985): Vasopressin in postmortem Alzheimer brain. *Ann. Neurol.*, 18:143–144.
71. Mazurek, M. F., Growdon, J. H., Beal, M. F., and Martin, J. B. (1986): CSF vasopressin concentration is reduced in Alzheimer's disease. *Neurology*, 36:1133–1137.
72. McKinney, M., Davies, P., and Coyle, J. T. (1982): Somatostatin in not co-localized in cholinergic neurons innervating the rat cerebral cortex-hippocampal formation. *Brain Res.*, 243:169–172.
73. Morrison, J. H., Rogers, J., Scherr, S., Benoit, R., and Bloom, F. E. (1985): Somatostatin immunoreactivity in neuritic plaques of Alzheimer's patients. *Nature*, 31:490–492.
74. Nakamura, S., and Vincent, S. R. (1985): Acetylcholinesterase and somatostatin-immunoreactivity coexist in human neocortex. *Neurosci. Lett.*, 61:183–187.
75. Naylor, S. L., Sakaguchi, A. Y., Shen, L., et al. (1983): Polymorphic human somatostatin gene is located on chromosome 3. *Proc. Natl. Acad. Sci. USA*, 80:2686–2689.
76. Nemeroff, C. B., Bissette, G., Busby, W. H., et al. (1983): Regional brain concentrations of neurotensin, thyrotropin releasing hormone and somatostatin in Alzheimer's disease. *Neurosci. Abstr.*, 9:1052.
77. Nemeroff, C. B., Widerlov, E., Bissette, G., et al. (1984): Elevated concentrations of CSF corticotropin-releasing factor-like immunoreactivity in depressed patients. *Science*, 226:1342–1344.
78. Nukina, N., and Ihara, Y. (1986): One of the antigenic determinants of paired helical filaments is related to tau protein. *J. Biochem.*, 99:1541–1544.
79. Okon, E., and Koch, Y. (1976): Localization of gonadotropin-releasing and thyrotropin-releasing hormone in human brain by radioimmunoassay. *Nature*, 263:345–347.
80. Perry, E. K., Blessed, G., Tomlinson, B. E., et al. (1981): Neurochemical activities in human temporal lobe related to aging with Alzheimer-type changes. *Neurobiol. Aging*, 2:251–256.
81. Perry, E. K., Perry, R. H., and Tomlinson, E. (1982): The influence of agonal status on some neurochemical activities of postmortem brain tissue. *Neurosci. Lett.*, 29:303–307.
82. Perry, R. H., Dockray, R., Dimaline, R., et al. (1981): Neuropeptides in Alzheimer's disease, depression and schizophrenia: post mortem analysis of vasoactive intestinal peptide and cholecystokinin in cerebral cortex. *J. Neurol. Sci.*, 51:465–472.
83. Price, D. L., Powers, R. E., Walker, L. C., Struble, R. G., et al. (1986): Corticotropin-releasing factor immunoreactivity in senile plaques. *Soc. Neurosci. Abstr.*, 12:98.
84. Raskind, M. A., Peskind, E. R., Lampe, T. L., Risse, S. C., Taborsky, G. J., and Dorsa, D. (1986): Cerebrospinal fluid vasopressin, oxytocin, somatostatin, and beta-endorphin in Alzheimer's disease. *Arch. Gen. Psychiatry*, 43:382–388.
85. Rasool, G., and Selkoe, D. (1986): Adrenocorticotropic hormone and melanocyte-stimulating hormone-like immunoreactive neurites in senile plaques. *J. Neuropathol. Exp. Neurol.*, 45:339 (abstract 66).
86. Roberts, G. W., Crow, T. J., and Polak, J. M. (1985): Location of neuronal tangles in somatostatin neurons in Alzheimer's disease. *Nature*, 314:92–94.
87. Rosenfeld, M. G., Mermod, J-J., Amara, S. G., et al. (1983): Production of a novel neuropeptide encoded by the calcitonin gene via tissue-specific RNA processing. *Nature*, 304:129–135.

88. Rossor, M. N., Emson, P. C., and Mountjoy, C. A. (1982): Neurotransmitters of the cerebral cortex in senile dementia of Alzheimer's type. *Exp. Brain Res.*, 5(Suppl.):133–157.
89. Rossor, M. N., Emson, P. C., Mountjoy, C. O., Roth, M., and Iversen, L. L. (1980): Reduced amounts of immunoreactive somatostatin in the temporal cortex in senile dementia of Alzheimer type. *Neurosci. Lett.*, 20:373–377.
90. Rossor, M. N., Garrett, N. J., and Johnson, A. I. (1982): A postmortem study of the cholinergic and GABA systems in senile dementia. *Brain*, 105:313–330.
91. Rossor, M. N., Iversen, L. L., Mountjoy, C. O., et al. (1980): Arginine vasopressin and choline acetyltransferase in brains of patients with Alzheimer type senile dementia. *Lancet*, 2:1367–1368.
92. Rossor, M. N., Iversen, L. L., Reynolds, G. P., Mountjoy, C. O., and Roth, M. (1984): Neurochemical characteristics of early and late onset types of Alzheimer's disease. *Br. Med. J.*, 288:961–964.
93. Rossor, M. N., Rehfeld, J. F., Emson, P. C., et al. (1981): Normal cortical concentration of cholecystokinin-like immunoreactivity with reduced choline acetyltransferase activity in senile dementia of Alzheimer type. *Life Sci.*, 29:405–410.
94. Rubinow, D. R., Gold, P. W., Post, R. M., et al. (1983): CSF somatostatin in affective illness. *Arch. Gen. Psychiatry*, 40:409–412.
95. Sakamoto, N., Michel, J. P., Kitahama, K., et al. (1985): Relationship between catecholamine, enkephalin, substance P and neurotensin immunoreactive neuronal systems in the infant human brain. *Neurosci. Abstr.*, 11:743.
96. Schmechel, D. E., Vickrey, B. G., Fitzpatrick, D., and Elde, R. P. (1984): GABAergic neurons of mammalian cerebral cortex: widespread subclass defined by somatostatin content. *Neurosci. Lett.*, 47:227–232.
97. Schwartz, W. J., and Reppert, S. M. (1985): Neural regulation of the circadian vasopressin rhythm in cerebrospinal fluid: a pre-eminent role for the suprachiasmatic nuclei. *J. Neurosci.*, 5:2771–2778.
98. Sharpless, N. S., Thal, L. J., Perlow, M. J., et al. (1984): Vasoactive intestinal peptide in cerebrospinal fluid. *Peptides*, 5:429–433.
99. Shen, L., Pictet, R. L., and Rutler, W. J. (1982): Human somatostatin I: sequence of the cDNA. *Proc. Natl. Acad. Sci. USA*, 79:4575–4579.
100. Soininen, H. S., Jolkonen, J. T., Reinikainen, K. J., Halonen, T. O., and Riekkinen, P. J. (1984): Reduced cholinesterase activity and somatostatin-like immunoreactivity in the cerebrospinal fluid of patients with dementia of the Alzheimer type. *J. Neurol. Sci.*, 63:167–172.
101. Somogyi, P., Hodgson, A. J., Smith, A. D., et al. (1984): Differential populations of GABAeric neurons in the visual cortex and hippocampus of the cat contain somatostatin or cholecystokinin immunoreactive material. *J. Neurosci.*, 4:2590–2603.
102. Sorensen, K. V. (1982): Somatostatin: localization and distribution in the cortex and the subcortical white matter of the human brain. *Neuroscience*, 7:1227–1232.
103. Sorensen, P. S., Gjerris, A., and Hammer, M. (1985): Cerebrospinal fluid vasopressin in neurological and psychiatric disorders. *J. Neurol. Neurosurg. Psychiatry*, 48:50–57.
104. Spokes, E. G. S. (1980): Neurochemical alterations in Huntington's chorea: a study of postmortem brain tissue. *Brain*, 103:179–210.
105. Struble, R. G., Kitt, C. A., Walker, L. C., Cork, L. C., and Price, D. L. (1984): Somatostatinergic neurites in senile plaques of aged non-human primates. *Brain Res.*, 324:394–396.
106. Struble, R. G., Powers, R. E., Casanova, M. F., et al. (1985): Multiple transmitter specific markers in senile plaques in Alzheimer's disease. *Neurosci. Abstr.*, 11:953.
107. Sulkava, R., Erkinjuntti, T., and Laatikainen, T. (1985): CSF beta-endorphin and beta-lipotropin in Alzheimer's disease and multi-infarct dementia. *Neurology*, 35:1057–1058.
108. Sundquist, J., Forsling, M. L., Olsson, J. E., and Akerlund, M. (1983): Cerebrospinal fluid arginine vasopressin in degenerative disorders and other neurological diseases. *J. Neurol. Neurosurg. Psychiatry*, 46:14–17.
109. Swaab, D. F., Fliers, E., and Partiman, T. S. (1985): The suprachiasmatic nucleus of the human brain in relation to sex, age and senile dementia. *Brain Res.*, 342:37–44.
110. Tang, F., Costa, E., and Schwartz, J. (1983): Increase of proenkephalin mRNA and enkephalin content of rat striatum after daily injection of haloperidol for 2 to 3 weeks. *Proc. Natl. Acad. Sci. USA*, 80:3841–3844.

111. Terry, R. D. (1986): The fine structure of neurofibrillary tangles in Alzheimer's disease. *J. Neuropathol. Exp. Neurol.*, 22:629-642.
112. Tomlinson, B. E., Irving, D., and Blessed, G. (1981): Cell loss in the locus coeruleus in senile dementia of Alzheimer type. *J. Neurol. Sci.*, 49:419–428.
113. Wikkelso, C., Fahrenkrug, J., Blomstrand, C., and Johansson, B. B. (1985): Dementia of different etiologies: vasoactive intestinal polypeptide in CSF. *Neurology,* 35:592–595.
114. Wood, J. G., Mirra, S. S., Pollock, N. J., and Binber, L. I. (1986): Neurofibrillary tangles of Alzheimer's disease store antigenic determinants with the axonal MAP tau. *Proc. Natl. Acad. Sci. USA,* 83:4040–4043.
115. Wood, P. L., Etienne, P., Lal, S., Gauthier, S., Cajal, S., and Nair, N. P. V. (1982): Reduced lumbar CSF somatostatin levels in Alzheimer's disease. *Life Sci.,* 31:2073–2079.
116. Yamamoto, T., and Hirano, A. (1985): Nucleus raphe dorsalis in Alzheimer's disease: neurofibrillary tangles and loss of large neurons. *Ann. Neurol.,* 17:573–577.
117. Yates, C. M., Fink, G., Bennie, J. G., et al. (1985): Neurotensin immunoreactivity in post-mortem brain is increased in Down's syndrome but not in Alzheimer-type dementia. *J. Neurol. Sci.,* 67:327–335.
118. Yates, C. M., Harmar, A. J., Rosie, R., et al. (1983): Thyrotropin-releasing hormone, luteinizing hormone-releasing hormone and substance P immunoreactivity in post-mortem brain from cases of Alzheimer-type dementia and Down's syndrome. *Brain Res.,* 258:45–52.

*Aging and the Brain,* edited by R. D. Terry.
Raven Press, New York © 1988.

# Aging, Neurotoxins, and Neurodegenerative Disease

## J. William Langston

*Institute for Medical Research, San Jose, California 95128*

At least two degenerative diseases of the human brain appear to require the fertile ground of an aging nervous system. These are, of course, Alzheimer disease and Parkinson disease. The reason these diseases favor the aged brain remains by and large a mystery, yet each has inspired intensive research efforts. Why? With Alzheimer disease, it was the realization that this disease process (or a similar one) might underlie the common occurrence of dementia in the aged population. This fact began to sink into the communal scientific consciousness after a seminal paper by Katzman in 1976 (38), pointing out the indistinguishability of the classical neuropathological features of Alzheimer disease in younger individuals and the neuropathological substrate of "senile dementia." In the case of Parkinson disease, the research renaissance that has bloomed during the last few years came about not as the result of careful scientific investigation, but rather, as the result of sloppy chemistry by a "kitchen chemist" trying to reap the financial rewards of the "designer drug" craze (42).

The purpose of this chaper is to step back for a moment to see how far we have come in regard to one of these two diseases, Parkinson disease, and assess the impact of recent work on future research into diseases that target the aging brain. Although the major thrust of this chapter is directed toward Parkinson disease, it should become obvious that many of the principles described could be applied to research in Alzheimer disease as well. A major thesis of this chapter is that neurotoxins provide a powerful tool for the study of aging and the neurodegenerative process. It is not unreasonable to hope that one or more of the approaches to be described could be instrumental in unlocking some of the secrets of these seemingly impenetrable diseases.

## IS PARKINSON DISEASE AGE-RELATED?

It may seem to be a strange way to begin a discussion of Parkinson disease, but in fact the issue of whether the disease is age-related is a matter of some controversy. Few would deny that Parkinson disease is rare before the age of 30 and typically has its onset after the age of 40. However, there is some debate as to whether the incidence of the disease reaches a peak in people in their late fifties or early sixties and then begins to decrease or whether it continues to increase in incidence during the later years of life. A study by Koller and colleagues (40), for example, showed that the incidence of Parkinson disease peaks at around 59 to 60 years of age, after which it declines rather precipitously. On the other hand, research by Kurland et al. (41), based on a community-controlled study, suggests that the incidence of the disease continues to increase throughout later life. There are several arguments that can be marshaled favoring the data of Kurland et al. First, studies such as the one carried out by Koller et al. (40), although providing important information, are based on data derived from referred patients. It could be argued that such patients, particularly when they are referred to a specialized movement disorders clinic, are highly selected and therefore may not be best for the collection of epidemiological data. For instance, the younger (and therefore the more atypical) a patient is, the more cautious his or her physician is apt to be in making a diagnosis, and hence the more likely the referral for a second opinion. Furthermore, younger patients, particularly those who are still employed, demand such consultation more frequently for reassurance regarding the diagnosis as well as for the best possible treatment if continued employability is at stake. In older patients a diagnosis of Parkinson disease is less likely to evoke diagnostic unease and usually does not threaten employability; therefore the diagnosis is probably more readily accepted without referral by a family practitioner. For example, it seems highly unlikely that a family physician would refer a nursing-home-bound 82-year-old with congestive heart failure to a distant specialty clinic just to confirm a diagnosis of early Parkinson disease. In summary, because the study by Kurland and colleagues (41) is based on a survey of all physicians and medical facilities in Rochester, Minnesota, it is therefore likely to better represent the actual incidence of the disease.

The issue is an important one. If it were proved for example, that the incidence of Parkinson disease peaks at age 60 and decreases thereafter, it would suggest that a window of increased vulnerability exists, the opening and closing of which is governed by age. This finding would have important implications in terms of underlying mechanisms and possibly etiology. If, on the other hand, it is simply a matter of increasing vulnerability with age, an entirely different set of considerations come into play. This issue is discussed later in this chapter when various hypotheses are being considered.

## AGING AND INCREASING NEURONAL VULNERABILITY

Although theories abound (6,13,14), none has yet proved decisive in explaining the predilection of either Parkinson or Alzheimer disease for the nervous system of aged individuals. For example, Selkoe and colleagues (72) have proposed that in Alzheimer disease age-related cross-linking of neuro-filaments with consequent accumulation of permanent, rigid fibrous polymers may lead to neuronal degeneration. However, it remains unclear why aging should cause neurofilaments to cross-link in the first place. Obviously, any observations providing answers to one or more of these questions could have an immense impact on the health of the aged population.

One of the current theories regarding the process of cellular aging in biological systems relates to the formation of potentially damaging free radicals that are produced through normal oxidative processes (15,31). To date, however, a mechanism that ties free radical generation directly to age-related neurodegenerative disease has not been convincingly demonstrated—although not for want of trying (3,13,29). For many reasons, the basal ganglia have beckoned as fertile ground to researchers interested in this area. It is because these structures appear to be vulnerable to the effects of aging, and there is reason to believe that they may be particularly susceptible to the effects of oxidative stress (3,13,47). For example, it has been known for some time that striatal dopamine in the human declines with aging (8), and there is evidence that a progressive loss of neurons in the substantia nigra occurs with aging as well (59). In regard to oxidative stress, dopamine has been proposed as a crucial factor (13). Eighty percent of the dopamine in the central nervous system (CNS) is located in the striatum (7). Oxidation of dopamine is likely to produce potentially damaging free radicals and quinones (46). In fact, Cohen (13) has proposed that the oxidation of dopamine, with resultant accumulation of damaging free radicals, could lead to premature senescence of dopaminergic neurons. It is of particular importance here that it has been known for some time that a variety of environmental neurotoxins (e.g., manganese) may damage basal ganglia structures, and, almost without exception, the proposed mechanism of action of these compounds involves the generation of free radicals (47).

Although these observations are of interest, none of these toxins is known to have effects that are linked to the aging process. However, recent discoveries relating to 1-methyl-4-phenyl-1,2,3,6-tetrahydropyridine (MPTP), a compound that is highly toxic to the nigrostriatal system of primates, appears to have changed this situation, perhaps dramatically.

## THE DISCOVERY OF MPTP: NEW CONCEPTS IN NEUROTOXICOLOGY

The story of the discovery of MPTP has been well chronicled elsewhere (42,52). In brief, this compound was first synthesized by Ziering and colleagues in 1947 (79); and although it was studied in some detail and made several appearances on the illicit drug scene (44), its actual biological effects were not clearly defined until an illicit chemist in northern California inadvertently made a batch of this compound and began selling it on the streets as "synthetic" heroin (48). The resulting parkinsonian syndrome that developed in heroin addicts self-administering this substance has been described in detail elsewhere (45,48). Suffice it to say that they exhibited full and unalloyed parkinsonism (2), responded to typical antiparkinsonian medications, and have even experienced the side effects typically encountered with long-term antiparkinsonian therapy (45). From the clinical standpoint then, the resemblance between MPTP-induced parkinsonism and Parkinson disease is remarkably close.

During the years since the discovery of MPTP, a great deal has been learned about the mechanism of action of this compound. It is highly toxic to the neurons of the zona compacta of the substantia nigra and a potent depletor of striatal dopamine in a wide variety of species (46). MPTP, a lipophilic substance, readily crosses the blood–brain barrier. Soon after systemic administration, it has been found to be widely distributed throughout the primate brain (50). We now know that MPTP is rapidly transformed in a process that involves monoamine oxidase B (MAO B) (10) to a pyridinium species known a 1-methyl-4-phenylpyridinium ion (MPP$^+$) (50,55). This biotransformation occurs throughout the body and CNS (50). If the biotransformation of MPTP to MPP$^+$ is blocked, large amounts of MPTP accumulate in the CNS (50,55), yet no toxicity is observed. These observations constitute strong evidence that MPTP itself is not toxic.

This discussion brings us to the first of the concepts to be presented here— that of a protoxin. This term is used to denote a nontoxic compound that, through the process of biotransformation, is coverted to a toxin. In the case of MPTP, this will have devastating consequences for the CNS because the protoxin (MPTP) crosses the blood–brain barrier, whereas the putative toxic metabolite MPP$^+$, as a charged compound, cannot (I. Irwin and J. W. Langston, *unpublished observations*). In short, this sequence of events circumvents the usually effective blood–brain barrier.

However, gaining access to the nervous system is just the beginning of a series of "deceptions." As already noted, MPTP itself does not appear to be toxic. For most xenobiotics there is a highly efficient metabolic machinery in place to handle exogenous compounds once they have gained entrance to the body. For the systemic circulation, this system resides primarily in the liver and is typified by the cytochrome P-450 mixed-function oxygenase system (5). However, the brain is largely devoid of this system. At first glance, this observation appears to be curious. However, viewed from one perspective, it does make sense. The brain can be envisioned as a system laden with millions of miniature biochemical vacuum pumps, designed for the reuptake of various neurotransmitters. Spewing the brain with a constant array of newly manufactured molecules from the cytochrome P-450 system could be risky indeed. One or more of these newly synthesized products of the detoxification process, if taken up by various neuronal systems, might prove toxic to those neurons.

Nature appears to have solved this problem by protecting the brain from xenobiotics with the construction of a blood–brain barrier, obviating the need for an extensive detoxification system within the CNS compartment. Obviously there is still a need for some type of detoxification process, however, and one appears to be monoamine oxidase. Although this enzyme has often been thought to play a role in the normal metabolism of various neurotransmitters, there is increasing evidence that this enzyme (particularly the B form, which resides primarily in the glia) may serve primarily a scavenger or detoxification function (76).

It was this line of reasoning that originally led Chiba and colleagues (10) to test the effects of MAO inhibitors on the biotransformation of MPTP to MPP$^+$. It is here also that the second deception of the system occurs, as all of the evidence to date suggests that it is MAO B, presumably in performing its role as a protective enzyme, that converts MPTP to its toxic metabolite (10,32,51,55,65), rather than detoxifying the molecule. To the best of this writer's knowledge, this action represents the first example of the brain's own enzymatic machinery converting a nontoxic compound to a selective neurotoxin. This precedent could have major implications in the study of neurodegenerative diseases should it prove to be a common occurrence.

However, even this situation probably would not be enough for the production of selective damage to the nigrostriatal system, as the biotransformation of MPTP to MPP$^+$ occurs throughout the CNS (50). For this a third deception appears necessary, which illustrates the potential dangers of having a reuptake system exposed to transformed xenobiotics. MPP$^+$, much to the surprise of most investigators, proved to be a high-affinity substrate for the dopamine reuptake system, equaling dopamine itself (11,34). Apparently, the uptake system recognizes MPP$^+$ as an appropriate substrate but is actually taking in a potentially lethal toxin. We have referred to it as the "Trojan horse" phenomenon.

This pathway to selective cellular destruction, when viewed in toto, appears to be novel. One might at first assume that this remarkable feat, which involves so many unexpected biological and chemical tricks, is a fluke, perpetrated by a unique coming together of a number of critical features in a single molecule, and one which therefore is unlikely to play a larger role in the biological scheme of things. This may very well be. However, four analogs of MPTP have already been discovered that have similar toxic effects (27,36,77,78), even though the search for such compounds is still in an early stage. It seems increasingly likely that an entire class of "catecholaminergic neurotoxins" may exist. Whether any of these will be found in the environment remains to be determined, of course. However, it could prove that rather than being an obscure pathway, this road to toxicity could be a veritable highway to the CNS—an Achilles heel of the brain, if you will. As was hinted at earlier, these concepts might also provide some clues that could link neuronal degeneration to the aging process itself—and it may be here that MPTP will provide the most unexpected yet valuable insights of all.

## THE AGING CONNECTION

There is now a rapidly accumulating body of evidence that the effects of MPTP vary with age. Not only do the effects of this compound seem to become more pronounced with age, but they appear to come closer to reproducing all of the features of Parkinson disease as well. In a way it seems almost too much to ask of an already highly satisfactory model, but there is at present little doubt that such a relation exists. As many of the studies have been carried out in rodents, it is first necessary to provide some background information regarding what constitutes youth or old age in these animals.

Fortunately, the C57B1/6J mouse, which is one of the most commonly used in MPTP-related studies, is one of the best studied and characterized rodents in regard to normal aging (20). According to numerous reports (9,18,19,23), 10- to 12-month-old animals can be defined as "mature," with full skeletal development and full brain and body weight, and are thus equivalent to a 20- to 30-year-old man. "Middle-aged" mice (presumably the equivalent of 40- to 50-year-old humans) are 18 to 20 months old, and senescent mice (the equivalent to 70- to 80-year-old humans) are 26 months old or more. The maximal life span of these mice appears to be around 30 months (62). The literature documents various manifestations of aging in mice that correspond to those seen in humans; they include decreases in bone density (28,66), blood dyscrasias (21), deficits in thermoregulation (22), and increases in tumor incidence (16,22).

Being thoroughly acquainted with the life cycle of the mouse, it will be immediately obvious in the following section that the first clues regarding the age-related effects of MPTP came not from studies of old animals but from young ones. Although this fact may at first seem puzzling, the explanation is relatively simple. Younger rodents are readily available and inexpensive; older ones are often much more difficult to obtain and require a considerable investment in time and money. Even though MPTP was being used to study a disease of aging, these time-honored factors were almost certainly at work in at least a few of the studies to be described.

The first objective evidence that the effects of MPTP increase with age came independently from three studies. Interestingly, one of these focused on the gut, rather than the brain. Fields (17) found that MPTP induced severe ulcers in 25% of 1-month-old rats but that the figure climbed to 50% in 2-month-old animals and to 80% in 3-month-old animals. At approximately the same time, Jarvis and Wagner (33) reported that 4-week-old rats were virtually immune to the effects of MPTP, whereas a 65% striatal dopamine reduction was seen in 4-month-old animals. It is also of note that all of the 1-year-old animals given MPTP in this study died, suggesting that the lethal effects of MPTP also increase with age. Ricaurte and colleagues (68) showed that MPTP, given intraperitoneally, produced cell death in the substantia nigra in older (8 months old) but not young (6–8 weeks old) C57B1/6J IMR mice, thus showing that the neurodegenerative effects of MPTP, in addition to the pharmacologic effects of the compound, were age-dependent. These investigators also showed that the effects of methamphetamine, another compound known to induce degeneration of nigrostriatal nerve terminals, were not age-dependent, suggesting that age-dependent neurotoxicity is not a universal phenomenon.

We have studied the biotransformation of MPTP to MPP$^+$ in some detail in an effort to gain insights into the possible mechanisms underlying these differential effects with aging (49). We found an almost linear correlation between the age of animals and the ability of the CNS to convert MPTP to MPP$^+$ (ages studied ranged from 6 weeks to 10 months). *In vivo* studies confirmed the increased efficiency of the neural tissue from older animals in converting MPTP to MPP$^+$; however, this change was not limited to the striatum but was seen in the frontal cortex as well.

One obvious explanation for these results relates to MAO B. This enzyme appears to be one of the few substances to increase with age in the brain and therefore could represent a key to a connection between aging, neurotoxins, and neuronal degeneration, particularly when considering the scheme outlined in detail above. Studies in humans (14,69,70) and monkeys have shown that MAO increases in the CNS with age. However, studies in the rat are conflicting (4,54,64). The only study of striatal MAO in C57B1/6JIMR mice we have located is that of Samorajski and Rolsten (71), which includes only two time points and shows no change with age. Clearly, more-detailed studies of MAO concentrations with age in the C57B1/6JIMR mouse are needed, but certainly the "MAO connection" seems plausible based on data from primates and, possibly, rats. It is also worth noting that several years ago Knoll (39) offered a somewhat similar suggestion, when he proposed that increasing concentrations of MAO-containing glia in the aging brain would lead to excessive catabolism of extraneuronal dopamine. One attractive feature of this hypothesis was that, if correct, this process would be amenable to therapeutic manipulation, as this biochemical deficit should be correctable with MAO inhibitor therapy. In a sense, we are now taking this concept one step further by suggesting that an increase of MAO B-containing glia might well be responsible for actual cell death (43).

As noted earlier, another concern regarding the aging studies described above is that they were done in young animals. The 1- to 10-month range in rodents represents the equivalent in terms of human years of approximately 3 to 30 years. In fact, it could be argued that these were developmental studies rather than studies of aging. It is important to extend all of this work to much older animals.

At least one group of investigators have clearly studied aged rodents. Gupta and colleagues (30), using catechol-fluorescence and immunohistochemistry to measure tyrosine hydroxylase (TH) activity, studied the effects of MPTP on various areas of the mouse brain. These investigators chose two age groups: 3 months and 2 years. The older group, again using the mouse-year analogy, would be the equivalent of human's in the sixth to seventh decades of life, a time when Parkinson disease is increasingly prevalent. The results were striking. Whereas MPTP induced loss of fluorescence and a marked diminution in TH staining in the substantia nigra of both groups, no such changes were seen in the ventral tegmental area or locus ceruleus of young animals. [Both of these areas, particularly the latter, are typically involved in Parkinson disease (24).] In the aged animals, however, MPTP induced a decrease in fluorescence and TH staining in both the locus ceruleus and ventral tegmental areas. Hence the effects of MPTP were not only more pronounced in aged animals, but they more closely resembled those findings seen in Parkinson disease. All of these studies suggest that exploring the effects of MPTP in aged primates could be a highly productive venture, and indeed, this has proven to be the case.

## PRIMATE STUDIES

Forno and colleagues (25) have recently reported the results of a study of primates which were, on the whole, approximately twice as old as those animals used in previous investigations. In five of six animals, unequivocal histological evidence of damage to the locus ceruleus was encountered (26). Similar findings have since been observed in an additional four animals (L. Forno et al., *unpublished observations.*) Because the absence of actual neuronal degeneration in the locus ceruleus has constituted one of the two major criticisms of the MPTP model, this finding is of particular interest in that it appears to bring the MPTP model much closer to Parkinson disease.

However, another feature of Parkinson disease, the Lewy body, has until recently eluded investigators using MPTP to study Parkinson disease. Lewy bodies are a cardinal feature of this disease, and inducing these structures has proved to be a major hurdle for those attempting to bring the MPTP model closer to Parkinson disease. It is here that the aging nervous system has provided the most fertile ground of all. In the Forno study (26), all three of the monkeys over the age of 15 years (approximately the equivalent of a 60- to 70-year-old human) were found to have also developed eosinophilic intra-neuronal inclusions as a result of exposure to MPTP. These inclusions bore a definite resemblance to Lewy bodies, and many of the structures even demon-strated the peripheral halo that is so typical of Lewy bodies. These inclusions have been seen in the locus ceruleus, substantia nigra, dorsal raphe, dorsal nucleus of the vagus, and nucleus basalis of Meynert (26). The latter finding is of particular interest for two reasons. First, it was in the nucleus basalis where Lewy himself first encountered these structures that bear his name (53). Secondly, the nucleus basalis is a cholinergic nucleus and one, of course, that has been the center of much investigation in regard to Alzheimer disease. It may be that another formidable barrier has been overcome in using MPTP to produce "extracatecholaminergic" lesions. This finding may also have implications for Alzheimer disease in view of the fact that in truly aged animals, MPTP appears to be evoking a degenerative process in this nucleus as well.

It should be cautioned that the inclusion bodies seen in aged primates have not yet been proved to be Lewy bodies; however, something of this nature occurring in a model that is already so close to Parkinson disease appears to be more than coincidental. Another interesting analogy between these structures and Lewy bodies is that both are seen in the nervous system of aged primates. Lewy bodies, whether they are incidental or associated with Parkinson disease, occur almost exclusively in aged humans. If, as suggested by the data presented in this chapter, MPTP can be used to induce most if not all of the pathological and neurochemical features of Parkinson disease in *aged* primates, including typical Lewy bodies, the implications could be far-reaching. For example, the closer the MPTP model comes to Parkinson disease, the greater the interest in the compound as an etiological agent for the disease. Such a finding would undoubtedly enhance the search for MPTP-like substances in the environment. We believe that a more general principle could be elaborated from these studies as well. A finding that the cytoskeletal properties of older neurons differ from younger ones to the point that they respond to injury in a morphologically different way could prove to be an important precedent. Perhaps the use of neurotoxins in aged animals will provide a key to the study of the classic neuropathological features of neurodegenerative disease (i.e., Lewy bodies in Parkinson disease; senile plaques and neurofibrillary tangles in Alzheimer disease). Indeed, neurotoxins have already been useful in inducing various forms of neurofibrillary tangles (61), though none has proved identical to those seen in Alzheimer disease. However, few if any of these studies using neurotoxins have been carried out in aged animals, particularly primates. It may be that a combined approach using these neurotoxins and the aged nervous system will prove to be a powerful tool for the study of one or both diseases.

Many of the MPTP-induced eosinophilic inclusions seen in the aged primate were not sharply demarcated and resemble intraneuronal swellings occasionally seen in Parkinson disease. In parkinsonian patients, these structures have often been thought to be Lewy bodies in their early phases of development (L. Forno, *personal communication*). We have now successfully carried out electron microscopy on several of these structures (L. Forno et al., *unpublished observations*) and found them to contain neurofilamentous structures. Once again, this observation appears to take us a step closer to a form of neurofilamentous degeneration, a finding of potential importance in regard to the mechanisms by which neurons degenerate in these age-related diseases.

## NEW HYPOTHESES

The data presented in this chapter provide the basis for a number of interesting hypotheses. We have previously suggested the possibility that Parkinson disease could be due to an environmental insult during early to mid-adult life in combination with the normal process of aging (6). It is generally accepted that an 80% loss of striatal dopamine is required for parkinsonian symptoms to develop (69). It has further been shown that approximately a 5 to 7% cell loss in nigral neurons occurs with each decade of life (8). Hence if a 50% striatal dopamine loss was incurred during midlife due to some type of external insult, e.g., a neurotoxin, the patient would likely remain asymptomatic. However, if the normal age-related loss continued, one would eventually expect to see a parkinsonian condition emerge later in life.

If the observations reviewed in this chapter prove to be correct, another hypothesis is suggested. It may be that there is constant exposure (perhaps low grade) to catecholaminergic neurotoxins throughout life. The young nervous system may be resistant or immune to these toxins, but as the aging process continues this resistance may be lost. As the aging nervous system becomes increasingly vulnerable (perhaps, as suggested above, because of the increasing concentration of MAO), these environmental toxins could begin to take their toll, eventually leading to an expression of clinically evident disease. Similar concepts could be applied to Alzheimer disease. Obviously, the debate about whether Parkinson disease actually continues to increase in old age has a major bearing on this hypothesis.

Another mechanism regarding the increasing vulnerability with age relates to the generation of free radicals, as noted at the beginning of the chapter. The oxidation of MPTP, or perhaps redox cycling between MPTP and its free radical (35), may play a role in MPTP neurotoxicity by generating an excess of free radicals. The evidence is currently divided on whether antioxidants protect against MPTP neurotoxicity. At least three groups have shown that it does (63,73,75). However, our group and two others (1,57) have been unable to reduplicate these findings, so the final answer is not yet in. Here again, however, we have a potential connection with the aging process and neurodegenerative phenomenon.

Another interesting hypothesis relates to regenerative capabilities of the nigrostriatal system. We have reported that young mice recover nearly completely from the dopamine-depleting effects of MPTP (68); older mice (8–10 months old), however, do not (67). This point raises yet another interesting possibility. Perhaps repeated exogenous assaults (e.g., toxins, infectious agents, trauma) occur throughout life, constantly taking their toll on particularly sensitive neuronal groups (e.g., catecholaminergic neurons). However, young neurons may be fully equipped to carry out a brisk reparative process. If, with age, this ability to repair decreases, the resulting neurodegenerative process could be secondary to failure to repair rather than a primary neurodegenerative event. It has been suggested that there may be certain pacemakers for aging (58). The catecholaminergic system may represent one of these pacemakers: hence, damage to this system could have consequences beyond just the dopaminergic and noradrenergic systems in the CNS. Again, if such a process were to be found at the heart of one or more neuro-degenerative diseases, therapeutic strategies could be developed to alter these pacemakers, in turn perhaps altering the aging process itself.

## FINAL THOUGHTS ON CHOOSING A MODEL

The use of toxins to study neurodegenerative disease is almost totally depen-dent on the use of biological models. The importance of choosing the correct model is enormous. The MPTP story illustrates this point as dramatically as any. Primates are exquisitely sensitive to the toxic effects of this compound, yet no one has successfully induced cell loss in the nigra of the rat, even when the compound was injected directly into the nigra itself (12). When it comes to aging, the issue of species variability becomes even more complex. Despite the many similarities between the aging process in the mouse and the human described earlier in this chapter, one can seriously question just how analo-gous a process that requires 9 days in the mouse could possibly be to one that requires 365 days in the human. In regard to the human, postmortem data have shown that the following events occur during the aging process: (a) striatal dopamine concentrations gradually decrease throughout life (8); (b) MAO concentrations increase (14,69); and (c) there may be an actual de-crease in the number of nigral neurons. The latter observation is based primar-ily on the report by McGeer and colleagues (59). Careful examination of their data, however, shows that if the single subject with a cell count of 100,000 is dropped, nigral cell counts remain relatively stable after the age of 30. Inter-estingly, the striking drop in tyrosine hydroxylase in the striatum, which was reported in this same study, occurred almost entirely during the first 30 years. Hence, it must be concluded that additional studies would be of value to confirm the widely held impression that nigral neurons decrease in number during the aging process.

What about the rodent? Most of the comments here focus on the C57B1/6JIMR mouse, as changes in the nigrostriatal system of these animals have been extensively studied. For example, reductions in striatal dopamine up-take (37), RNA (9), catecholamine histofluorescence (60), and spiroperidol binding (74) have all been reported in aged animals.

However, when it comes to studies of striatal dopamine concentrations, the data are surprisingly limited. For example, in Finch's original study (19), only two time points were examined (young maturity and senescence). We have been unable to find a study with multiple time points throughout the aging cycle in this species of mouse. Furthermore, observations from our own laboratory show that dopamine concentrations actually increase through the first 4 months of life, then remain stable throughout the next 2 years (J. W. Langston et al., *unpublished observations*). As noted earlier, there are few data regarding changes in MAO concentrations with age in this species.

Another area where the rodent appears to differ clearly from the human relates to neuromelanin. This poorly characterized substance has intrigued parkinsonologists for years. It has never been observed in the mouse but is seen in higher species, particularly the primate. The closer one comes to the human, the more likely neuromelanin is to be encountered (56). Neuromelanin is not present at birth but may accumulate in sufficient quantities to be visualized by the end of the second year of life. Hence, the presence of neuromelanin is clearly a differentiating factor between aging nigral neurons in rodents and primates.

All of this discussion lends a cautionary note to investigators planning to use the rodent for the study of neurodegenerative diseases of aging. It may be that certain neurodegenerative processes require years (in absolute terms) to become manifest. In view of the foregoing, two conclusions appear to be appropriate. First, if C57B1/6JIMR mice are to become a mainstay for age-related research, further characterization of normal changes that accompany the aging process are in order (including studies of MAO concentrations, antioxidant capabilities, and cell counts). Secondly, even if all of these issues are worked out, it is likely that a certain number of studies will still have to be done in aged primates. Rodents simply may not live long enough to develop some of the degenerative disorders we encounter far too often in aged humans.

## ACKNOWLEDGMENTS

This work was supported in part by the United Parkinson Foundation, the Retirement Research Foundation, the Institute for Medical Research, and NIEHS grant R01 ES03697-03.

## REFERENCES

1. Baldessarini, R. J., Kula, N. S., Francoeur, D., and Finklestein, S. P. (1986): Antioxidants fail to inhibit depletion of striatal dopamine by MPTP. *Neurology*, 36:735.
2. Ballard, P. A., Tetrud, J. W., and Langston, J. W. (1985): Permanent human parkinsonism due to 1-methyl-4-phenyl-1,2,3,6-tetrahydropyridine (MPTP): seven cases. *Neurology*, 35:949–956.
3. Barbeau, A. (1984): Etiology of Parkinson's disease: a research strategy. *Can. J. Neurol. Sci.*, 11:24–28.
4. Benedetti, M. S., and Keane, P. E. (1980): Differential changes in monoamine oxidase A and B activity in the aging rat brain. *J. Neurochem.*, 35:1026–1032.
5. Brodie, B. B., Gillette, J. R., and LaDu, B. N. (1958): Enzymatic metabolism of drugs and other foreign compounds. *Annu. Rev. Biochem.*, 27:427–454.

6. Calne, D. B., and Langston, J. W. (1983): On the aetiology of Parkinson's disease. *Lancet,* 2:1457–1459.
7. Carlsson, A. (1959): The occurrence, distribution and physiologic role of catecholamines in the nervous system. *Pharmacol. Rev.,* 11:490–493.
8. Carlsson, A., and Winblad, B. (1976): Influence of age and time interval between death and autopsy on dopamine and 3-methyoxytyramine levels in human basal ganglia. *J. Neural Transm.,* 38:271–276.
9. Chaconas, G., and Finch, C. E. (1973): The effect of ageing on RNA/DNA ratios in brain regions of the C57B1/6J male mouse. *J. Neurochem.,* 21:1469–1473.
10. Chiba, K., Trevor, A., and Castagnoli, N., Jr. (1984): Metabolism of the neurotoxic tertiary amine, MPTP, by brain monoamine oxidase. *Biochem. Biophys. Res. Commun.,* 120:574–578.
11. Chiba, K., Trevor, A. J., and Castagnoli, N., Jr. (1985): Active uptake of MPP+, a metabolite of MPTP, by brain synaptosomes. *Biochem. Biophys. Res. Commun.,* 128: 1229–1232.
12. Chiueh, C. C., Markey, S. P., Burns, R. S., Johannessen, J. N., Pert, A., and Kopin, I. J. (1984): Neurochemical and behavorial effects of systemic and intranigral administration of n-methyl-4-phenyl-1,2,3,6-tetrahydropyridine in the rat. *Eur. J. Pharmacol.,* 100:189–194.
13. Cohen, G. (1983): The pathobiology of Parkinson's disease: biochemical aspects of dopamine neuron senescence. *J. Neural Transm.,* 19(Suppl.):89–103.
14. Cote, L. J., and Kremzner, L. T. (1983): Biochemical changes in normal aging in human brain. In : *The Dementias,* edited by R. Mayeux and W. G. Rosen, pp. 19–30. Raven Press, New York.
15. Dormandy, T. L. (1983): An approach to free radicals. *Lancet,* 2:1010–1014.
16. Ewing, L. L. (1967): Effect of ageing on testicular metabolism in the rabbit. *Am. J. Physiol.,* 212:1261–1267.
17. Fields, J. Z. (1985): Aging and a novel neurotoxin 1-methyl-4-phenyl-1,2,5,6-tetrahydropyridine elicit deficits in brain dopamine tracts and increases in duodenal ulcers. *Dig. Dis. Sci.,* 30(4):374.
18. Finch, C. E. (1971): Comparative biology of senescence: some evolutionary and developmental considerations. In: *Animal Models for Biomedical Research, Vol. 4,* pp. 47–67. National Academy of Sciences, Washington, D. C.
19. Finch, C. E. (1973): Catecholamine metabolism in the brains of ageing male mice. *Brain Res.,* 52:261–276.
20. Finch, C. E. (1978): Age-related changes in brain catecholamines: a synopsis of findings in C57B1/6J mice and other rodent models. *Adv. Exp. Med. Biol.,* 113:15–39.
21. Finch, C. E., and Foster, J. R. (1973): Hematologic and serum electrolyte values of the C57B1/6J male mouse in maturity and senescence. *Lab. Anim. Sci.,* 23:339–359.
22. Finch, C. E., Foster, J. R., and Mirsky, A. E. (1969): Ageing and the regulation of cell activities during exposure to cold. *J. Gen. Physiol.,* 54:690–712.
23. Finch, C. E., Jonec, V., Hody, G., Walker, J. P., Morton-Smith, W., Alper, A., and Dougher, G. J. (1975): Aging and the passage of L-tyrosine, L-dopa, and inulin into mouse brain slices in vitro. *J. Gerontol.,* 30:33–40.
24. Forno, L. S. (1982): Pathology of Parkinson's disease. In: *Movement Disorders,* edited by C. D. Marsden and S. Fahn, pp. 25–40. Butterworth, London.
25. Forno, L. S., DeLanney, L. E., Irwin, I., and Langston, J. W. (1986): Neuropathology of MPTP-treated monkeys: comparison with the neuropathology of human idiopathic Parkinson's disease. In: *MPTP: A Neurotoxin Producing a Parkinsonian Syndrome,* edited by S. P. Markey, N. Castagnoli Jr., A. J. Trevor, and I. J. Kopin, pp. 119–140. Academic Press, New York.
26. Forno, L. S., Langston, J. W., DeLanney, L. E., Irwin, I., and Ricaurte, G. A. (1986): Locus ceruleus lesions and eosinophilic inculsions in MPTP-treated monkeys. *Ann. Neurol.,* 20:449–455.
27. Fuller, R. W., and Hemrick-Luecke, S. K. (1986): Persistent depletion of striatal dopamine in mice by m-hydroxy-MPTP. *Res. Commun. Chem. Pathol. Pharmacol.,* 53:167–172.
28. Garn, S., Rohman, C. G., and Watner, B. (1967): Bone loss as a general phenomenon in man. *Fed. Proc.,* 26:1729–1736.

29. Graham, D. G. (1978): Oxidative pathways for catecholamines in the genesis of neuro-melanin and cytotoxic quinones. *Mol. Pharmacol.,* 14:633–643.
30. Gupta, M., Gupta, B. K., Thomas, R., Bruemmer, V., Sladek, J. R., Jr., and Felten, D. L. (1986): Aged mice are more sensitive to 1-methyl-4-phenyl-1,2,3,6-tetrahydropyridine treatment than young adults. *Neurosci. Lett.,* 70:326–331.
31. Halliwell, B., and Gutteridge, J. M. (1984): Lipid peroxidation, oxygen radicals, cell damage, and antioxidant therapy, *Lancet,* 2:1396–1397.
32. Heikkila, R. E., Manzino, L., Cabbat, F. S., and Duvoisin, R. C. (1984): Protection against the dopaminergic neurotoxicity of 1-methyl-4-phenyl-1,2,5,6-tetrahydropyridine by monoamine oxidase inhibitors. *Nature,* 311:467–469.
33. Jarvis, M. F., and Wagner, G. C. (1985): Age-dependent effects of 1-methyl-4-phenyl-1,2,3,6-tetrahydropyridine (MPTP). *Neuropharmacology,* 24:581–583.
34. Javitch, J. A., D'Amato, R. J., Strittmatter, S. M., and Snyder, S. H. (1985): Parkinsonism-inducing neurotoxin, n-methyl-4-phenyl-1,2,3,6-tetrahydropyridine: uptake of the metabolite n-methyl-4-phenylpyridine by dopamine neurons explains selective toxicity. *Proc. Natl. Acad. Sci. USA,* 82:2173–2177.
35. Johannessen, J. N., Bacon, J. P., Markey, C. J., Chiueh, C. C., and Markey, S. P. (1986): Striatal dopamine depletion by an aminated analog of MPTP. *Soc. Neurosci. Abstr.,* 12:758.
36. Johannessen, J. N., Chiueh, C. C., Burns, R. S., and Markey, S. P. (1985): Differences in the metabolism of MPTP in the rodent and primate parallel differences in sensitivity to its neurotoxic effects. *Life Sci.,* 36:219–224.
37. Jonec, V., and Finch, C. E. (1975): Ageing and dopamine uptake by subcellular fractions of the C57B1/6J male mouse brain. *Brain Res.,* 91:197–215.
38. Katzman, R. (1976): The prevalence and malignancy of Alzheimer's disease. *Arch. Neurol.,* 33:217–218.
39. Knoll, J. (1981): The pharmacology of selective MAO inhibitors. In: *Monoamine Oxidase Inhibitors—The State of the Art,* edited by M. B. H. Youdim and E. S. Paykel, pp. 45–61 Wiley, Chichester.
40. Koller, W., O'Hara, R., Weiner W., Lang, A., Nutt, J., Agid Y., Bonnet, A. M., and Jankovic, J. (1987): Relationship of aging to Parkinson's disease. In: *Advances in Neurology, Vol. 45, Parkinson's Disease,* edited by M. D. Yahr and K. J. Bergmann, pp. 317–322. Raven Press, New York.
41. Kurland, L. T., Hauser, W. A., Okazaki, H., and Nobrega, F. T. (1969): Epidemiologic studies of parkinsonism with special reference to the cohort hypothesis. In: *Third Symposium on Parkinson's Disease,* edited by F. S. Livingstone, pp. 12–16. Churchill Livingstone, Edinburgh.
42. Langston, J. W. (1985): The case of the tainted heroin. *Sciences,* 25:34–40.
43. Langston, J. W. (1986): MPTP: A neurodegenerative neurotoxin of aging? In: *Proc. 4th Cong. Hung. Pharmacol. Soc. Budapest,* Vol. 3, Sec. 5, *Dopamine, Ageing and Diseases,* edited by L. Kerecsen and L. Gyorgy, pp. 55–60. Akademei Kiado Publishing House of the Hungarian Academy of Science, Budapest.
44. Langston, J. W. (1987): MPTP: The promise of a new neurotoxin. In: *Movement Disorders,* 2, edited by C. D. Marsden and S. Fahn, pp. 73–90. Butterworth, London
45. Langston, J. W., and Ballard, P. A. (1984): Parkinsonism induced by 1-methyl-4-phenyl-1,2,3,6-tetrahydropyridine (MPTP): implications for treatment and the pathogenesis of Parkinson's disease. *Can. J. Neurol. Sci.,* 11:160–165.
46. Langston, J. W., and Irwin, I. (1986): MPTP current concepts and controversies. *Clin. Neuropharmacol.,* 9:485–507.
47. Langston, J. W., and Irwin, I. (1987): Neurotoxins, parkinsonism and Parkinson's disease. *Pharmacol. Ther.,* 32 (Special Issue: *Parkinsonism*):19–49.
48. Langston, J. W., Ballard, P. A., Tetrud, J. W., and Irwin, I. (1983): Chronic parkinsonism in humans due to a product of meperidine-analog synthesis. *Science,* 219:979–980.
49. Langston, J. W., Irwin, I., and DeLanney, L. E. (1987): The biotransformation of MPTP and disposition of MPP$^+$: the effects of aging. *Life Sci.,* 40:749–754.
50. Langston, J. W., Irwin, I., Langston, E. B., and Forno, L. S. (1984): 1-Methyl-4-phenylpyridinium ion (MPP$^+$): identification of a metabolite of MPTP, a toxin selective to the substantia nigra. *Neurosci. Lett.,* 48:87–92.
51. Langston, J. W., Irwin, I., Langston, E. B., and Forno, L. S. (1984): Pargyline prevents MPTP-induced parkinsonism in primates. *Science,* 225:1480–1482.

52. Lewin, R. (1984): Trail of ironies to Parkinson's disease. *Science*, 224:1083–1085.
53. Lewy, F. H.(1982): Paralysis agitans. I. Pathologische anatomie. In: *Handbuch der Neurologie*, edited by M. Lewandowsky, pp. 920–933. Springer, Berlin.
54. Mantle, T. J., Garret, N. J., and Tipton, K. F. (1976): The development of monoamine oxidase in rat liver and brain. *FEBS Lett.*, 64:227–230.
55. Markey, S. P., Johannessen, J. N., Chiueh, C. C., Burns, R. S., and Herkenham, M. A. (1984): Intraneuronal generation of a pyridinium metabolite may cause drug-induced parkinsonism. *Nature*, 311:464–467.
56. Marsden, C. D. (1961): Pigmentation in the nucleus substantiae nigrae of mammals. *J. Anat.*, 95:256–261.
57. Martinovits, G., Melamed, E., Cohen, O., Rosenthal, J., and Uzzan, A. (1986): Systemic administration of antioxidants does not protect mice against the dopaminergic neurotoxicity of 1-methyl-4-phenyl-1,2,5,6-tetrahydropyridine (MPTP). *Neurosci. Lett.*, 69:192–197.
58. Marx, J. (1974): Aging research. II. Pacemakers for aging? *Science*, 186:1196–1197.
59. McGeer., P. L., McGeer, E. G., and Suzuki, J. S. (1977): Aging and extrapyramidal function. *Arch. Neurol.*, 34:33–35.
60. McNeill, T. H., Koek, L. L., and Haycock, J. W. (1984): Age-correlated changes in dopaminergic nigrostriatal perikarya of the C57B1/6NNia mouse. *Mech. Ageing Dev.*, 24:293–307.
61. Miller, C., Haugh, M., Kahn, J., and Anderton, B. (1986): The cytoskeleton and neurofibrillary tangles in Alzheimer's disease. *Trends in Neurosciences*, 9(2):76–81
62. Myers, D. D. (1978): Review of disease patterns and life span in aging mice: genetic and environmental interactions. In: *Birth Defects*, 14:41–53.
63. Perry, T. L., Yong, V. W., Clavier, R. M., Jones, K., Wright, J. M., Foulks, J. G., and Wall, R. A. (1985): Partial protection from the dopaminergic neurotoxin n-methyl-4-phenyl-1,2,3,6-tetrahydropyridine by four different antioxidants in the mouse. *Neurosci. Lett.*, 60:109–114.
64. Prange, A. J., White, J. E., Lipton, M. A., and Kinkead, A. M. (1967): Influence of age on monoamine oxidase and catechol-O-methyltransferase in rat tissues. *Life Sci.*, 6:581–586.
65. Ramsay, R. R., Salach, J. I., Dadgar, J., and Singer, T. P. (1986): Inhibition of mitochondrial NADH dehydrogenase by pyridine derivatives and its possible relation to experimental and idiopathic parkinsonism. *Biochem. Biophys. Res. Commun.*, 135:269–275.
66. Rao, G. V. G., Ts'ao, K., and Draper, H. H. (1972): The effect of fluoride on some physical and chemical characteristics of the bones of ageing mice. *J. Gerontol.*, 27:183–187.
67. Ricaurte, G. A., DeLanney, L. E., Irwin, I., and Langston, J. W. (1987): Older dopaminergic neurons do not recover from the effects of MPTP. *Neuropharmacology*, 26:97–99.
68. Ricaurte, G. A., Irwin, I., Forno, L. S., DeLanney, L. E., Langston, E. B., and Langston, J. W. (1987): Aging and MPTP-induced degeneration of dopaminergic neurons in the substantia nigra. *Brain Res.*, 403:43–51.
69. Riederer, P., and St. Wuketich, S. (1976): Time course of nigrostriatal degeneration in Parkinson's disease. *J. Neural Transm.*, 38:277–301.
70. Robinson, D. S., Davis, J. M., Nies, A., Ravaris, C. L., and Sylwester, D. (1971): Relation of sex and aging to monoamine oxidase activity of human brain, plasma, and platelets. *Arch. Gen. Psychiatry*, 24:536–539.
71. Samorajski, T., and Rolsten, C. (1973): Age and regional differences in the chemical composition of brains of mice, monkeys and humans. *Prog. Brain Res.*, 40:253–265.
72. Selkoe, D. J., Ihara, Y., and Salazar, F. J. (1982): Alzheimer's disease: insolubility of partially purified paired helical filaments in sodium dodecyl sulfate and urea. *Science*, 215:1243–1245.
73. Sershen, H., Mason, M. F., Hashim, A., and Lajthe, A. (1985): Effect of n-methyl-4-phenyl-1,2,3,6-tetrahydropyridine (MPTP) on age-related changes in dopamine turnover and transporter function in the mouse striatum. *Eur. J. Pharmacol.*, 113:135–136.
74. Severson, J. A., and Finch, C. E. (1980): Reduced dopaminergic binding during aging in the rodent striatum. *Brain Res.*, 192:147–162.
75. Wagner, G. C., Jarvis, M. F., and Carelli, R. M. (1985): Ascorbic acid reduced the dopamine depletion induced by MPTP. *Neuropharmacology*, 24:1261–1262.
76. Westlund, K. N., Denney, R. M., Kochersperger, L. M., Rose, R. M., and Abell, C. W. (1985): Distinct monoamine oxidase A and B populations in primate brain. *Science*, 230:181–183.

77. Wilkening, D., Vernier, V. G., Arthaud, L. E., Treacy, G., Kenny, J. P., Nickolson, V. J., Clark, R., Smith, D. H., Smith, C., and Boswell, G. (1986): A Parkinson-like neurologic deficit in primates is caused by a novel 4-substituted piperidine. *Brain Res.*, 368:239–246.
78. Youngster, S. K., Duvoisin, R. C., Hess, A., Sonsalla, P. K., Kendt, M. V., and Heikkila, R. E. (1986): 1-Methyl-4-phenyl-(2'-methylphenyl)-1,2,3,6-tetrahydropyridine [2'CH3MPTP] is a more potent dopaminergic neurotoxin than MPTP in mice. *Eur. J. Pharmacol.*, 122:283–287.
79. Ziering, A., Berger, L., Heineman, S. D., and Lee, J. (1947): Piperidine derivatives. III. 4-Ayrlpiperidines. *J. Org. Chem.*, 12:894–903.

*Aging and the Brain,* edited by R. D. Terry.
Raven Press, New York © 1988.

# Protein Chemistry of Neurofibrillary Tangles and Amyloid Plaques in Alzheimer Disease: Relation to the Cytoskeleton

## Dennis J. Selkoe

*Department of Neurology (Neuroscience), Harvard Medical School; and Center for Neurologic Diseases, Brigham and Women's Hosptial, Boston, Massachusetts 02115*

Research on the biological basis of Alzheimer disease (AD) has accelerated rapidly in the years since it became widely appreciated that dementia of the Alzheimer type is the most common cause of intellectual failure in late life. To observers outside the relatively small but growing field of AD biological research, the studies that have been undertaken have often appeared to be highly diverse and lacking a common thread or unified scientific rationale. Such a variety of seemingly unrelated experimental approaches may be expected when research is undertaken on a complex human brain disorder for which there is little preexisting knowledge regarding mechanism or etiology.

Most of the biological investigations of AD have sought to address one or more of three broad questions: (a) What is the initiating event(s) or cause(s) of progressive age-related neuronal degeneration of the Alzheimer type? (b) Regardless of the cause(s), what are the mechanisms of progressive neuritic and perikaryal degeneration; that is, what is the sequence of molecular alterations that precede neuronal loss? (c) What are the functional characteristics of the neurons that are selectively affected in AD? In particular, what are their neurotransmitter specificities?

Since the discovery of the marked loss of presynaptic cholinergic activity in AD cerebral cortex by three independent research groups in 1976, the third question posed above has received the most experimental attention. It has become clear that several neurotransmitter and neuromodulator substances are altered in cortical and subcortical structures in AD brain. In particular, studies have demonstrated that altered cortical neurites present in neuritic (senile) plaques in cerebral cortex are derived from neurons of varying transmitter specificities and that other dystrophic neurites not organized into discrete plaques are widely scattered in the cortex. These findings have complicated the search for an effective replacement therapy that would provide transmitter precursors or postsynaptic agonists.

The first broad area of inquiry, that involving the search for causative factors, has received increasing attention but is difficult to address directly given the complexity of the disease, its clinical variability, and the lack of strong leads at present. Causative factors such as an unconventional infectious agent, a specific toxin, or some other environmental exposure have not yet become apparent. One initiating factor that is clearly operative in many cases of AD is a genetic predisposition. In certain families the disease appears as an autosomal dominant trait. Recessive or sex-linked forms of transmission have not been clearly documented thus far. The mounting evidence of a genetic factor causing the disease in a significant portion of victims is an important development and is discussed further in the following pages. Epidemiological investigation of AD as regards distribution in various populations, genetic predisposition, and environmental factors should be actively pursued.

Given the difficulty of approaching causative factors directly, efforts to understand the macromolecular alterations that occur prior to neuronal death in AD are accelerating. Much of the effort in this area of research has focused on understanding the basis for the striking structural alterations of neurons, their processes, and their external milieu that are so apparent in Alzheimer brain tissue. It is this area of study, lying between the initiating factors and the ultimate loss of neurotransmitter/neuromodulator function, that is the subject of the present discussion. It should be emphasized that investigations in this area are not viewed as addressing the primary cause of the disease; rather, the protein chemical changes observed are thought to be an effect of the initiating process. However, understanding some of the molecular events underlying widespread neuritic degeneration (and possible regeneration) may provide clues to more fundamental events that precede the classical filamentous lesions in AD. Furthermore, the characterization of structural protein abnormalities leads directly to the identification and study of genes encoding these proteins. In this regard, one wishes to know if any of the protein alterations could be linked directly or indirectly to the gene or family of genes responsible for autosomal dominant AD.

## STRUCTURE AND BIOCHEMISTRY OF PAIRED HELICAL FILAMENTS AND RELATED INTRANEURONAL FIBERS

Before the current biochemical and immunochemical data about the filaments found in neurofibrillary tangles and certain altered neurites in the cerebral cortex can be discussed, the complexity of these fibrous changes at the ultrastructural level should be recalled. Ever since the original electron microscopic descriptions of the abnormal fibers found in both neuronal perikarya [neurofibrillary tangles (NFTs)] and neurites were first described in 1963 (25,54), it has been known that neurons and their processes in AD may contain a variety of ultrastructurally distinguishable fibers. In addition to classical paired helical filaments (PHFs), which are the most commonly observed fibrous element in the neuritic and perikaryal lesions, straight filaments varying in diameter from 10 to 20 nm, often around 15 nm, can occur (32,51,60,64). Certain neurites and cell bodies may contain mixtures of PHFs and straight filaments. Some filaments having diameters close to those of normal neurofilaments (~10 nm) may also be seen. In our experience, certain cases of clinically and light microscopically typical AD have been associated with perikaryal and neuritic filaments that are almost entirely straight, with few if any visible PHFs (D. J. Selkoe, *unpublished observations*). Such cases may show ready disaggregation of the tangles in gentle or harsh solvents; this fact may explain the observation of Iqbal and colleagues that certain AD cases have a high percentage of "soluble" tangles (21). It is not yet clear whether the individual straight filaments comprising such tangles are solubilized into subunit polypeptides or are only disaggregated and therefore no longer microscopically visible by solvent treatment; certainly, some straight filaments can be recovered in sodium dodecyl sulfate (SDS)-insoluble pellets in these cases.

In addition to recognizing bundles containing PHFs and/or abnormal straight filaments in the neurites of senile plaques, antibodies to such fibers can detect the antigens in fine cortical neurites that are widely dispersed in the cerebral cortex and not organized into neuritic plaques. This immunochemical evidence of a more widespread "random" alteration of neurites is in accordance with early electron microscopic studies of AD cerebral cortex. Thus the histopathological concept of AD as "plaque and tangle disease" is a simplification. A more widespread and complex disruption of the neuritic architecture of cortical and subcortical structures is actually observed.

Neurofibrillary tangles are also found in another morphological form, i.e., bundles of abnormal filaments lacking associated neuronal structure and apparently lying free in the extracellular neuropil. Such presumed extracellular tangles, referred to as ghost tangles or tombstones, are particularly prevalent in certain brain regions, e.g., entorrhinal cortex, parahippocampal gyrus, and nucleus basalis. It is generally believed that these structures represent the fibrous residua of once-intraneuronal tangles. One may further speculate that parts or all of these extracellular fibrous masses are slowly catabolized and disappear, as long-surviving cases of AD often demonstrate only moderate numbers of ghost tangles in addition to classical intraneuronal NFTs. Alzheimer himself and other early observers of the morphological changes in AD described the putative transition of neuronal tangles into extracellular fibrous masses. This morphological change is accompanied by an immunochemical transition in which the amount of PHF-reactive antigens is substantially decreased in extracellular compared to intraneuronal tangles (see below).

The issue of extracellular transition forms of NFTs needs to be borne in mind when attempts are made to quantitate the number of NFTs in a particular nucleus or a cortical zone in comparison to other parameters, e.g., degree of clinical dysfunction and extent of neurotransmitter loss. Not all tangles that have existed in a neuronal population are detectable at one sampling point (i.e., at the time of biopsy or autopsy). If a certain small percentage of all neurons in a nuclear structure such as the locus ceruleus display tangles in an AD brain specimen, it may be inferred that a considerably higher percentage of perikarya have been affected over the entire course of the disease to date. The same considerations presumably apply to smaller bundles of PHFs and/or straight filaments found in senile plaques.

## NEUROFILAMENT AND MICROTUBULE-ASSOCIATED PROTEINS

The earliest immunochemical studies (17,63) showed that proteins present in crude microtubule-enriched fractions shared antigens with PHFs and related fibers in NFTs. It soon became apparent that tubulin itself was not the cross-reacting antigen. Unfortunately, the precise peptides that did cross-react with PHFs in these fractions were not established until recently. Work carried out independently in several laboratories during the past 1 to 2 years has now shown that the family of microtubule-associated phosphoproteins designated "tau" are antigenic constituents of PHFs (4,15,28,38,59) and are the antigens responsible, at least in part, for the cross-reaction of PHFs with microtubule-enriched fractions (15). Prior to this discovery, another microtubule-associated protein, designated MAP 2, had been implicated as a component of PHFs, or at least an associated protein, on immunochemical grounds (27,36). Thus at least two microtubule-associated proteins (MAPs) that are heat-stable (do not precipitate upon heating), tau and MAP 2, appear to be implicated in the composition of the abnormal fibers.

The other category of cross-reacting cytoskeletal proteins that have been documented is the family of neurofilament proteins. Among the three principal neurofilament subunits, the two higher-molecular-weight forms [approximately 145 and 200 kilodaltons (KD)] have been found to share epitopes with PHFs and related fibers in AD (1,2,5,9,20,33,40,43,45,53). Although several laboratories have reported polyclonal or monoclonal neurofilament antibodies that label the fibers of NFTs at the light or electron microscopic levels, the interpretation of these findings has been called into question by data demonstrating the cross-reaction of several of these antibodies with phosphorylated tau proteins (39). The latter study demonstrated that antibodies to phosphorylated neurofilament epitopes that recognize the fibers of NFTs also react with tau proteins. Following *in vitro* dephosphorylation of neurofilament and tau proteins, these neurofilament antibodies no longer recognize either protein; nor do they recognize dephosphorylated NFTs in tissue sections. In contrast, several neurofilament monoclonal antibodies that recognize neurofilament proteins, whether phosphorylated or dephosphorylated, do not cross-react with tau and do not stain tangles. These results

suggest that at least some of the cross-reaction between neurofilament proteins and polypeptides of the PHFs may be due to conserved phosphorylated
epitopes that are found on the higher-molecular-weight neurofilament proteins and on tau proteins. Independent evidence for the presence of
neurofilament epitopes not shared with tau proteins is now required. These
new results by no means exclude the presence of neurofilament protein sequences in the PHFs; they only call into question the interpretation of previous immunochemical data linking these two kinds of fiber.

In agreement with the work just summarized is the evidence arising from
antibodies prepared directly against isolated PHFs. The observation of the
relatively high degree of insolubility of many if not most PHFs has led to
methods of preparing PHFs in highly enriched but not purified form (see
below). Polyclonal antibodies to such PHF preparations were observed to
show no reaction with neurofilament proteins; furthermore, immunoblots of
AD and normal aged human brain homogenates failed to reveal any specific
cross-reacting antigens with such PHF antibodies (3,18). A partial explanation for this lack of a cross-reacting normal antigen is provided by the discovery of tau antigens in PHFs. It appears that the amount and stability of tau
proteins in aged normal and AD postmortem brain samples was such that the
cross-reactive tau proteins were not readily detectable in Western blots.
When heat-stable MAP fractions were prepared from young or adult brain
(particularly fetal brain), the cross-reaction of antibodies to PHFs with the tau
proteins was detected (e.g., 28). However, the situation is more complex than
these new findings imply. Extensive absorption of polyclonal PHF antibodies
with heat-stable MAP fractions much enriched in tau and MAP 2 abolish the
staining of these proteins on immunoblots but do not completely eliminate the
staining of PHF-containing structures in brain sections. Moreover, antibodies
against native tau recognize most if not all NFTs and altered neurites but seem
not to react well with the extracellular or ghost tangles found in AD brain.
These results suggest that epitopes other than those shared with normal tau
are present in the fibers of tangles and altered neurites. Whether these other,
as yet unidentified proteins are highly modified from tau protein or represent
entirely distinct polypeptides is not yet clear. It seems likely, however, that
some protein constituents unrelated to tau will be found incorporated into, or
at least closely associated with, PHFs. Thus the nature of the principal subunit
protein of PHF is not yet known. The above statements are also supported by
characterization of monoclonal antibodies raised against isolated NFTs; some
of these antibodies fail to recognize tau proteins, neurofilaments, or any other
specific brain protein examined to date (62).

Even the tau proteins that are now known to be associated with or incorporated into PHFs have characteristics that distinguish them from normal tau in
the mammalian brain. First, the tau protein in AD brain lesions is highly
stable to fixation, even with conventional formaldehyde fixatives. In contrast,
normal tau-containing structures, i.e., axons in fixed postmortem human

brain are not labeled by tau antibodies or by PHF antisera (which contain tau antibodies). Second, the tau proteins associated with PHFs appear to resist *in vitro* proteolytic digestion, e.g., by the nonspecific enzyme proteinase K (37). In contrast, normal mammalian brain tau is completely degraded by this enzyme. Third, the tau associated with PHFs may be abnormally phosphorylated (16,19,39). This altered phosphorylation state may arise following conformational changes of the tau protein that occur when PHFs are formed in the neuronal cytoplasm, or it may precede the incorporation of tau into PHFs. At this juncture, it appears that the tau protein that finds its way into PHFs is considerably altered from its native state.

The various immunochemical results summarized above indicate the difficulty of using antibodies to dissect the composition of these pathological structures. Direct protein chemical approaches have been seriously hampered by the fact that at least a major portion of PHFs and other altered filaments found in AD brain are insoluble in common protein solvents (49). Even heating in strong detergents, e.g., SDS, or exposure to chaotrophic salts such as urea, guanidine hydrochloride, or lithium bromide fails to depolymerize quantitatively PHFs into their subunits (14,49,61). Iqbal and colleagues have observed modest amounts of soluble 50 to 60-KD polypeptides associated with certain PHF-enriched fractions if harsh extraction procedures are not used to prepare the PHFs (and therefore they are less purified). PHF fractions prepared by more extensive detergent extraction have been found to lack these associated soluble polypeptides in gel electrophoretic studies (49,50). One interpretation is that less harsh preparative methods allow the co-purification of soluble, mid-molecular-weight polypeptides, presumably tau proteins (15), that either represent partial precursors of the PHFs or at least are closely associated proteins. Despite this observation, the precise identity of most of the protein comprising PHFs is not apparent from electrophoretic studies, as a large amount of PHF-immunoreactive protein remains insoluble and gel excluded (14,19,21).

These considerations point out the problem of fully purifying paired helical filaments. Their insolubility as well as the fact that their dimensions are similar to amyloid filaments found abundantly in most if not all cases of AD have so far precluded the biochemical purification of PHFs to homogeneity. So long as PHF-enriched fractions are heterogeneous, it will be difficult to determine the precise identity and stoichiometry of the subunit polypeptides making up the fibers. Further attempts to develop a full PHF purification procedure are clearly necessary.

In lieu of such methods, attempts have been made proteolytically to digest PHF-enriched fractions and compare the derived fragments to known proteins by both immunochemical and protein-sequence techniques. Such studies indicate that characteristic peptide fragments derived from PHFs are closely related if not identical to the tau proteins (37). Therefore all currently available data, taken in aggregate, indicate a prominent role for phosphorylated tau proteins in the antigenic structure of PHFs and related straight fibers.

It should be mentioned that the straight filaments that are found in certain NFTs in AD brain as well as the straight filaments comprising the characteristic Pick bodies in Pick disease are recognized by both PHF antibodies and antibodies to neurofilament or microtubule-associated proteins that label PHFs (6,41,44). This cross-reactivity of filaments showing different fine structures suggests that certain cytoskeletal proteins can be assembled into pathological fibers that appear distinct but may be closely related at the protein level. To what extent there are subtle protein compositional differences in these filaments has yet to be determined.

## SIGNIFICANCE OF NFT AND RELATED INTRANEURONAL FILAMENTS

On the basis of comparative studies of neuronal fibers occurring in a variety of presumably unrelated neurodegenerative disorders, it can be said that the various conclusions about PHFs summarized in the preceding section apply equally to the NFTs in a number of human neuropathological conditions (e.g., 8,21). Thus there is no current evidence that AD per se involves a special or unique neuronal cytoskeletal reorganization not seen in other human brain disorders. More likely, progressive protein alteration and formation of abnormal filamentous structures in neuronal cytoplasm may represent a somewhat nonspecific response of certain classes of human neurons to a variety of insults. To date, no specific antigenic or other biochemical characteristics of PHF-bearing neurons in AD have been identified to distinguish them from tangle-bearing neurons found in normal aging, Guam Parkinson–dementia complex, other rare degenerative diseases (8), and even in certain virus or slow virus disorders. One thus needs to question if understanding the detailed molecular origin of PHFs and associated fibers will provide important insights into the initiating factors that trigger widespread neuritic and perikaryal degeneration in AD.

## PROTEIN CHEMISTRY AND IMMUNOCHEMISTRY OF AMYLOID FILAMENTS IN AD

In contrast to the relative nonspecificity of NFTs in human brain disorders, the neuritic plaques with their characteristic amyloid cores appear to be a considerably more specific marker for AD. For all intents and purposes, the neuritic plaque is observed in only three conditions: normal aging, AD, and the Alzheimer-type degenerative process occurring in middle-aged and older patients with Down syndrome. The numerous pathological conditions showing abundant NFTs (e.g, Guam Parkinson–dementia complex, post-encephalitic Parkinson disease, dementia pugilistica) do not display neuritic plaques, except in cases where the affected patient was old enough to be expected to have age-related neuritic plaque formation.

In addition to the relative specificity of neuritic plaques for AD, the widespread diffuse disruption of cortical neurites referred to earlier may also be more characteristic of AD than of other degenerative disorders displaying just NFTs. Therefore the events leading to the morphological alteration and presumed degeneration (and/or regeneration) of innumerable cortical neurites having a variety of transmitter specificities is an important area for further study in AD.

As is well known, neuritic plaques have several morphological components: a peripheral rim of altered neurites (both axonal terminals and dendrites), a central core of extracellular amyloid filaments, and increased numbers of microglial cells and astrocytes. Some but not all of the plaque neurites contain PHFs and/or related straight filaments; many neurites also contain abnormal numbers of mitochondria and lysosomes. A major point of debate has been the frequency of amyloid deposition in the center of neuritic plaques. By light microscopy, many plaques appear to lack amyloid cores. However, published and unpublished observations from several laboratories indicate that most if not all plaques do contain at least small amounts of extracellular amyloid filaments. In this regard, the study of Miyakawa and colleagues is particularly informative (34). In six cases of AD studied by this group, all neuritic plaques that were subjected to serial electron microscopic sectioning revealed not only amyloid filaments in the centers of the plaques but an amyloid-bearing capillary associated with each plaque. The amyloid was apparently found outside the basement membrane at certain points along the extent of the capillary. In earlier studies of the ultrastructure of the neuritic plaque, Wisnewski and Terry had also observed wisps of amyloid (a few filaments) in virtually all neuritic plaques examined in biopsied AD cortex (57). The amount of amyloid in a senile plaque has been used as a criterion to judge the age or "maturity" of the plaque. Very primitive or primitive plaques have been considered to be those that contain altered neurites and glial cells but no light microscopically detectable amyloid. So-called mature plaques contain a halo of neurites and glial cells surrounding a compacted amyloid star. Advanced or "burned out" plaques are those that contain abundant amyloid deposits but few if any demonstrable neurites. Obviously, the order of development of these various forms of senile plaques is impossible to establish with certainty in a nondynamic discipline such as histopathology. However, this classification of plaque types has been rather widely accepted. Regardless of whether it is fully accurate, the hypothesis does not answer the question of whether the amyloid filaments are present prior to neuritic degeneration or form as a consequence of alterations in neurites and glial cells. The fact that many plaques are spherical or cylindrical on serial sectioning and have altered neurites of varying transmitter types might suggest that random neurites present in the vicinity of a nidus for plaque formation (e.g., an extracellular amyloid deposit) become involved in the neuritic plaque in a nonspecific fashion. However, this model of a secondary neuritic degeneration surrounding an initial local glial or microvascular abnormality remains to be proved. Further studies confirming the intriguing findings of Miyakawa et al. (34) will be particularly important.

Several investigators have pointed to the presence of amyloid-bearing capillaries, arterioles, and small arteries in the cerebral cortex and amyloidotic small arteries in the meningeal space in many cases of AD (10,13,24,29,34,56). The presence of microvascular amyloid has been used by authors to propose an early role for localized vascular amyloid deposits in the genesis of senile plaques and perhaps other degenerative changes in AD brain. Glenner has indicated that a high percentage (above 90%) of cases of AD that he examined had some degree of vascular amyloid deposition (10). In our own series of randomly received autopsy brains, we have observed widely varying vascular amyloidosis in all cases of AD that were carefully examined by Congo red staining (24). Thioflavin S fluorescence histochemistry may be an even more sensitive technique to detect minor amounts of amyloid deposition. Theories about the pathogenesis of the lesions of AD need to incorporate the microvascular amyloidosis that is now so commonly observed in AD. Nevertheless, further quantitative morphometric studies attempting to correlate the precise amount and location of capillary amyloid deposits with neuritic pathology, particularly senile plaques, are sorely needed.

A number of immunohistochemical studies have been carried out on the amyloid cores of senile plaques. The results of these studies have been heterogeneous and sometimes conflicting (7,22,23,42,46,52,55). In view of the limitations of immunohistochemistry on amyloid deposits, direct protein chemical approaches have been conducted. Methods to partially enrich or highly purify amyloid cores are now available (31,47). The isolated amyloid core fractions derived from these procedures display the characteristic insolubility of amyloid filaments found in all other known human amyloidoses. However, the solubility of the meningeal vascular amyloid deposits in guanidine hydrochloride, a solvent commonly used to solubilize nonneural amyloid deposits, is not shared with the compacted amyloid cores found in senile plaques (31,47). The more chaotrophic salt guanidine thiocyanate or formic acid can solubilize in considerable part the purified amyloid cores. Two laboratories have reported the release by these solvents of one or more hydrophobic, low-molecular-weight proteins from the cores that have a characteristic amino acid composition (31,47). These analyses indicate a composition highly similar to that previously reported by Glenner and Wong for a meningeal vascular amyloid protein found in vessel fractions from AD but not control meninges (11,12). In the case of the vascular amyloid protein isolated by the latter authors, an unambiguous amino acid sequence representing the first 28 N-terminal amino acids was obtained. In the case of amyloid cores, one laboratory reported an apparently similar sequence but containing considerable N-terminal heterogeneity (31), whereas another laboratory was unable to obtain unambiguous, reproducible sequences from purified amyloid core fractions devoid of vascular amyloid deposits (47). Our laboratory has found that vascular amyloid from meningeal arteries can be isolated by the procedure of Glenner and Wong (11) or by a modified version of the SDS extraction technique used to prepare cores (47) but containing the addition of collagenase; the low-molecular-weight amyloid protein (4–7 KD) solubilized from the meningeal vascular deposits is sequencible, and its sequence is highly similar if not identical to that published by Glenner and Wong (L. Duffy et al., *unpublished data*). The difficulty of sequencing the protein(s) of tissue deposits of amyloid (i.e., senile plaque cores) and their greater insolubility in guanidine hydrochloride suggests that the compacted amyloid cores of neuritic plaques may have undergone some further modifications from the amyloid found in blood vessel walls.

Immunohistochemical studies using antibodies raised either to the native low-molecular-weight amyloid-derived proteins or to synthetic peptides having the sequence reported by Glenner and Wong have generally indicated that vascular amyloid deposits and senile plaque cores are antigenically indistinguishable (31,47,58). One group has found that certain anti-amyloid peptide antibodies also recognize some neurofibrillary tangles (30). This result has never been observed in our own laboratory using antibodies to either the synthetic peptide or the native amyloid protein (47), nor have Wong et al. reported such cross-reactivity between tangles and amyloid (30). Masters et al. have further reported (30) that PHF-enriched fractions contain a protein having the same sequence (but even greater N-terminal heterogeneity) as the amyloid core proteins and the vascular amyloid sequenced by Glenner and Wong. An important caveat in this regard is the possibility of contamination by varying amounts of amyloid filaments in PHF-enriched fractions; certainly it has been observed in fractions prepared by our method. So long as mixed fiber fractions are used either for amino acid analyses, sequencing, or immunization, the precise relation of PHFs to extraneuronal amyloid filaments will not be possible to determine.

Several observations about the biology of AD and other neurofibrillary degenerations tend to favor the notion of distinct protein origins for intracellular PHFs and extracellular amyloid filaments in AD. A number of neurological disorders display abundant NFTs, including extracellular NFTs, but show no amyloidosis and no senile plaque formation whatsoever. These include Guam Parkinson–dementia complex, postencephalitic Parkinson disease, certain variants of Hallervorden-Spatz disease, dementia pugilistica, and even Pick disease, in which the Pick body filaments cross-react with PHFs but no amyloidosis is seen. Furthermore, extensive numbers of ghost tangles can be found in some areas of AD brain, e.g., parahippocampus, that display no extracellular amyloid filaments. Subcortical nuclei such as the nucleus basalis or the locus ceruleus can also show large numbers of NFTs, both intra- and extraneuronal, but no local amyloid deposition. Importantly, extensive amyloid filaments that are immunochemically indistinguishable from those in the neuritic plaque cores are found in the walls of the meningeal artery outside the brain; this locus makes it less likely that the amyloid in question derives from neuronal cells inside the brain. All polyclonal and monoclonal antibodies reported to date that recognize NFTs, with one exception (31), have not been reported to stain the amyloid cores of senile plaques. Absorption of a mixed PHF antiserum that also contains antibodies against amyloid using purified, sonicated plaque cores causes abolition of the core staining but no significant change in the staining of NFTs and PHF-bearing plaque neurites. The amyloid filaments are 4 to 9 nm in diameter, unpaired, and have an ultrastructure clearly distinct from that of PHFs. The former are found extracellularly, whereas the latter clearly arise intraneuronally.

Perhaps the most compelling argument to date for the apparently distinct origins of amyloid filaments and PHFs in AD comes from comparative studies of microvascular and senile plaque amyloid deposits in other aged mammals (48). We have used a panel of antibodies produced against amyloid filaments and their constituent proteins from human (AD) central nervous system to demonstrate complete cross-reaction with cerebral and microvascular amyloid deposits in five other species of aged mammals, including monkey, orangutan, bear, and dog. The 28-amino-acid peptide, representing the only currently known protein sequence in AD amyloid, was detectable in the cortical and cerebrovascular amyloid of all aged mammals examined. These results demonstrate the conservation among several aged mammalian species of the amyloid proteins associated with cortical degeneration in AD. The findings have implications for theories about the pathogenesis of neuritic degeneration in AD and indicate that aged primates provide biochemically relevant models for certain principal features of AD. Moreover, the absence of PHFs or other perikaryal fibrous inclusions by either microscopy or immunocytochemistry in all of these nonhuman mammals and the presence of immunochemically indistinguishable amyloid deposits would further complicate the hypothesis that amyloid in AD derives from intraneuronal PHFs and actually represents the same protein. However, further detailed studies of PHF-derived proteins in comparison to the proteins of amyloid filaments are required to settle fully the relation of these two kinds of insoluble, $\beta$-pleated sheet fibers in AD brain.

It should be mentioned at this juncture that x-ray diffraction analyses on partially purified PHFs and on amyloid cores purified by fluorescence-activated cell sorting have been carried out (26). The diffraction patterns demonstrate intramolecular spacings that are consistent with the presence of cross-$\beta$-pleated sheet structure in these fibers. The work with PHFs needs to be confirmed when a method of complete purification of these fibers is achieved. The present data support the widely assumed notion that both PHFs and amyloid filaments in AD and aged brain are organized in a cross-$\beta$-

pleated sheet confirmation, given their characteristic tinctorial properties with Congo red and thioflavin. What is particularly unusual in the case of AD is that one form of amyloid-like $\beta$-pleated sheet fiber, i.e., the PHFs, occurs intraneuronally, whereas virtually all human and animal amyloid deposits described in neural and non-neural organs to date have been extracellular. Furthermore, the PHFs have a fine structure quite distinct from that of conventional extracellular amyloid filaments in various organs. It may therefore be appropriate not to refer to PHFs as amyloid fibers per se.

## APPROACHES TO POSSIBLE EXTRACEREBRAL ORIGINS OF AD AMYLOID PROTEINS

In view of the apparent lack of a rigorous relation between the PHFs and the extracellular amyloid filaments in AD and normal aged brain, we have attempted to determine if extracerebral proteins contribute to the amyloid deposits seen in meningeal and parenchymal blood vessels and senile plaques. We have used several polyclonal AD amyloid antibodies to screen human plasmas and have observed several cross-reacting polypeptides in both normal and AD plasma. The most consistent and strongly reacting plasma proteins have approximate molecular weights of 95, 88, 47 to 49, and 32 KD, although other faintly reactive proteins are seen with certain amyloid antisera at higher molecular weights. The specificity of this cross-reaction was determined by absorbing the amyloid antisera recognizing these plasma proteins with either amyloid core fractions or with identically prepared fractions from normal aged cerebral cortex lacking amyloid. These results unequivocally showed that only the amyloid-bearing fractions abolished the staining of these proteins by amyloid antisera; control absorption did nothing. The possibility that the amyloid cores were nonspecifically absorbing antibodies in our antisera was eliminated by showing that extensive absorption of a PHF-specific antiserum with amyloid cores did not alter its staining of NFTs in AD brain sections or of tau proteins on immunoblots. Absorption of the amyloid antisera with total plasma proteins eliminated the staining of the aforementioned plasma proteins on blots and diminished but did not abolish the staining of amyloid deposits in cerebral vessels and plaque cores. Absorption of a mixed antiserum containing both PHFs and amyloid antibodies with large amounts of tau protein essentially abolished the staining of neurofibrillary tangles in plaque neurites but did not significantly decrease the staining of amyloid filaments or the reaction of the antiserum on the indicated plasma proteins. All of these analyses were carried out in blinded fashion. Our results indicate that certain plasma proteins present in normal and AD blood share epitopes with the amyloid filaments in blood vessels and plaque cores in AD and aged brain.

We have also used affinity purification of polyclonal antibodies on nitrocellulose strips containing the plasma proteins of interest. Such affinity-purified antibodies recognize the plasma protein to which they were bound as well as amyloid in vessels and plaque cores in AD brain sections. In contrast, antibodies bound to areas of an immunoblot not containing immunoreactive plasma proteins produce no staining of AD amyloid deposits.

We are now in the process of attempting to purify certain of the immuno-reactive plasma proteins, particularly those at ~95 and ~88 KD, which appear to be the most immunoreactive bands. Rigorous determination of the relation of these plasma proteins to the amyloid filaments in AD brain requires identification and sequencing of the proteins, the preparation of oligopeptides and then antibodies to these oligopeptides, and the demonstration that these peptides are indeed contained within the amyloid filaments in AD brain. At present, we can state only that there are cross-reactive plasma proteins detectable with amyloid antibodies but not with PHF antibodies and other hyperimmune sera.

Even if a precise relation of a plasma protein to amyloid in AD can be rigorously demonstrated, this finding does not preclude the possibility of considerable local processing of an amyloid precursor in perithelial, micro-glial, or other brain cells and/or the addition of amyloid protein constituents deriving solely from the nervous system. Nonetheless, this early work raises the intriguing possibility that the amyloid deposition so commonly observed in AD brain and to a much lesser extent in normal aging derives *in part* from an extracerebral source. Such a model would have some analogy to other known amyloidoses, including some that affect the nervous system, e.g., familial amyloidotic polyneuropathy in certain ethnic groups. In the latter autosomal dominant disorders, single amino acid substitutions in a normal plasma protein precursor (transthyretin or prealbumin) have been demonstrated in the amyloid filaments that form deposits in peripheral nerves. There are a number of forms of amyloidosis in humans, some of which may represent primary disorders at the gene or protein level whereas others are clearly a secondary reactive phenomenon. Into which category the amyloid of AD falls is presently unknown.

## MOLECULAR GENETIC APPROACHES
## TO THE FIBROUS LESIONS OF AD

Progress in the immunochemistry and protein chemistry of altered intra- and extraneuronal filaments in AD and aged brain now enables the application of specific molecular biological techniques to this complex disorder. Human cDNAs encoding microtubule-associated proteins that have been implicated in NFT formation, i.e., MAP 2 (35) and tau, have now been isolated from expression libraries. The cDNAs will be sequenced and can also be used in Northern analysis and *in situ* hybridization studies to answer the question of whether the message for MAP 2 and/or tau is altered in AD brain compared to non-AD brain and in tangle-bearing versus non-tangle-bearing neurons. Several laboratories are currently attempting to isolate cDNAs encoding amyloid-related proteins in AD, and this task should soon be accomplished. Such work is important in determining the precise tissue and cellular origin of the protein(s) comprising amyloid in AD and aged brain, its level of expression in various tissues during aging, and its relation to other amyloidogenic proteins, including those apparently neuronal proteins that comprise the PHFs.

## CONCLUSION

The various approaches summarized in this chapter do not necessarily address the question of the cause(s) of age-related neuronal degeneration of the Alzheimer type. However, it is likely that further progress in understanding the origin and nature of amyloid proteins and the deciphering of the complete composition of PHFs will provide major clues to what kind of cellular process underlies these lesions. Particularly important will be the use of cloned DNAs encoding these proteins in more dynamic studies of PHFs and amyloid filament formation in the brain and/or in nonneural organs. The finding of immunochemically closely similar amyloid deposits in several aged mammals provides an attractive system for controlled, longitudinal experiments of senile plaque and microvascular amyloid deposition during the aging process. With the increasing number of investigators concentrating on this line of biological research in AD, the probability of significant developments over the next several years is high. One can hope that this work will lead to a better understanding of the genetic basis of AD in those families displaying autosomal dominant forms of the disorder and in patients with Down syndrome.

## REFERENCES

1. Anderton, B. H., Breinburg, D., Downes, M. J., Green, P. J., Tomlinson, B. E., Ulrich, J., Wood, J. N., and Kahn J. (1982): Monoclonal antibodies show that neurofibrillary tangles and neurofilaments share antigenic determinants. *Nature,* 298:84–86.
2. Autilio-Gambetti, L., Gambetti, P., Crane, R. C. (1983): Paired helical filaments: relatedness to neurofilaments shown by silver staining and reactivity with monoclonal antibodies. In: *Banbury Report 15: Biological Aspects of Alzheimer's Disease,* pp. 117–124, edited by R. Katzman. Cold Spring Harbor Laboratory, New York.
3. Brion, J. P., Couck, A. M., Passareiro, E., and Flament-Durand, J. (1985): Neurofibrillary tangles of Alzheimer's disease: an immunohistochemical study. *J. Submicrosc. Cytol.,* 17:89–96.
4. Brion, J. P., van den Bosch de Aguilar, P., and Flament-Duran, J. (1985): In: *Advances in Applied Neurological Science: Senile Dementia of the Alzheimer Type,* edited by J. Traber and W. H. Gispens, pp. 164–174. Springer, Berlin.
5. Cork, L. C., Sternberger, N. H., Sternberg, C. A., Casanova, M. F., Struble, R. G., and Price, D. C. (1986): Phosphorylated neurofilament antigens in neurofibrillary tangles in Alzheimer's disease. *J. Neuropathol. Exp. Neurol.,* 455:56–64.
6. Dickson, D. W., Kress, Y., Crowe, A., and Yen, S-H. (1985): Monoclonal antibodies to

Alzheimer's neurofibrillary tangles. 2. Demonstration of a common antigenic determinant between ANT and neurofibrillary degeneration in progressive supranuclear palsy. *Am. J. Pathol.*, 120:292–303.

7. Eikelenbloom, P., and Stam, F. C. (1982): Immunoglobulins and complement factors in senile plaques: an immunoperoxidase study. *Acta Neuropathol. (Berl.)*, 57:239–242.
8. Feldman, R. G., Chandler, K. A., Levy, L. L., Glaser, G. H. (1963): Familial Alzheimer's disease. *Neurology*, 13:811–824.
9. Gambetti, P., Velasco, M. E., Dahl, D., Bignami, A., Roessmann, U., and Sindely, S. D. (1980): Alzheimer neurofibrillary tangles: an immunohistochemical study. In: *Aging of the Brain and Dementia*, edited by L. Amaducci, A. N. Davison, and P. Antuono. Raven Press, New York.
10. Glenner, G. G. (1983): Alzheimer's disease: multiple cerebral amyloidosis. In: *Banbury Report 15: Biological Aspects of Alzheimer's Disease*, edited by R. Katzman, pp. 137–144. Cold Spring Harbor Laboratory, New York.
11. Glenner, G. G., and Wong, C. W. (1984): Alzheimer's disease: initial report of the purification and characterization of a novel cerebrovascular amyloid protein. *Biochem. Biophys. Res. Commun.*, 120:885–890.
12. Glenner, G. G., and Wong, C. W. (1984): Alzheimer's disease and Down's syndrome: sharing of a unique cerebrovascular amyloid fibril protein. *Biochem. Biophys. Res. Commun.*, 122:1131–1135.
13. Glenner, G. G., Henry, J. H., and Fujihara, S. (1981): Congophilic angiopathy in the pathogenesis of Alzheimer's degeneration. *Ann. Pathol.*, 1:120–129.
14. Gorevic, P., Goni, F., Pons-Estel, B., Alvarez, F., Peress, R., and Frangione, B. (1986): Isolation and partial characterization of neurofibrillary tangles and amyloid plaque core in Alzheimer's disease: immunohistological studies. *J. Neuropathol. Exp. Neurol.*, 45:647–664.
15. Grundke-Iqbal, I., Iqbal, K., Quinlan, M., Turg, Y-C., Zaidi, M. S., and Wisniewski, H. M. (1986): Microtubule-associated protein tau: a component of Alzheimer paired helical filaments. *J. Biol. Chem.*, 261:6084–6089.
16. Grundke-Iqbal, I., Iqbal, K., Turg, Y-C., Quinlan, M., Wisniewski, H. M., and Binder, L. I. (1986): Abnormal phosphorylation of the microtubule-associated protein tau in Alzheimer cytoskeletal pathology. *Proc. Natl. Acad. Sci. USA*, 83:4913–4917.
17. Grundke-Iqbal, I., Johnson, A. B., Terry, R. D., Wisniewski, H. M., and Iqbal, K. (1979): Alzheimer neurofibrillary tangles: antiserum and immunohistochemical staining. *Ann. Neurol.*, 6:532–537.
18. Ihara, Y., Abraham, C., and Selkoe, D. J. (1983): Antibodies to paired helical filaments in Alzheimer's disease do not recognize normal brain proteins. *Nature*, 304:727–730.
19. Ihara, Y., Nukina, N., Miura, R., and Ogawarra, M. (1986): Phosphorylated tau protein is integrated into paired helical filaments in Alzheimer's disease. *J. Biochem.*, 99:1807–1810.
20. Ihara, Y., Nukina, N., Sugita, H., and Toyokura, V. (1981): Staining of Alzheimer's neurofibrillary tangles with antiserum against 200K component of neurofilament. *Proc. Jpn. Acad.*, 57:152–156.
21. Iqbal, K., Zaidi, T., Thompson, C. H., Merz, P. A., and Wisniewski, H. M. (1984): Alzheimer paired helical filaments: bulk isolation, solubility and protein composition. *Acta Neuropathol. (Berl.)*, 62:167–177.
22. Ishii, T., and Haga, S. (1984): Immuno-electron-microscopic localization of complements in amyloid fibrils of senile plaques by means of fluorescent antibody technique. *Acta Neuropathol. (Berl.)*, 32:157–162.
23. Ishii, T., Haga, S., and Shimizu, F. (1975): Identification of components of immunoglobulins in senile plaques by means of fluorescent antibody technique. *Acta Neuropathol. (Berl.)*, 32:157–162.
24. Joachim, C. L., Morris, J., and Selkoe, D. J. (1986): Autopsy neuropathology in 76 cases of clinically diagnosed Alzheimer's disease. *Neurology*, 36(Suppl. 1):226 (abstract).
25. Kidd, M. (1963): Paired helical filaments in electron microscopy of Alzheimer's disease. *Nature*, 197:192–193.
26. Kirschner, D. A., Abraham, C., and Selkoe, D. J. (1986): X-ray diffraction from intraneuronal paired helical filaments and extraneuronal amyloid fibers in Alzheimer disease indicates cross-$\beta$ conformation. *Proc. Natl. Acad. Sci. USA*, 83:503–507.
27. Kosik, K. S., Duffy, L. K., Dowling, M. M., Abraham, C., McCluskey, A., and Selkoe,

D. J. (1984): Microtubule-associated protein 2: monoclonal antibodies demonstrate the selective incorporation of certain epitopes into Alzheimer neurofibrillary tangles. *Proc. Natl. Acad. Sci. USA,* 81:7941–7945.

28. Kosik, K. S., Joachim, C. L., and Selkoe, D. J. (1986): The microtubule-associated protein, tau, is a major antigenic component of paired helical filaments in Alzheimer's disease. *Proc. Natl. Acad. Sci. USA,* 83:4044–4048.

29. Mandybur, T. I. Cerebral amyloid angiopathy: the vascular pathology and complications. *J. Neuropathol. Exp. Neurol.,* 45:79–90.

30. Masters, C. L., Multhaup, G., Simms, G., Pottigiesser, J., Martins, R. N., and Beyreuther, K. (1985): Neuronal origin of a cerebral amyloid: neurofibrillary tangles of Alzheimer's disease contain the same protein as the amyloid of plaque cores and blood vessels. *EMBO J.,* 4:2757–2763.

31. Masters, C. L., Simms, G., Weinman, N. A., Multhaup, G., McDonald, B. L., Beyreuther, K. (1985): Amyloid plaque protein in Alzheimer's disease and Down's syndrome. *Proc. Natl. Acad. Sci. USA,* 82:4245–4249.

32. Metuzals, J., Montpetit, V., and Clapin, D. F. (1981): Organization of the neurofilamentous network. *Cell Tissue Res.,* 214:455–482.

33. Miller, C. J., Brion, J-P., Calvert, R., Chin, T. K., Eagles, P. A. M., Downes, M. J., Flament-Durand, J., Haugh, M., Kahn, J., Probst, A., Ulrich, J., and Anderton, B. H. (1986): Alzheimer's paired helical filaments share epitopes with neurofilament sidearms. *EMBO J.,* 5:269–276.

34. Miyakawa, T., Shimoji, A., Kuramoto, R., and Higuchi, Y. (1982): The relationship between senile plaques and cerebral blood vessels in Alzheimer's disease and senile dementia: morphological mechanism of senile plaque production. *Virchows Arch. [Cell Pathol.],* 40:121–129.

35. Neve, R., Selkoe, D. J., Kurnit, D. M., and Kosik, K. S. (1987): A cDNA for a human microtubule-associated protein 2 epitope in the Alzheimer neurofibrillary tangle. *Molec. Brain Res.,* 1:193–196.

36. Nukina, N., and Ihara, Y. (1983): Immunocytochemical study on senile plaques in Alzheimer's disease. II. Abnormal dendrites in senile plaques as revealed by antimicrotubule-associated proteins (MAPs) immunostaining. *Proc. Jpn. Acad.,* 59:288–292.

37. Nukina, N., and Ihara, Y. (1985): Proteolytic fragments of Alzheimer's paired helical filaments. *J. Biochem.,* 98:1715–1718.

38. Nukina, N., and Ihara, Y. (1986): One of the antigenic determinants of paired helical filaments is related to tau protein. *J. Biochem.,* 99:1541–1544.

39. Nukina, N., and Selkoe, D. J. (1987): Recognition of Alzheimer paired helical filaments by monoclonal neurofilament antibodies is due to crossreaction with tau protein. *Proc. Natl. Acad. Sci. USA ,* 84:3415–3419.

40. Perry, G., Rizzuto, N., Autilio-Gambetti, L., and Gambetti, P. (1985): Alzheimer's paired helical filaments contain cytoskeletal components. *Proc. Natl. Acad. Sci. USA,* 82:3916–3920.

41. Perry, G., Stewart D., Autilio-Gambetti, L., and Gambetti, P. (1986): Pick body straight filaments contain neurofilament and microtubule elements. *J. Neuropathol. Exp. Neurol.,* 45:332(abstract).

42. Powers J. M., Schlaepfer, W. W., Willingham, M. C., and Hall, B. J. (1981): An immunoperoxidase study of senile cerebral amyloidosis with pathogenic considerations. *J. Neuropathol. Exp. Neurol.,* 40:592–612.

43. Rasool, C. G., and Selkoe, D. J. (1984): Alzheimer's disease: exposure of neurofilament immunoreactivity in SDS-insoluble paired helical filaments. *Brain Res.,* 322:194–198.

44. Rasool, C. G., and Selkoe, D. J. (1985): Sharing of specific antigens by degenerating neurons in Pick's disease and Alzheimer's disease. *N. Engl. J. Med.,* 312:700–705.

45. Rasool, C. G., Abraham, C., Anderton, B. H., Haugh, M. C., Kahn, J. and Selkoe, D. J. (1984): Alzheimer's disease: immunoreactivity of neurofibrillary tangles with anti-neurofilament and anti-paired helical filament antibodies. *Brain Res.,* 310:249–260.

46. Rowe, I. F., Nensson, O., Lewis, P. D., Candy, J., Tennent, G. A., and Pepys, M. B. (1984): Immunohistochemical demonstration of amyloid P component in cerebrovascular amyloidosis. *Neuropathol. Appl. Neurobiol.,* 10:53–61.

47. Selkoe, D. J., Abraham, C. R., Podlisny, M. B., and Duffy, L. K. (1986): Isolation of low-

molecular-weight proteins from amyloid plaque fibers in Alzheimer's disease. *J. Neurochem.*, 146:1820–1834.

48. Selkoe, D. J., Bell, D., Podlisny, M. B., Cork, L. C., and Price, D. L. (1987): Conservation of brain amyloid proteins in several aged mammals and in humans with Alzheimer's disease. *Science*, 235:873–877.

49. Selkoe, D. J., Ihara, Y., and Salazar, F. J. (1982): Alzheimer's disease: insolubility of partially purified helical filaments in sodium dodecyl sulfate and urea. *Science*, 215:1243–1245.

50. Selkoe, D. J., Ihara, Y., Abraham, C., Rasool, C. G., and McCluskey, A. H. (1983): Biochemical and immunocytochemical studies of Alzheimer paired helical filaments. In: *Banbury Report 15: Biological Aspects of Alzheimer's Disease*, edited by R. Katzman, pp. 125–134. Cold Spring Harbor Laboratory, New York.

51. Shibayama, H., and Kitoh, J. (1978): Electron microscopic structure of Alzheimer's neurofibrillary changes in a case of atypical senile dementia. *Acta Neuropathol. (Berl.)*, 41:229–234.

52. Shirahama, T., Skinner, M., Westermark, P., Rubinow, A., Cohen, A. S., Brun, A., and Kemper, T. L. (1982): Senile cerebral amyloid: prealbumin as a common constituent in the neuritic plaque, in the neurofibrillary tangles, and in the microangiopathic lesion. *Am. J. Pathol.*, 197:41–50.

53. Sternberger, N. H., Sternberger, L. A., and Ulrich, J. (1985): Aberrant neurofilament phosphorylation in Alzheimer's disease. *Proc. Natl. Acad. Sci. USA*, 82:4274–4276.

54. Terry, R. D. (1963): The fine structure of neurofibrillary tangles in Alzheimer's disease. *J. Neuropathol. Exp. Neurol.* 22:629–642.

55. Torack, R. M., and Lynch, R. G. (1981): Cytochemistry of brain amyloid in adult dementia. *Acta Neuropathol. (Berl.)*, 53:189–196.

56. Vanley, C. T., Aguilar, M. J., Kleinhenz, R. J., and Lagios, M. D. (1981): Cerebral amyloid angiopathy. *Hum. Pathol.*, 12:609–616.

57. Wisniewski, H. M., and Terry, R. D. (1973): Reexamination of the pathogenesis of the senile plaque. *Prog. Neuropathol.* 2:1–26.

58. Wong, C. W., Quaranta, V., and Glenner, G. G. (1985): Neuritic plaques and cerebrovascular amyloid in Alzheimer disease are antigenically related. *Proc. Natl. Acad. Sci. USA*, 82:8729–8732.

59. Wood, J. G., Mirra, S. S., Pollock, N. J., and Binder, L. I. (1986): Neurofibrillary tangles of Alzheimer's disease share antigenic determinants with the axonal microtubule-associated protein tau. *Proc. Natl. Acad. Sci. USA*, 83:4040–4043.

60. Yagashita, S., Itoh, T., Nan, W., and Amano, N. (1981): Reappraisal of the fine structure of Alzheimer's neurofibrillary tangles. *Acta Neuropathol. (Berl.)*, 54:239–246.

61. Yen, S-H., and Kress, Y. (1983): The effect of chemical reagents or proteases on the ultrastructure of paired helical filaments. In: *Banbury Report 15: Biological Aspects of Alzheimer's Disease*, edited by R. Katzman, pp. 155–165. Cold Spring Harbor Laboratory, New York.

62. Yen, S-H., Crowe, A., and Dickson, D. W. (1985): Monoclonal antibodies to Alzheimer's neurofibrillary tangles. I. Identification of polypeptides. *Am. J. Pathol.*, 120:282–291.

63. Yen, S-H., Gaskin, F., and Terry, R. D. (1981): Immunocytochemical studies of neurofibrillary tangles. *Am. J. Pathol.* 104:77–89.

64. Yoshimura, N. (1984): Evidence that paired helical filaments originate from neurofilaments. *Clin. Neuropathol.*, 3:22–27.

*Aging and the Brain*, edited by R. D. Terry.
Raven Press, New York © 1988.

# Amyloidogenic $A_4$ Protein Subunit: Clues to the Pathogenesis of the Neurofibrillary Tangle, Alzheimer Plaque, and Congophilic Angiopathy

Colin L. Masters and *Konrad Beyreuther

*Neuromuscular Research Institute, Department of Pathology, University of Western Australia, Western Australia 6009, and Department of Neuropathology, Royal Perth Hospital, Perth, Western Australia 6001; and *Institute of Genetics, University of Cologne, D-5000 Cologne 41, Federal Republic of Germany*

> One cannot pretend that the structures blackened here by silver possess any morphological relationship to the neurofibrils normally present in these cells.
> *Max Bielschowsky (13) on the Alzheimer neurofibrillary tangle*

There are three forms of amyloid protein deposition in the brain in Alzheimer disease (AD): the intracellular neurofibrillary tangle (NFT) and extracellular amyloid deposits comprising the Alzheimer plaque core (APC) and congophilic angiopathy (ACA) (Table 1). Present accounts of the structure of the NFT in AD tend to substantiate Bielschowsky's opinion, based as it was on the argyrophilic properties of the fibrillar material that is deposited in the soma of neurons and in neurites around the periphery of the plaque. However, if the NFT does not have its origin from normal neurofilaments, is it derived from some modified component of the cytoskeleton or from some completely unrelated macromolecule? Our studies (96,97; *unpublished data*) support the latter possibility, whereas those of other investigators (5,6,21,28,48–50,55–60,62,66–71,74,82,83,103,108,113,115,118,119,125–127, 137,142,148,160,163–165) indicate that a variety of modified normal cytoskeletal proteins (e.g., tau, MAP2, NF-H, M) are the major protein subunits of the NFT. In fact, it is possible that both theories may turn out to be correct: the $A_4$ protein subunit we have described as the major protein component of the NFT may be decorated with normal cytoskeletal components.

In this chapter we review the currently available evidence on the morphology, biochemistry, and immunochemistry of the amyloid protein depositions in AD. Because these amyloid deposits form the pathognomonic basis of AD, it hardly needs stressing that an understanding of their molecular pathogenesis is a prerequisite for an understanding of the cause of AD. Because AD occupies a pivotal position in relation to certain other chronic degenerative

TABLE 1. *Structural basis of AD*

---

*Pathognomonic light microscopic changes*
   Intracellular fibrillar amyloid deposits
      Neurofibrillary tangles (NFTs) composed of paired helical filaments (PHFs) and single
         "straight" filaments.
      NFTs accumulate within neuronal soma and in presynaptic axonal terminals surround-
         ing the plaque (neuritic degeneration, dystrophic neurites, regenerative neurites).
   Extracellular fibrillar amyloid deposits
      Infiltration then condensation of amyloid, leading to crystalline amyloid plaque cores
         (APCs) either of the *amorphous* or *compact* type, usually with surrounding neuritic
         degeneration.
      Amyloid congophilic angiopathy (ACA) with or without surrounding neuritic degenera-
         tion.

*Associated changes*
   Possibly a more extensive and subtle neuritic change caused by the deposition of the $A_4$
      protein affecting synapses throughout the neuropil.
   Neuronal loss and gliosis in areas affected by amyloid deposition.
   Granulovacuolar degeneration in hippocampal pyramidal cells.
   Hirano body formation.

---

diseases of the central nervous system (Fig. 1; Table 2), it is likely that this understanding of the pathogenesis of the AD amyloid proteins will have wide ramifications.

## MORPHOLOGICAL STUDIES OF AMYLOID DEPOSITIONS IN AD

The classic morphological descriptions of the NFT, APC, and ACA at both light and electron microscopic levels are still subject to reinterpretation and controversy. For example, it is not clear whether the paired helical filament (PHF) is the only structural component to the NFT or single straight filaments (SSFs) coexist with the PHF. Observations on the straight filaments of the NFT in progressive supranuclear palsy (105) have shown that these straight filaments may have a protofilamentous substructure similar to that of the PHF of AD (PHF-AD). These studies also have shown an apparent continuity within single straight and PHFs. These observations are of more than passing interest, as our (96) biochemical studies indicate that the same protein subunit is the major component of the intracellular PHF and the extracellular SSF.

The extracellular SSFs (i.e., the amyloid fibrils in the APC and ACA) also show a twisted periodic substructure, suggesting at least two protofilamentous domains within the individual fibril (101,109). Such twisted bifilar helices are now accepted as the rule for most types of amyloid fibril, whether of systemic or cerebral origin, natural or synthetic. The globular nature of the subunits visualized by high-resolution electron microscopy (29,155,157,158) may allow the differences between PHFs and SSFs to be explained on the basis of the

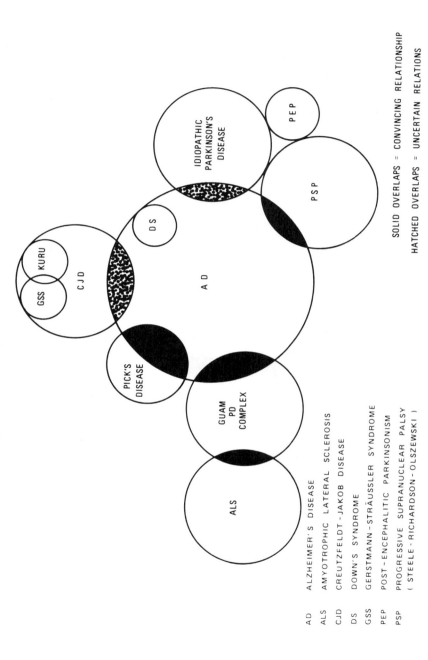

SOLID OVERLAPS = CONVINCING RELATIONSHIP

HATCHED OVERLAPS = UNCERTAIN RELATIONS

AD    ALZHEIMER'S DISEASE

ALS   AMYOTROPHIC LATERAL SCLEROSIS

CJD   CREUTZFELDT-JAKOB DISEASE

DS    DOWN'S SYNDROME

GSS   GERSTMANN-STRÄUSSLER SYNDROME

PEP   POST-ENCEPHALITIC PARKINSONISM

PSP   PROGRESSIVE SUPRANUCLEAR PALSY
      ( STEELE-RICHARDSON-OLSZEWSKI )

**FIG. 1.** Interrelations between Alzheimer disease and several other chronic neurological disorders. There is now definitive biochemical evidence that the NFTs in the Guam Parkinson–dementia (PD) complex is the same as in AD (Fig. 3), but the biochemical nature of the NFTs in Pick disease and progressive supranuclear palsy has yet to be determined. Similar membrane glycoproteins are now known to form the basis of the amyloid depositions in AD and the unconventional virus diseases. The basis of the dementing process in idiopathic Parkinson disease is still subject to controversy.

TABLE 2. *Conditions in which cerebral amyloid depositions occur*

---

A. *As intracellular neurofibrillary tangles*
  1. As an essential component of the disease process
     a. Alzheimer disease (including aged Down syndrome)
     b. Progressive supranuclear palsy (Steele-Richardson-Olszewski)
     c. Guam amyotrophic lateral sclerosis/parkinsonism–dementia complex
     d. Dementia pugilistica
     e. Pick disease
  2. Reported to occur in a proportion of cases and at a level above that expected as a coincidental finding
     a. Virus-induced: subacute sclerosing panencephalitis
     b. Toxin-induced: lead, manganese poisoning
     c. Diffuse metabolic: tuberous sclerosis, neuroaxonal dystrophy, Spatz disease, Cockayne's syndrome
     d. Localized malformative: meningoangiomatosis (61)
  3. Isolated case reports where the association may be only coincidental: herpes and rabies virus infection; Creutzfeldt-Jakob disease; amyotrophic lateral sclerosis; chronic tuberculosis; scarlet fever; hereditary spastic spinal paresis; familial cerebellar ataxia; storage disease; lipofuscinosis; ganglioglioma

B. *As extracellular amyloid plaques and/or angiopathy*
  1. Alzheimer disease (including aged Down syndrome)
  2. Unconventional virus disease (including scrapie, kuru, Creutzfeldt-Jakob disease, and Gerstmann-Sträussler syndrome)
  3. Icelandic hereditary congophilic angiopathy and other related forms of familial and sporadic primary cerebrovascular amyloidosis
  4. Localized amyloidosis (amyloidoma)
  5. Postirradiation change and arteriovenous malformation

---

packing density of the basic building blocks of the fibrils. These globular domains may also help exclude the possibility that the amyloid fibrils are built from $\alpha$-helical coiled rods that coalesce through side-to-side interactions, as seen in all classes of intermediate filaments. However, the globular substructure may also be artifactual in nature, and in any event such morphological approaches do not lead to a direct understanding of the nature of the amyloid filaments.

There is even less agreement on some of the fundamental morphological changes that are associated with the Alzheimer plaque (156). The nature of the neuritic change surrounding the extracellular amyloid deposits (41,51,156) has not been resolved in terms of a reactive change or a "dystrophic" degenerative process that in some fashion is associated with deposition of the amyloid. The most pressing question is whether the cell that generates the amyloid fibril can be identified on a purely structural basis (53). Suggestions that adjacent cells such as microglia, astrocytes, and pericytes are involved in the process of amyloidogenesis have been based on structural associations, which may turn out to be only coincidental (134). We still favor a neuronal origin of the amyloid fibril (96) in which its deposition in the extracellular space causes a reactive change not only in neuronal processes but also of an astrocytic and microglial/macrophage nature. We now have evidence of a gradual process of infiltration, condensation, and finally crystallization of the $A_4$ amyloidogenic subunit as the basic process underlying the pathogenesis of the plaque. Structural studies aimed at elucidating the temporal sequence in the formation of the plaque may contribute to this concept. Thus the "amorphous" plaque cores first defined by von Braunmühl may represent the phase of condensation of the $A_4$. There is some biochemical evidence that the amorphous APC is more soluble than the crystalline APC-AD, that the subunit $A_4$ is proportionally of greater full-length chain (97), and that the amorphous APC is more prevalent in relatively younger patients with Down syndrome than in those with AD (1,97). Associated with the more obvious NFT/APC lesions of AD are more subtle ultrastructural changes reflecting plasticity of synapses (44) and whatever proves to be the earliest morphological change as a result of the disturbance of the processing of the $A_4$ precursor.

It would be helpful to have more detailed studies of the type presented by Ulrich (152) in which an attempt has been made to evaluate the earliest morphological changes associated with AD. It appears that NFTs develop before plaques, consistent with our hypothesis on the neuronal origin of the amyloid proteins. More important, however, are some topographic studies on the distribution of NFTs and plaques (37,65,106,117,129), which should dispel any notion on the hematogenous origin of the plaque, as has been proposed by Glenner and Wong (48–50) and Selkoe et al. (138–140). These critical topographic studies point clearly to the unique distribution of lesions in AD: the probable olfactory origin of the disease process and the primary involvement of corticocortical association cortex. These concepts will prove to be most fruitful in the development of hypotheses on the evolution of the AD process.

Finally, the remarkable observations on the plaques in the cortex of aged normal monkeys (149) show clearly for the first time that "neuritic" plaques can develop in the absence of NFTs. Because the nonhuman primate plaque amyloid may also be composed of the $A_4$ subunit (D. J. Selkoe, *this volume*), it will be of great interest to learn of the biochemical and morphological lesions that form the basis of this "neuritic" change.

## BIOCHEMICAL STUDIES OF AMYLOID DEPOSITIONS IN AD

Because the amyloid deposits (NFTs, APCs, and ACAs) are the only pathognomonic features of AD, it has always been obvious that a direct biochemical analysis of their composition would be required as the first step in understanding AD. Austin and colleagues (110,111) appear to be the first to have attempted isolation of the APCs for biochemical analysis, with subsequent attempts being directed at the isolation and purification of the NFTs by groups led by Iqbal and Selkoe. The initial studies of Selkoe (137) led to the

isolation of myelin basic protein as a contaminant of "neurofilament preparations" (141). The relative insolubility of NFTs in 0.2 M NaOH, sodium
dodecyl sulfate (SDS), and urea (142) then led Selkoe to postulate that NFTs
were the result of cross-linked neurofilaments (139). We have now shown that
the major protein subunit is soluble in 0.2 M NaOH and in SDS and urea if
first solubilized in formic acid (96,97), and the presence of cross-linked proteins in NFTs has not yet been confirmed biochemically. Cross-linking of
proteins, as originally proposed by Ishii et al. (74), may still be involved in the
pathogenesis of the NFT, but not through the transglutaminase mechanisms
postulated by Selkoe. Other investigators have found that NFTs or PHFs
prepared by different methods are soluble in SDS (70,71,136) but have been
unable to identify the major protein subunit. Iqbal et al. (70,71) identified
several major bands (45 KD, 57 KD, 62 KD) in their SDS-soluble "PHF"
preparations, in addition to components of different size (50 KD and 45–70
KD) identified immunologically (58,60). The chemical identity of these proteins has not been determined, although it is possible that they represent a
species of proteins sharing a tau epitope (see below) that have either co-
purified with or decorate the surface of the NFT. Similarly, proteolytic cleavage of "PHF" preparations may release peptides of 10, 26, and 36 KD (114),
but it has not yet been shown that these proteolytic fragments are integral
components of the intracellular NFT. Under most conditions, NFTs are resistant to proteolysis (96,162), and again it is possible that the fragments detected by Nukina and Ihara (114) are the NFT-associated proteins with tau/
MAP2 epitopes.

Our strategy in the analysis of the AD amyloid proteins was first to purify
the APCs, which we now realize are the most crystalline forms of the plaque
amyloid. Other attempts at APC purification had yielded amino acid composi-
tions and elemental analyses (2,110,111,130,140), but we (96,97) were able to
identify definitively the major structural unit of the APC amyloid filament as
the $A_4$ protein using solubility profiles, gel electrophoresis (Figs. 2 and 3), gel
filtration (high performance liquid chromatography, HPLC), amino acid analysis, and N-terminal protein sequence. Subsequent confirmation of our findings has come through immunochemical studies, construction of amyloidogenic synthetic peptides corresponding to the $A_4$ sequence, and most recently
molecular cloning of the gene for $A_4$ (75a). Using similar techniques, we are
able to show that the $A_4$ molecule is the major identifiable protein species
present in purified preparations of NFTs obtained from cases of AD, aged
individuals with Down syndrome, and in the Guam parkinsonism–dementia
complex (60a,96) (Fig. 3).

The basic features of the $A_4$ of APCs and NFTs may be summarized as
follows. The subunit mass is 4.5 KD, and the full-length protein consists of
only 42 or 43 residues. The $A_4$ monomer readily aggregates into dimers (9
KD), tetramers (18 KD), and higher oligomeric species. The solubility of

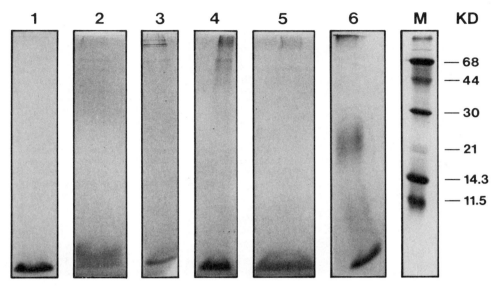

**FIG 2.** Comparison of NFT and APC protein isolated by procedures employing a protease step (lanes 1, 3, 4) with those isolated without protease treatment (lanes 2, 5). APC proteins (lanes 1 and 4, 3 $\mu$g each, corresponding to 3 × 10$^4$ cores, two cases) and NFT proteins (lane 3, I $\mu$g, corresponding to 10$^5$ tangles) were prepared according to our methods (96,97) using a pepsin digestion step. APC proteins (lane 5, 2 $\mu$g) and NFT proteins (lane 2, I$\mu$g) were prepared without protease treatment using a combination of the procedure of Ihara et al. (66) and our procedure (steps that follow pepsin treatment of our methods) (96,97). Lane 6 is synthetic A$_4$ (42 residues) (4 $\mu$g). Lane M shows marker proteins. The proteins were extracted with formic acid, lyophilized, redissolved in Laemmli sample buffer containing 6 M urea, and heated for 30 min at 37°C before loading on the gel (15% w/v). The proteins were stained with Coomassie brilliant blue R.

the A$_4$ fibrils in both APCs and NFTs is dramatically altered after treatment of the native amyloid fibrils with concentrated formic acid. The nature of this formic acid-sensitive aggregation is presently under investigation. The aggregational properties of both the native A$_4$ monomer and the synthetic peptides corresponding to the 42 residues in the A$_4$ sequence show a dependence on pH, concentration, and ionic strength. So far, we have been unable to demonstrate the presence of carbohydrate or the effect of any other form of posttranslational modification (e.g., phosphorylation or acylation).

Sequencing of A$_4$ from both APC and NFT preparations has proved difficult because of the presence of ragged N-termini. We have been able to show that this raggedness is not the result of the proteolysis used during purification of the NFTs and APCs (unpublished data derived from N-terminal sequencing of APC and NFT using protease-free methods; see Fig. 2). Because NFT-A$_4$ tends to show a greater degree of N-terminal raggedness than the APC, we have interpreted this as evidence of *in situ* processing and have postulated that

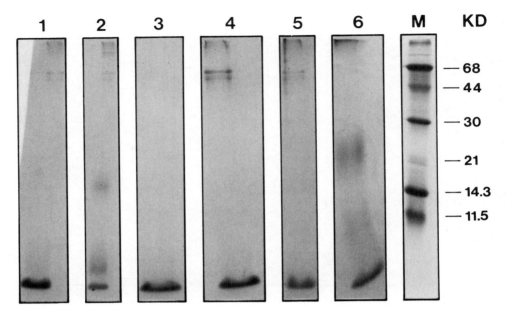

**FIG. 3.** SDS-PAGE of amyloid plaque cores (APC) from various AD cases (lanes 1–4) and of neurofibrillary tangles (NFT) from a case of Guam Parkinson–dementia complex (Guam PD) (lane 5). APC proteins of four AD cases (lane 1: case 1, $5 \times 10^4$ cores; lane 2: case 2, $1.5 \times 10^4$ cores; lane 3: case 3, $3 \times 10^4$ cores; lane 4: case 4, $3 \times 10^4$ cores) and NFTs of the Guam PD case ($2 \times 10^5$ NFTs) were isolated using our procedure that includes a pepsin digestion step. Lane 6 is snythetic $A_4$ (2 $\mu$g) containing 42 residues. Marker proteins are shown in lane M. APC and NFTs were extracted with formic acid at 20°C for 60 min, lyophilized, dissolved in sample buffer containing 6 M urea, and treated for 30 min at 37°C. Electrophoresis was according to Laemmli using a 15% (w/v) polyacrylamide slab gel. Coomassie brilliant blue R was used for staining.

the NFT is deposited earlier than the APC. Of course it may also be that the intracellular NFT is exposed to more proteolytic events than the extracellular APC, in which case chronological interpretations of the differences in raggedness become unnecessary. A similar (if not identical) species of protein is the major component of the ACA (3,49,50,96,159), but the homogeneity of the N-terminal state of ACA-$A_4$ has not yet been determined. In addition to showing that the amyloid comprising the APCs (97) and NFTs (*unpublished data*) of aged individuals with Down syndrome (DS) is composed from the same $A_4$ subunit as found in AD, we have demonstrated that the APC-DS had less ragged N-termini than the APC-AD. This finding may correlate with the observations on the relative states of condensation/crystallization of the amorphous versus compact forms of APCs found in DS and AD.

Table 3 provides a first-order approximation of the number of molecules of $A_4$ present in an NFT/APC, and an estimate of the number of cells required to produce such structures within the time constraints of 5 to 10 years (the

TABLE 3. *Estimation of the number of neurons involved in the production of NFTs and APCs*

| Measurement | NFTs | APCs |
|---|---|---|
| Protein content[a] | $1.0 \pm 0.10 \times 10^{-8}$ mg | $1.0 \pm 0.15 \times 10^{-7}$ mg |
| No. of $A_4$ molecules[b] | $1.3 \pm 0.13 \times 10^{9}$ | $1.3 \pm 0.2 \times 10^{10}$ |
| Required rate of synthesis for $A_4$[c] | $4-8$ $A_4$/sec | $41-82$ $A_4$/sec |
| Steady-state level of $A^4$-precursor mRNA[d] | 35–69 molecules | 346–692 molecules |
| Neurons involved[e] | 1 | 10 |

[a]Determined by quantitative amino acid analyses of hydrolysates obtained with $10^5$ NFT and $10^4$ APC particles, respectively.
[b]Based on the relative molecular mass of 4,500 for the $A_4$ monomer.
[c]Values are calculated for a time span of 10 to 5 years for NFT or APC formation.
[d]Assumed rate of protein synthesis: 5 residues added to the chain per second, per mRNA (8.4 sec for the 42 residues of $A_4$), and a period of 10 to 5 years.
[e]Under the assumption of a common neuronal $A_4$ precursor for NFTs and APCs.

estimated duration of disease). Some of the basic features of the $A_4$ subunit in the NFT/APC in AD have been confirmed in other laboratories (3,78,140), although requests for independent confirmation of the N-terminal sequence (4) have not yet been met. Such independent confirmation of the protein sequence of $A_4$ is desirable, even though we now know the sequence predicted from the structure of the $A_4$ gene, as variant $A_4$ proteins may still exist (and even form the basis of familial AD).

Derivation of the protein sequence of $A_4$ has allowed comparison of anti-sera (polyclonal and monoclonal) to the native and synthetic $A_4$ molecules, the mapping of relevant epitopes, and the development of immunochemical assays and purification protocols. We have shown (96) that a major epitope for APC/ACA resides between residues 10 and 23 on the $A_4$ molecule, and that a minor epitope for NFT is to be found in the N-terminal region. These results have been confirmed (3,159) for the APC/ACA epitope. The NFT epitope we have discovered is exposed only on a subpopulation of all NFTs present in the AD brain (estimate of 10%) and is found only in NFTs in the cell soma in neocortical areas of the brain. The NFTs in the pyramidal cells of the hippocampus and associated "ghost tangles" do not present this epitope. A full determination of all epitopes on NFTs and APCs/ACAs is clearly of importance for the development of immunodiagnostic procedures (99).

Biophysical approaches to the structure of the AD amyloid filaments holds great promise. Although x-ray diffraction studies on the native $A_4$ polymers has shown a cross-$\beta$ conformation (79), our strategy has been to pursue the structure of the amyloid filaments using infrared spectroscopy, magnetic resonance imaging (MRI), negative stain electron microscopy, and gel filtration of the synthetic and native $A_4$ molecules. Preliminary results show an amyloid fibril built from antiparallel arrays of the $A_4$ monomer.

We are now intensively engaged in the search for the precursor that gives rise to the $A_4$. The gene sequence of the $A_4$ precursor ($PA_4$) shows that it is typical of a glycosylated membrane receptor (75a). Two basic strategies are being followed. Western blotting using antisera generated to the native and synthetic $A_4$ molecules is being used to characterize and isolate immunoreactive protein species. cDNA probes for the $A_4$ gene will provide unambiguous evidence of where the precursor is being produced and will open up many techniques for studying the natural biology of the precursor.

## IMMUNOCYTOCHEMICAL APPROACHES TO IDENTIFICATION OF CEREBRAL AMYLOID PROTEINS IN AD

An enormous variety of antigenic determinants on tangles, plaques, and congophilic vessels have been defined by immunocytochemical methods (Tables 4 and 5). There are two lessons to be learned by perusing the literature on this subject: (a) Immunocytochemistry is a useful adjunct to support preconceived ideas on the composition of the amyloid fibrils (i.e., that NFTs are composed of neurofilaments and that APCs are composed of immunoglobulin); and (b) the limitations of immunocytochemistry are not generally appreciated. One consoling feature has been that it is possible to immunize an animal with either NFTs or APCs and produce a respectable antiserum that reacts

TABLE 4. *Antigens suggested to be present in the deposits of amyloid proteins in AD*

Neurofibrillary tangles (NFTs) and neurites surrounding plaques
    Neurofilament triplet subunits, heavy and medium (NF-H,M) with and without
        "phosphorylated epitopes"
    Microtubule proteins (tubulins)
    Microtubule-associated proteins (MAP2, tau)
    Other cytoskeletal components (e.g., vimentin)
    Various neuropeptides (somatostatin, neuropeptide Y)
    Cystatin C ($\gamma$-trace)
    PrP protein (scrapie-associated fibril, intracellular)
    NFT-specific antigen
    $A_4$ epitope as defined by antibodies to native and synthetic molecules

Alzheimer plaque core (APC) and congophilic angiopathy (ACA)
    Immunoglobulin (IgG and light chains)
    Complement ($C1_q$, $C_4$, $C_3$)
    Serum AA protein
    Serum amyloid P component
    Transthyretin (prealbumin)
    Other serum proteins
    Cystatin C ($\gamma$-trace)
    PrP protein (scrapie-associated fibrils, extracellular)
    APC/ACA specific antigens
    $A_4$ epitope as defined by antibodies to native and synthetic peptides

TABLE 5. *Checklist for the nonspecific nature of the "PHF-related antigen" as demonstrated by its sharing of epitopes with diverse structures*

| | |
|---|---|
| Neurofibrillary tangles and neurites surrounding plaque cores | Alzheimer disease |
| | Progressive supranuclear palsy (Steele-Richardson-Olszewski |
| | Guam parkinsonism–dementia complex |
| | Postencephalitic parkinsonism |
| Lewy body | Idiopathic Parkinson disease |
| Pick body | Pick disease |
| Axonal spheroids | Amyotrophic lateral sclerosis |
| | Neuroaxonal dystrophy |
| Torpedoes of Purkinje cells | Diverse conditions |
| Neurofilament aggregates | Experimental aluminum and IDPN neurotoxicity |
| | Inhibitors of microtubule assembly |
| Dystrophic dendrites | Deafferented Purkinje cells in conditions such as Menkes disease and olivary neurons in crossed cerebellar atrophy |

either with NFTs or APCs/ACAs. There is only one possible solid conclusion to be derived from this welter of literature: NFTs and APCs/ACAs contain different epitopes. Herein lies the paradox, as the biochemistry of the NFT shows that it is built from the same $A_4$ monomer as contained in the APCs/ACAs. Nevertheless, some plausible explanations are emerging to account for this paradoxical state.

The greatest immunocytochemical effort has been placed in the study of the presence of neurofilament (NF) antigens (triplet proteins NF-H,M,L) in NFTs. As soon as polyclonal and monoclonal antibodies to the NF antigens became available, researchers applied them to the AD brain, with positive results (5,6,34,39,42,43,68,74,103). The monoclonal antibodies appeared to be reacting with phosphorylated epitopes (28,62,148), and the notorious propensity for monoclonals to recognize trivial shared epitopes was temporarily put aside (89,161). Bignami et al. (14) found that not all NFTs were NF-immunoreactive, and Autilio-Gambetti et al. (7) defined a highly charged domain that may be responsible for both the argyrophilic histochemical reactivity and the phosphorylated epitope defined by monoclonal antibodies. Other studies showed that a wide variety of structural lesions in neurons (both natural and experimental) would show similar positive immunoreactivity (Table 4) (32,33,40,42,43,108,122,144,151). Then it became apparent that many of the antibodies that were supposedly NF-specific were reacting in a fashion that mimicked antibodies to microtubules and their associated proteins (57,59,60,82,114,115,118,163–165), culminating in the observations that an epitope shared with the tau protein is easily demonstrable on the NFT

(21,35,55,56,67,83,115,160). The most readily acceptable explanation is that the major epitope present on the surface of the NFT is shared between NF-H,M, MAP2, and tau, and that this epitope in some manner is influenced by treatment with alkaline phosphatase. The precise chemical identification of this major epitope is still unknown. But recent data suggest a unifying principle in the discovery of ubiquitin epitopes on the NFT.

In our hands, a certain proportion of NFTs contain an epitope that is recognized by antisera to the N-terminal region of $A_4$ (96). How this relates to the major "tau" epitope is uncertain, but there is still reason to believe that the most important NFT epitope is yet to be defined, as many workers in this field have generated antibodies to the native NFT that cannot be absorbed by antigens such as NF-H, M, MAP2, and tau (20,58,60,66,119,120,125–127,153; *unpublished data* from our laboratories). Such antibodies, loosely referred to as "anti-PHF," are thought of as recognizing a specific NFT determinant and fail to cross-react with "any normal brain component." More work is required with these classes of antibodies before one can accept the concept of a serological definition of a specific NFT determinant. At present, it still appears that the "tau" epitope is a major surface antigen of the NFT, and there is no compelling evidence that this epitope is structurally a component of the intracellular amyloid filament itself. The situation is somewhat analogous to the presence of the serum amyloid P component in the deposition of the systemic amyloids of the AA type.

The picture is now much clearer when we review the antigenic composition of the extracellular APCs and ACAs. Although some conflicting data exist on the presence of immunoglobulins and other serum proteins (Table 4) (38,52,72,73,75,76,80,81,86,90,121,133,134,145,150), biochemical data on the composition of the major protein species of the APC/ACAs (96,97) suggest that these other contenders defined immunocytochemically are at best minor components or the result of the postmortem leakage of serum proteins into the brain parenchyma. The determination of the amino acid sequence of $A_4$ has permitted the precise definition of the major structural epitopes of the extracellular amyloid through the use of antibodies to synthetic peptides (3,96,159) and has allowed us to visualize the widespread extracellular amyloid deposition as a process of initial infiltration, followed by condensation and then crystallization into APC and ACA.

## OTHER THEORIES ON THE PATHOGENESIS AND CAUSE OF AD

Our approach to the unraveling of AD has been based on the assumption that the protein amyloid depositions are of primary significance. The nonproteinaceous components of the amyloid, including metals such as aluminum and silicon (23,96,111), obviously deserve attention, although it appears at this stage that these cations are present in the NFTs and APCs as secondary phenomena (possibly attracted by the overall negative charge present on the amyloid filaments). The vast literature on neurotransmitter and neuropeptide alterations in AD serves to illustrate the difficulty inherent in the application of technologies for which there was no *a priori* justification. If it transpires that the precursor of the $A_4$ amyloid is indeed a neurotransmitter receptor molecule or is in some other way involved in neurotransmitter function, a more fruitful avenue of research will become apparent.

As a derivative of the concept that the neuronal cytoskeleton in some fashion is specifically altered in AD, morphological (53) and biochemical (69) evidence for microtubule anomalies has been presented. It is too early to judge the relevance of these observations, just as it is for our particular theory on the role of oxidative stress and free radical formation (93).

## PATHOGENESIS OF AD: RELATION TO UNCONVENTIONAL VIRUS DISEASES (SCRAPIE, KURU, CREUTZFELDT-JAKOB DISEASE, GERSTMANN-STRÄUSSLER SYNDROME)

From the time Creutzfeldt-Jakob disease (CJD) was shown to be caused by an unconventional virus, the expectation increased that other chronic degenerative neurological diseases would have a similar etiology. Of all these other diseases AD stood out as a prime candidate, not only because of its clinical, epidemiological, and genetic overlap with CJD (94) but particularly in the occurrence of amyloid deposits was a common pathogenesis most suspected (95). Although the nature of the infectious agent is still hotly disputed (30,31,92,131,132), our strategy of studying the nature of the amyloid deposits in AD (94,97) has been vindicated by the discoveries of Prusiner and colleagues of the PrP protein and its contribution to infectivity and amyloid formation in the unconventional virus diseases.

The PrP protein (16,98), as initially purified, had a mass of 27 to 30 KD but is now recognized as a glycoprotein of mass 33 to 35 KD. Numerous studies from independent laboratories have produced remarkably similar results (8,12,15,17,18,26,63,64,91,107,123,135,143,146) that are consistent with contentions that: (a) PrP is the major molecule that co-purifies with infectivity. (b) It is the major structural component of the scrapie-associated filament (SAF)/amyloid rod (9,19,36,100,102,124). (c) The PrP is the major constituent of the extracellular amyloid plaque found in a certain proportion of cases of the unconventional virus diseases (K. Beyreuther and C. L. Masters, *unpublished data;* 11,81). (d) Molecular cloning of the PrP gene (10,25, 84,85,87,116,128,147,154) shows that PrP is a highly conserved host-encoded glycoprotein present in many tissues and species, that the disease-associated form of PrP, which readily aggregates to form the protease-resistant SAF/amyloid rods, is probably the result of a posttranslational modification, and that the brain-derived PrP is of neuronal origin. (e) The gene for PrP is tightly linked to *Sinc,* the gene that controls the incubation period of scrapie in mice, and it is possible that PrP is in fact the *Sinc* gene product (24). (f) PrP accumulates in the extracellular space not only as plaques (22) but also as congophilic angiopathy (47,77).

The relatedness of PrP to the precursor that gives rise to $A_4$ is now becoming readily apparent. Both are membrane glycoproteins, which in some fashion are probably posttranslationally modified to form an altered protein with an amyloidogenic propensity. In the case of PrP, the cleavage product that forms the extracellular amyloid fibril contains at least one of the transmembrane hydrophobic domains, which is similar to the transmembrane hydrophobic domain of the $A_4$ cleavage product. It is possible that these regions of PrP and $A_4$ are the principal domains that confer amyloidogenicity. The questions now to be answered concern the manner in which the infectious agent is related to PrP and the precursor of $A_4$. At this time, the balance of evidence points toward a modified form of PrP being used by the infectious agent as a structural component. If so, it is possible that a similar process is occurring in AD, although it is still conceivable that a completely different noninfectious process is operating in AD.

## PRIMARY AMYLOID CEREBRAL ANGIOPATHY

There is a rare disease entity, usually of a familial nature (although we have data now on one sporadic case), in which amyloid deposits are restricted to the cerebral vasculature, causing either widespread parenchymal degeneration or spontaneous hemorrhage. Studies have elucidated the biochemical nature of this amyloid as being related to cystatin C (27,45,46,54), and the basis for its amyloidogenicity lies either in an amino acid substitution or as a cleavage product from a modified precursor. Although a completely different class of protein molecule than either PrP or $A_4$, it is likely that the cystatin C is of neuronal origin (88), and its relevance to AD lies in this fact: Here is another example of a neuronally derived protein giving rise to a restricted form of cerebral amyloidoses. Hypotheses on the hematogenous origin of brain-restricted amyloidoses (48–50,138,140,156) may not prove necessary.

## ACKNOWLEDGMENTS

Our studies are supported by grants from the National Health and Medical Research Council of Australia and the Deutsche Forschungsgemeinschaft. Ms. Gail Della Torre typed the manuscript.

# REFERENCES

1. Allsop, D., Kidd, M., Landon, M., and Tomlinson, A. (1986): Isolated senile plaque cores in Alzheimer's disease and Down's syndrome show differences in morphology. *J. Neurol. Neurosurg. Psychiatry,* 49:886–892.
2. Allsop, D., Landon, M., and Kidd, J. (1983): The isolation and amino acid composition of senile plaque core protein. *Brain Res.,* 259:348–352.
3. Allsop, D., Landon, M., Kidd, M., Lowe, J. S., Reynolds, G. P., and Gardner, A. (1986): Monoclonal antibodies raised against a subsequence of senile plaque core protein react with plaque cores, plaque periphery and cerebrovascular amyloid in Alzheimer's disease. *Neurosci. Lett.,* 68:252–256.
4. Anderton, B., and Miller, C. (1986): Proteins in a twist: are neurofibrillary tangles and amyloid in Alzheimer's disease composed of the same protein? *Trends Neurosci.,* 9:337–338.
5. Anderton B. H., Breinburg, D., Downes, M. J., Green, P. J., Tomlinson, B. E., Ulrich, J., Wood, J. N., and Kahn, J. (1982): Monoclonal antibodies show that neurofibrillary tangles and neurofilaments share antigenic determinants. *Nature,* 298:84–86.
6. Anderton, B. H., Calvert, R., Probst, A., and Kahn, J. (1984): Antibody studies of neurofilaments and neurofibrillary tangles. *J. Submicrosc. Cytol.,* 16:63–64.
7. Autilio-Gambetti, L., Crane, R., and Gambetti, P. (1986): Binding of Bodian's silver and monoclonal antibodies to defined regions of human neurofilament subunits: Bodian's silver reacts with a highly charged unique domain of neurofilaments. *J. Neurochem.,* 46:366–370.
8. Barry, R. A., and Prusiner, S. B. (1986): Monoclonal antibodies to the cellular and scrapie prion proteins. *J. Infect. Dis.,* 154:518–521.
9. Barry, R. A., McKinley M. P., Bendheim, P. E., Lewis, G. K., DeArmond, S. J., and Prusiner, S. B. (1985): Antibodies to the scrapie protein decorate prion rods. *J. Immunol.,* 135:603–613.
10. Basler, K., Oesch, B., Scoff, M., Westaway, D., Wälchli, M., Groth, D. F., McKinley, M. P., Prusiner, S. B., and Weissmann, C. (1986): Scrapie and cellular PrP isoforms are encoded by the same chromosomal gene. *Cell.,* 46:417–428.
11. Bendheim, P. E., Barry, R. A., DeArmond, S. J., Stites, D. P., and Prusiner, S. B. (1984): Antibodies to a scrapie prion protein. *Nature,* 310:418–421.
12. Bendheim, P. E., Bockman, J. M., McKinley, M. P., Kingsbury, D. T., and Prusiner, S. B. (1985): Scrapie and Creutzfeldt-Jakob disease prion proteins share physical properties and antigenic determinants. *Proc. Natl. Acad. Sci. USA,* 82:997–1001.
13. Bielschowsky, M. (1932): Histopathology of nerve cells. In: *Cytology and Cellular Pathology of the Nervous System,* edited by W. Penfield, Vol. 1, pp. 145–188. Hafner, New York (facsimile reprint 1965).
14. Bignami, A., Selkoe, D. J., and Dahl, D. (1984): Amyloid-like (congophilic) neurofibrillary tangles do not react with neurofilament antisera in Alzheimer's cerebral cortex. *Acta Neuropathol. (Berl.),* 64:243–250.
15. Bockman, J. M., Kingsbury, D. T., McKinley, M. P., Bendheim, P. E., and Prusiner, S. B. (1985): Creutzfeldt-Jakob disease prion proteins in human brains. *N. Engl. J. Med.,* 312:73–78.
16. Bolton, D. C., McKinley, M. P., and Prusiner, S. B. (1982): Identification of a protein that purifies with the scrapie prion. *Science,* 218:1309–1311.
17. Bolton, D. C., McKinley, M. P., and Prusiner, S. B. (1984): Molecular characteristics of the major scrapie prion protein. *Biochemistry,* 23:5898–5906.
18. Bolton, D. C., Meyer, R. K., and Prusiner, S. B. (1985): Scrapie PrP 27–30 is a sialoglycoprotein. *J. Virol.,* 53:596–606.
19. Braig, H. R., and Diringer, H. (1985): Scrapie: concept of a virus-induced amyloidosis of the brain. *EMBO J.,* 4:2309–2312.
20. Brion, J. P., Couck, A. M., Passareiro, E., and Flament-Durand, J. (1985): Neurofibrillary tangles of Alzheimer's disease: an immunohistochemical study. *J. Submicrosc. Cytol.,* 17:89–96.
21. Brion, J. P., van den Bosch de Aguilar, P., and Flament-Durand, J. (1985): Senile dementia of the Alzheimer type: morphological and immunocytochemical studies. In: *Senile Dementia of the Alzheimer Type. Early Diagnosis, Neuropathology and Animal Models,* edited by J. Traber and W. H. Gispen, pp. 164–174. Springer Verlag, Berlin.

22. Bruce, M. E., and Dickinson, A. G. (1985): Genetic control of amyloid plaque production and incubation period in scrapie-infected mice. *J. Neuropathol. Exp. Neurol.*, 44:285–294.
23. Candy, J. M., Oakley, A. E., Klinowski, J., Carpenter, T. A., Perry, R. H., Atack, J. R., Perry, E. K., Blessed, G., Fairbairn, A., and Edwardson, J. A. (1986): Aluminosilicates and senile plaque formation in Alzheimer's disease. *Lancet*, 1:354–357.
24. Carlson, G. A., Kingsbury, D. T., Goodman, P. A., Coleman, S., Marshall, S. T., DeArmond, S., Westaway, D., and Prusiner, S. B. (1986): Linkage of prion protein and scrapie incubation time genes. *Cell*, 46:503–511.
25. Chesebro, B., Race, R., Wehrly, K., Nishio, J., Bloom, M., et al. (1985): Identification of scrapie prion protein-specific mRNA in scrape-infected and uninfected brain. *Nature*, 315:331–333.
26. Cho, H. J. (1986): Antibody to scrapie-associated fibril protein identifies a cellular antigen. *J. Gen. Virol.*, 67:243–253.
27. Cohen, D. H., Feiner, H., Jensson, O., and Frangione, B. (1983): Amyloid fibril in hereditary cerebral hemorrhage with amyloidosis (HCHWA) is related to the gastroentero-pancreatic neuroendocrine protein, gamma trace. *J. Exp. Med.*, 158:623–628.
28. Cork, L. C., Sternberger, N. H., Sternberger, L. A., Casanova, M. F., Struble, R. G., and Price, D. L. (1986): Phosphorylated neurofilament antigens in neurofibrillary tangles in Alzheimer's disease. *J. Neuropathol. Exp. Neurol.*, 45:56–64.
29. Crowther, R. A., and Wischik, C. M. (1985): Image reconstruction of the Alzheimer paired helical filament. *EMBO J.*, 4:3661–3665.
30. Czub, M., Braig, H. R., Blode, H., and Diringer, H. (1986): The major protein of SAF is absent from spleen and thus not an essential part of the scrapie agent. *Acta Virol (Praha)*, 91:383–386.
31. Czub, M., Braig, H. R., Blode, H., and Diringer, H. (1986): Pathogenesis of scrapie: study of the temporal development of clinical symptoms, of infectivity titres and scrapie associated fibrils in brains of hamsters infected intraperitoneally. *J. Gen. Virol.*, 67:2005–2009.
32. Dahl, D., and Bignami, A. (1978): Immunochemical cross-reactivity of normal neurofibrils and aluminum-induced neurofibrillary tangles: immunofluorescence study with anti-neurofilament serum. *Exp. Neurol.*, 58:74–80.
33. Dahl, D., Bignami, A., Bich, N. T., and Chi, N. H. (1980): Immunohistochemical characterization of neurofibrillary tangles induced by mitotic spindle inhibitors. *Acta Neuropathol. (Berl.)*, 51:165–168.
34. Dahl, D., Selkoe, D. J., Pero, R. T., and Bignami, A. (1982): Immunostaining of neurofibrillary tangles in Alzheimer's senile dementia with a neurofilament antiserum. *J. Neurosci.*, 2:113–119.
35. Delacourte, A., and Defossez, A. (1986): Alzheimer's disease: tau proteins, the promoting factors of microtubule assembly, are major components of paired helical filaments. *J. Neurol. Sci.*, 76:173–186.
36. Diringer, H., Gelderblom, H., Hilmert, H., Özel, M., Edelbluth, C., and Kimberlin, R. H. (1983) Scrapie infectivity, fibrils and low molecular weight protein. *Nature*, 306:476–478.
37. Duyckaerts, C., Hauw, J-J., Bastenaire, F., Piette, F., Poulain, C., Rainsard, V., Javoy-Agid, F., and Berthaux, P. (1986): Laminar distribution of neocortical senile plaques in senile dementia of the Alzheimer type. *Acta Neuropathol. (Berl.)*, 70:249–256.
38. Eikelenboom, P., and Stam, F. C. (1982): Immunoglobulins and complement factors in senile plaques. *Acta Neuropathol. (Berl.)*, 57:239–242.
39. Elovaara, I., Paetau, A., Lehto, V-P., Dahl, D., Virtanen, I., and Palo, J. (1983): Immunocytochemical studies of Alzheimer neuronal perikerya with intermediate filament antisera. *J. Neurol. Sci.*, 62:315–326.
40. Forno, L. S., Sternberger, L. A., Sternberger, N. H., Strefling, A. M., Swanson, K., and Eng, L. (1986): Reaction of Lewy bodies with antibodies to phosphorylated and non-phosphorylated neurofilaments. *Neurosci. Lett.*, 64:253–258.
41. Friede, R. L. (1965): Enzyme histochemical studies of senile plaques. *J. Neuropathol. Exp. Neurol.*, 24:477–491.
42. Gambetti, P., Autilio-Gambetti, L., Perry, G., Shecket, G., and Crane, R. C. (1983): Antibodies to neurofibrillary tangles of Alzheimer's disease raised from human and animal neurofilament fractions. *Lab. Invest.*, 49:430–435.

43. Gambetti, P., Shecket, G., Ghetti, B., Hirano, H., and Dahl, D. (1983): Neurofibrillary changes in human brain: an immunocytochemical study with a neurofilament antiserum. *J. Neuropathol. Exp. Neurol.*, 42:69–79.

44. Geddes, J. W., Monaghan, D. T., Cotman, C. W., Lott, I. T., Kim, R. C., Chui, H. C. (1985): Plasticity of hippocampal circuitry in Alzheimer's disease. *Science*, 230:1179–1181.

45. Ghiso, J., Jensson, O., and Frangione, B. (1986): Amyloid fibrils in hereditary cerebral hemorrhage with amyloidosis of the Icelandic type is a variant of γ-trace basic protein (cystatin C). *Proc. Natl. Acad. Sci. USA*, 83:2974–2978.

46. Ghiso, J., Pans-Estel, B., and Frangione, B. (1986): Hereditary cerebral amyloid angiopathy: the amyloid fibrils contain a protein which is a variant of cystatin C, an inhibitor of lysosomal cysteine proteases. *Biochem. Biophys. Res. Commun.*, 136:548–554.

47. Gilmour, J. S., Bruce, M. E., and Mackellar, A. (1985): Cerebrovascular amyloidosis in scrapie-affected sheep. *Neuropathol. Appl. Neurobiol.*, 11:173–183.

48. Glenner, G. G. (1985): Alzheimer's disease: the pathology, the patient and the family. In: *Senile Dementia of the Alzheimer Type*, edited by J. T. Hutton and A. D. Kenny, pp. 275–291. Alan R. Liss, New York.

49. Glenner, G. G., and Wong, C. W. (1984): Alzheimer's disease: initial report of the purification and characterization of a novel cerebrovascular amyloid protein. *Biochem. Biophys. Res. Commun.*, 120:885–890.

50. Glenner, G.G., and Wong, C. W. (1984): Alzheimer's disease and Down's syndrome: sharing of a unique cerebrovascular amyloid fibril protein. *Biochem. Biophys. Res. Commun.*, 122:1131–1135.

51. Gonatas, N. K., Anderson, W., and Evangelista, I. (1967): The contribution of altered synapses in the senile plaque: an electron microscopic study in Alzheimer's dementia. *J. Neuropathol. Exp. Neurol.*, 26:25–39.

52. Goust, J-M., Magnum, M., and Powers, J. M. (1984): An immunologic assessment of brain-associated IgG in senile cerebral amyloidosis. *J. Neuropathol. Exp. Neurol.*, 43:481–488.

53. Gray, E. G. (1986): Spongiform encephalopathy: a neurocytologist's viewpoint with a note on Alzheimer's disease. *Neuropathol. Appl. Neurobiol.*, 12:149–172.

54. Grubb, A., Jensson, O., Gudmundsson, G., Arnason, A., Löfberg, H., and Malm, J. (1984): Abnormal metabolism of γ-trace alkaline microprotein: the basic defect in hereditary cerebral hemorrhage with amyloidosis. *N. Engl. J. Med.*, 311:1547–1549.

55. Grundke-Iqbal, I., Iqbal, K., Quinlan, M., Tung, Y-C., Zaidi, M. S., and Wisniewski, H. M. (1986): Microtubule associated protein tau: a component of Alzheimer paired helical filaments. *J. Biol. Chem.*, 261:6084–6089.

56. Grundke-Iqbal, I., Iqbal, K., Tung, Y-C., Quinlan, M., Wisniewski, H. M., and Binder, L. I. (1986): Abnormal phosphorylation of the microtubule-associated protein τ (tau) in Alzheimer cytoskeletal pathology. *Proc. Natl. Acad. Sci. USA*, 83:4913–4917.

57. Grundke-Iqbal, I., Iqbal, K., Tung, Y-C., Wang, G. P., and Wisniewski, H. M. (1985): Alzheimer paired helical filaments: cross-reacting polypeptide/s normally present in brain. *Acta Neuropathol. (Berl.)*, 66:52–61.

58. Grundke-Iqbal, I., Iqbal, K., Tung, Y-C., and Wisniewski, H. M. (1984): Alzheimer paired helical filaments: immunochemical identification of polypeptides. *Acta Neuropathol. (Berl.)*, 62:259–267.

59. Grundke-Iqbal, I., Johnson, A. B., Terry, R. D., Wisniewski, H. M., and Iqbal, K. (1979): Alzheimer neurofibrillary tangles: antiserum and immunohistological staining. *Ann. Neurol.*, 6:532–537.

60. Grundke-Iqbal, I., Johnson, A. B., Wisniewski, H. M., Terry, R. D., and Iqbal, K. (1979): Evidence that Alzheimer neurofibrillary tangles originate from neurotubules. *Lancet*, 1:578–580.

60a. Guiroy, D. C., Miyazaki, M., Multhaup, G., Fischer, P., Garruto, R. M., Beyreuther, K., Masters, C. L. Simms, G., Gibbs, C. J., Jr., and Gajdusek, D. C. (1987): Amyloid of neurofibrillary tangles of Guamanian parkinsonism–dementia and Alzheimer disease share identical amino acid sequence. *Proc. Natl. Acad. Sci. USA*, 84:2073–2077.

61. Halper, J., Scheithaner, B. W., Okazaki, H., and Laws, E. R., Jr. (1986): Meningo-angiomatosis: a report of six cases with special reference to the occurrence of neurofibrillary tangles. *J. Neuropathol. Exp. Neurol.*, 45:426–446.

62. Haugh, M. C., Probst, A., Ulrich, J., Kahn, J., and Anderton, B. H. (1986): Alzheimer neurofibrillary tangles contain phosphorylated and hidden neurofilament epitopes. *J. Neurol. Neurosurg. Psychiatry*, 49:1213–1220.
63. Hilmert, H., and Diringer, H. (1984): A rapid and efficient method to enrich SAF-protein from scrapie brains of hamsters. *Biosci. Rep.*, 4:165–170.
64. Hope, J., Morton, L. J. D., Farquhar, C. F., Multhaup, G., Beyreuther, K., and Kimberlin, R. H. (1986): The major polypeptide of scrapie-associated fibrils (SAF) has the same size, charge distribution and N-terminal protein sequence as predicted for the normal brain protein (PrP). *EMBO J.*, 5:2591–2597.
65. Hyman, B. T., Van Hoesen, G. W., Kromer, L. J., and Damasio, A. R. (1986): Perforant pathway changes and the memory impairment of Alzheimer's disease. *Ann. Neurol.*, 20:472–481.
66. Ihara, Y., Abraham, C., and Selkoe, D. J. (1983): Antibodies to paired helical filaments in Alzheimer's disease do not recognize normal brain proteins. *Nature*, 304:727–730.
67. Ihara, Y., Nukina, N., Miura, R., and Ogawara, M. (1986): Phosphorylated tau protein is integrated into paired helical filaments in Alzheimer's disease. *J. Biochem. (Tokyo)*, 99:1807–1810.
68. Ihara, Y., Nukina, N., Sugita, H., and Toyokura, Y. (1981): Staining of Alzheimer's neurofibrillary tangles with antiserum against 200K component of neurofilament. *Proc. Jpn. Acad.*, 57(B):152–156.
69. Iqbal, K., Grundke-Iqbal, I., Zaidi, T., Merz, P. A., Wen, G. Y., Shaikh, S. S., Wisniewski, H. M., Alafuzoff, I., and Winblad, B. (1986): Defective microtubule assembly in Alzheimer's disease. *Lancet*, 2:421–426.
70. Iqbal, K., Grundke-Iqbal, I., Zaidi, T., Ali, N., and Wisniewski, H. M. (1986): Are Alzheimer neurofibrillary tangles insoluble polymers? *Life Sci.*, 38:1695–1700.
71. Iqbal, K., Zaidi, T., Thompson, C. H., Merz, P. A., and Wisniewski, H. M. (1984): Alzheimer paired helical filaments: bulk isolation, solubility, and protein composition. *Acta Neuropathol. (Berl.)*, 62:167–177.
72. Ishii, T., and Haga, S. (1976): Immuno-electron microscopic localization of immunoglobulins in amyloid fibrils of senile plaques. *Acta Neuropathol. (Berl.)*, 36:243–249.
73. Ishii, T., and Haga, S. (1984): Immuno-electron-microscopic localization of complements in amyloid fibrils of senile plaques. *Acta Neuropathol. (Berl.)*, 63:296–300.
74. Ishii, T., Haga, S., and Tokutake, S. (1979): Presence of neurofilament protein in Alzheimer's neurofibrillary tangles (ANT): an immunofluorescent study. *Acta Neuropathol. (Berl.)*, 48:105–112.
75. Ishii, T., Sato, M., Haga, S., Shimoda, T., Kato, K., and Saito, T. (1986): A monoclonal antibody to amyloid in the brains of patients with Alzheimer's disease. *Neuropathol. Appl. Neurobiol.*, 12:441–445.
75a. Kang, J., Lemaire, H-G., Unterbeck, A., Salbaum, J. M., Masters, C. L., Grzeschik, K-H., Multhaup, G., Beyreuther, K., and Müller-Hill, B. (1987): The precursor of Alzheimer's disease amyloid A4 protein resembles a cell-surface receptor. *Nature*, 325:733–736.
76. Katenkamp, D., Stiller, D., and Thos, K. (1970): Untersuchungen zum immunhistochemischen Verhalten der senilen Plaques des menschlichen Gehirnes. *Virchows Arch. [A]*, 351:333–339.
77. Keohane, C., Peatfield, R., and Duchen, L. W. (1985): Subacute spongiform encephalopathy (Creutzfeldt-Jakob disease) with amyloid angiopathy. *J. Neurol. Neurosurg. Psychiatry*, 48:1175–1178.
78. Kidd, M., Allsop, D., and Landon, M. (1985): Senile plaque amyloid, paired helical filaments, and cerebrovascular amyloid in Alzheimer's disease are all deposits of the same protein. *Lancet*, 1:278.
79. Kirschner, D. A., Abraham, C., and Selkoe, D. J. (1986): X-ray diffraction from intraneuronal paired helical filaments and extraneuronal amyloid fibers in Alzheimer disease indicates cross-β conformation. *Proc. Natl. Acad. Sci. USA*, 83:503–507.
80. Kitamoto, T., Tateishi, J., Hikita, H., and Takeshita, I. (1985): A new method to classify amyloid fibrils. *Acta Neuropathol. (Berl.)*, 67:272–278.
81. Kitamoto, T., Tateishi, J., Tashima, T., Takeshita, I., Barry, R. A., DeArmond, S. J., and Prusiner, S. B. (1986): Amyloid plaques in Creutzfeldt-Jakob disease stain with prion protein antibodies. *Ann. Neurol.*, 20:204–208.
82. Kosik, K. S., Duffy, L. K., Dowling, M. M., Abraham, C., McCluskey, A., and Selkoe,

D. J. (1984): Microtubule-associated protein 2: monoclonal antibodies demonstrate the selective incorporation of certain epitopes into Alzheimer neurofibrillary tangles. *Proc. Natl. Acad. Sci. USA*, 81:7941–7945.

83. Kosik, K. S., Joachim, C. L., and Selkoe, D. J. (1986): Microtubule-associated protein tau ($\tau$) is a major antigenic component of paired helical filaments in Alzheimer disease. *Proc. Natl. Acad. Sci. USA*, 83:4044–4048.

84. Kretzschmar, H. A., Prusiner, S. B., Stowring, L. E., and DeArmond, S. J. (1986): Scrapie prion proteins are synthesized in neurons. *Am. J. Pathol.*, 122:1–5.

85. Kretzschmar, H. A., Stowring, L. E., Westaway, D., Stubblebine, W. H., Prusiner, S. B., and DeArmond, S. J. (1986): Molecular cloning of a human prion protein cDNA. *DNA*, 5:315–324.

86. Linke, R. P. (1982): Immunohistochemical identification and cross reactions of amyloid fibril proteins in senile heart and amyloid in familial polyneuropathy: lack of reactivity with cerebral amyloid in Alzheimer's disease. *Clin. Neuropathol.*, 1:172–182.

87. Locht, C., Chesebro, B., Race, R., and Keith, J. M. (1986): Molecular cloning and complete sequence of prion protein cDNA from mouse brain infected with the scrapie agent. *Proc. Natl. Acad. Sci. USA*, 83:6372–6376.

88. Löfberg, H., Grubb, A. O., and Brun, A. (1981): Human brain cortical neurons contain $\gamma$-trace: rapid isolation, immunohistochemical and physicochemical characterization of human $\gamma$-trace. *Biomed. Res.*, 2:298–306.

89. Luca, F. C., Bloom, G. S., and Vallee, R. B. (1986): A monoclonal antibody that cross-reacts with phosphorylated epitopes on two microtubule-associated proteins and two neurofilament polypeptides. *Proc. Natl. Acad. Sci. USA*, 83:1006–1010.

90. Mann, D.M.A., Davies, J. S., Hawkes, J., and Yates, P. O. (1982): Immunohistochemical staining of senile plaques. *Neuropathol. Appl. Neurobiol.*, 8:55–61.

91. Manuelidis, L., Valley, S., and Manuelidis, E. E. (1985): Specific proteins associated with Creutzfeldt-Jakob disease and scrapie share antigenic and carbohydrate determinants. *Proc. Natl. Acad. Sci. USA*, 82:4263–4267.

92. Marsh, R. F., Dees, C., Castle, B. E., Wade, W. F., and German, T. L. (1984): Purification of the scrapie agent by density gradient centrifugation. *J. Gen. Virol.*, 65:415–421.

93. Martins, R. N., Harper, C. G., Stokes, G. B., and Masters, C. L. (1986): Increased cerebral glucose-6-phosphate dehydrogenase activity in Alzheimer's disease may reflect oxidative stress. *J. Neurochem.*, 46:1042–1045.

94. Masters, C. L., Gajdusek, D. C., and Gibbs, C. J., Jr. (1981): The familial occurrence of Creutzfeldt-Jakob and Alzheimer's disease. *Brain*, 104:535–558.

95. Masters, C. L., Gajdusek, D. C., and Gibbs, C. J., Jr. (1981): Creutzfeldt-Jakob disease virus isolation from the Gertsmann-Sträussler syndrome: with an analysis of the various forms of amyloid plaque deposition in the virus-induced spongiform encephalopathies. *Brain*, 104:559–587.

96. Masters, C. L., Multhaup, G., Simms, G., Pottgiesser, J., Martins, R. N., and Beyreuther, K. (1985): Neuronal origin of a cerebral amyloid: neurofibrillary tangles of Alzheimer's disease contain the same protein as the amyloid of plaque cores and blood vessels. *EMBO J.*, 4:2757–2763.

97. Masters, C. L., Simms, G., Weinman, N. A., Multhaup, G., McDonald, B. L., and Beyreuther, K. (1985): Amyloid plaque core protein in Alzheimer disease and Down syndrome. *Proc. Natl. Acad. Sci. USA*, 82:4245–4249.

98. McKinley, M. P., Bolton, D. C., and Prusiner, S. B. (1983): A protease-resistant protein is a structural component of the scrapie prion. *Cell*, 35:57–62.

99. Mehta, P. D., Thal, L., Wisniewski, H. M., Grundke-Iqbal, I., and Iqbal, K. (1985): Paired helical filament antigen in CSF. *Lancet*, 2:35.

100. Merz, P. A., Somerville, R. A., Wisniewski, H. M., Manuelidis, L., Manuelidis, E. E, (1983): Scrapie-associated fibrils in Creutzfeldt-Jakob disease. *Nature*, 306:474–476.

101. Merz, P. A., Wisniewski, H. M., Somerville, R. A., Bobin, S. A., Masters, C. L., and Iqbal, K. (1983): Ultrastructural morphology of amyloid fibrils from neuritic and amyloid plaques. *Acta Neuropathol. (Berl.)*, 60:113–124.

102. Meyer, R. K., McKinley, M. P., Bowman, K. A., Braunfeld, M. B., Barry, R. A., and Prusiner, S. B. (1986): Separation and properties of cellular and scrapie prion proteins. *Proc. Natl. Acad. Sci. USA*, 83:2310–2314.

103. Miller, C. C. J., Brion, J-P., Calvert, R., Chin, T. K., Eagles, P. A. M., Downes, M. J.,

Flament-Durand, J., Haugh, M., Kahn, J., Probst, A., Ulrich, J., and Anderton, B. H. (1986): Alzheimer's paired helical filaments share epitopes with neurofilament side arms. *EMBO J.*, 5:269–276.

104. Miyakawa, T., Katsuragi, S., Watanabe, K., Shimoji, A., and Ikeuchi, Y. (1986): Ultrastructural studies of amyloid fibrils and senile plaques in human brain. *Acta Neuropathol. (Berl.)*, 70:202–208.

105. Montpetit, V., Clapin, D. F., and Guberman, A. (1985): Substructure of 20nm filaments of progressive supranuclear palsy. *Acta Neuropathol. (Berl.)*, 68:311–318.

106. Morrison, J. H., Scherr, S., Lewis, D. A., Campbell, M. J., Bloom, F. E., Rogers, J., and Benoit, R. (1986): The laminar and regional distribution of neocortical somatostatin and neuritic plaques: implications for Alzheimer's disease as a global neocortical disconnection syndrome. In: *The Biological Substrates of Alzheimer's Disease*, edited by A. B. Scheibel, A. F. Wechsler, and M. A. B. Brazier, pp. 115–131. UCLA Forum in Medical Sciences No. 27. Academic Press, New York.

107. Multhaup, G., Diringer, H., Hilmert, H., Prinz, H., Heukeshoven, J., and Beyreuther, K. (1985): The protein component of scrapie-associated fibrils is a glycosylated low molecular weight protein. *EMBO J.*, 4:1495–1501.

108. Nakazato, Y., Sasaki, A., Hirato, J., and Ishida, Y. (1984): Immunohistochemical localization of neurofilament protein in neuronal degenerations. *Acta Neuropathol. (Berl.)*, 64:30–36.

109. Narang, H. K. (1980) High-resolution electron microscopic analysis of the amyloid fibril in Alzheimer's disease. *J. Neuropathol. Exp. Neurol.*, 39:621–631.

110. Nikaido, T., Austin, J., Rinehart, R., Trueb, L., Hutchinson, J., Stukenbrok, H., and Miles, B. (1971): Studies in ageing of the brain. I. Isolation and preliminary characterization of Alzheimer plaques and cores. *Arch. Neurol.*, 25:198–211.

111. Nikaido, T., Austin, J., Trueb, L., and Rinehart, R. (1972): Studies in ageing of the brain. II. Microchemical analyses of the nervous system in Alzheimer patients. *Arch. Neurol.*, 27:549–554.

112. Nukina, N., and Ihara, Y. (1983): Immunocytochemical study on senile plaques in Alzheimer's disease. I. Preparation of an antimicrotubule-associated proteins (MAPs) antiserum and its specificity. *Proc. Jpn. Acad.*, 59(ser B):284–287.

113. Nukina, N., and Ihara, Y. (1983): Immunocytochemical study on senile plaques in Alzheimer's disease. II. Abnormal dendrites in senile plaques as revealed by antimicrotubule-associated proteins (MAPs) immunostaining. *Proc. Jpn. Acad.*, 59(serB):288–292.

114. Nukina, N., and Ihara, Y. (1985): Proteolytic fragments of Alzheimer's paired helical filaments. *J. Biochem. (Tokyo)*, 98:1715–1718.

115. Nukina, N., and Ihara, Y. (1986): One of the antigenic determinants of paired helical filaments is related to tau protein. *J. Biochem. (Tokyo)*, 99:1541–1544.

116. Oesch, B., Westaway, D., Wälchli, M., McKinley, M. P., Kent, S. B. H., Aebersold, R., Barry, R. A., Tempst, P., Teplow, D. B., Hood, L. E., Prusiner, S. B., and Weissmann, C. (1985): A cellular gene encodes scrapie PrP 27–30 protein. *Cell*, 40:735–746.

117. Pearson, R. C. A., Esiri, M. M., Hiorns, R. W., Wilcock, G. K., and Powell, T. P. S. (1985): Anatomical correlates of the distribution of the pathological changes in the neocortex in Alzheimer disease. *Proc. Natl. Acad. Sci. USA*, 82:4531–4535.

118. Perry, G., Rizzuto, N. Autilio-Gambetti, L., and Gambetti, P. (1985): Paired helical filaments from Alzheimer disease patients contain cytoskeletal components. *Proc. Natl. Acad. Sci. USA*, 82:3916–3920.

119. Perry, G., Selkoe, D. J., Block, B. R., Stewart, D., Autilio-Gambetti, L., and Gambetti, P. (1986): Electron microscopic localization of Alzheimer neurofibrillary tangle components recognized by an antiserum to paired helical filaments. *J. Neuropathol. Exp. Neurol.*, 45:161–168.

120. Persuy, P., Defossez, A., Delacourte, A., Tramu, G., Bouchez, B., and Arnott, G. (1985): Anti-PHF antibodies: an immunohistochemical marker of the lesions of the Alzheimer's disease: characterization and comparison with Bodian's silver impregnation. *Virchows Arch. [Pathol. Anat.]*, 407:13–23.

121. Powers, J. M., Sullivan, L., and Rosenthal, C. J. (1982): Permanganate oxidation of senile cerebral amyloid and its relationship to AA protein. *Acta Neuropathol. (Berl.)*, 58:275–278.

122. Probst, A., Anderton, B. H., Ulrich, J., Kohler, R., Kahn, J., and Heitz, P. U. (1983): Pick's disease: an immunocytochemical study of neuronal changes: monoclonal antibodies

show that Pick bodies share antigenic determinants with neurofibrillary tangles and neurofilaments. *Acta Neuropathol. (Berl.)*, 60:175–182.

123. Prusiner, S. B., Groth, D. F., Bolton, D. C., Kent, S. B., and Hood, L. E. (1984): Purification and structural studies of a major scrapie prion protein. *Cell*, 38:127–134.

124. Prusiner, S. B., McKinley, M. P., Bowman, K. A., Bolton, D. C., Bendheim, P. E., Groth, D. F., and Glenner, G. G. (1983): Scrapie prions aggregate to form amyloid-like birefringent rods. *Cell*, 35:349–358.

125. Rasool, C. G., Abraham, C., Anderson, B. H., Haugh, M., Kahn, J., and Selkoe, D. J. (1984): Alzheimer's disease: immunoreactivity of neurofilament tangles with anti-neurofilament and anti-paired helical filament antibodies. *Brain Res.*, 310:249–260.

126. Rasool, C. G., and Selkoe, D. J. (1984): Alzheimer's disease: exposure of neurofilament immunoreactivity in SDS-insoluble paired helical filaments. *Brain Res.*, 322:194–198.

127. Rasool, C. G., and Selkoe, D. J. (1985): Sharing of specific antigens by degenerating neurons in Pick's disease and Alzheimer's disease. *N. Engl. J. Med.*, 312:700–705.

128. Robakis, N. K., Devine-Gage, E. A., Jenkins, E. C., Kascsak, R. J., Brown, W. T., Krawczun, M. S., and Silverman, W. P. (1986): Localization of a human gene homologous to the PrP gene on the p arm of chromosome 20 and detections of PrP-related antigens in normal human brain. *Biochem. Biophys. Res. Commun.*, 140:758–765.

129. Rogers, J., and Morrison, J. H. (1985): Quantitative morphology and regional and laminar distributions of senile plaques in Alzheimer's disease. *J. Neurosci.*, 5:2801–2808.

130. Roher, A., Wolfe, D., Palutke, M., and KuKuruga, D. (1986): Purification, ultrastructure, and chemical analysis of Alzheimer disease amyloid plaque core protein. *Proc. Natl. Acad. Sci. USA*, 83:2662–2666.

131. Rohwer, R. G. (1984): Scrapie infectious agent is virus-like in size and susceptibility to inactivation. *Nature*, 308:658–662.

132. Rohwer, R. G. (1984): Virus-like sensitivity of the scrapie agent to heat inactivation. *Science*, 223:600–602.

133. Rowe, I. F., Jensson, O., Lewis, P. D., Candy, J., Tennent, G. A., and Pepys, M. B. (1984): Immunhistochemical demonstration of amyloid P component in cerebro-vascular amyloidosis. *Neuropathol. Appl. Neurobiol.*, 10:53–61.

134. Rozemuller, J. M., Eikelenboom, P., and Stam, F. C. (1986): Role of microglia in plaque formation in senile dementia of the Alzheimer type: an immunohistochemical study. *Virchows. Arch. [Cell Pathol.]*, 51:247–254.

135. Rubenstein, R., Kascsak, R. J., Merz, P. A., Papini, M. C., Carp, R. I., Robakis, N. K., and Wisniewski, H. M. (1986): Detection of scrapie-associated fibril (SAF) proteins using anti-SAF antibody in non-purified tissue preparations. *J. Gen. Virol.*, 67:671–681.

136. Rubenstein, R., Kascsak, R. J., Merz, P. A., Wisniewski, H. M., Carp. R. I., and Iqbal, K. (1986): Paired helical filaments associated with Alzheimer disease are readily soluble structures. *Brain Res.*, 372:80–88.

137. Selkoe, D. J. (1980): Altered protein composition of isolated human cortical neurons in Alzheimer disease. *Ann. Neurol.*, 8:468–478.

138. Selkoe, D. J. (1986): Altered structural proteins in plaques and tangles: what do they tell us about the biology of Alzheimer's disease? *Neurobiol. Aging*, 7:425–432.

139. Selkoe, D. J., Abraham, C., and Ihara, Y. (1982): Brain transglutaminase: in vitro crosslinking of human neurofilament proteins into insoluble polymers. *Proc. Natl. Acad. Sci. USA*, 79:6070–6074.

140. Selkoe, D. J., Abraham, C. R., Podlinski, M. B., and Duffy, L. K. (1986): Isolation of low-molecular-weight proteins from amyloid plaque fibers in Alzheimer's disease. *J. Neurochem.*, 46:1820–1834.

141. Selkoe, D. J., Brown, B. A., Salazar, F. J., and Marotta, C. A. (1981): Myelin basic protein in Alzheimer disease neuronal fractions and mammalian neurofilament preparations. *Ann. Neurol.*, 10:429–436.

142. Selkoe, D. J., Ihara, Y., and Salazar, F. J. (1982): Alzheimer's disease: insolubility of partially purified paired helical filaments in sodium dodecyl sulfate and urea. *Science*, 215:1243–1245.

143. Shinagawa, M., Munekata, E., Doi, S., Takahashi, K., Goto, H., and Sato, G. (1986): Immunoreactivity of a synthetic pentadecapeptide corresponding to the N-terminal region of the scrapie prion protein. *J. Gen. Virol.*, 67:1745–1750.

144. Shinoba, R. A., Eng, L. F., Sternberger, L. A., Sternberger, N. H., and Urich, H. (1987): The cytoskeleton of the human cerebellar cortex: an immunohistochemical study of normal and pathological materials. *Brain Res. (in press)*.
145. Shirahama, T., Skinner, M., Westermark, P., Rubinow, A., and Cohen, A. S. (1982): Senile cerebral amyloid: prealbumin as a common constituent in the neuritic plaque, in the neurofibrillary tangle, and in the microangiopathic lesion. *Am. J. Pathol.,* 107:41–50.
146. Sklaviadis, T., Manuelidis, L., and Manuelidis, E. E. (1986): Characterization of major peptides in Creutzfeldt-Jakob disease and scrapie. *Proc. Natl. Acad. Sci. USA,* 83:6146–6150.
147. Sparkes, R. S., Simon, M., Cohn, V. H., Fournier, R. E. K., Lem, J., Klisak, I., Heinzman, C., Blatt, C., Lucerno, M., Mohandas, T., DeArmond, S. J., Westaway, D., Prusiner, S. B., and Weiner, L. P. (1986): Assignment of the human and mouse prion protein genes to homologous chromosomes. *Proc. Natl. Acad. Sci. USA,* 83:7378–7362.
148. Sternberger, N. H., Sternberger, L. A., and Ulrich, J. (1985): Aberrant neurofilament phosphorylation in Alzheimer disease. *Proc. Natl. Acad. Sci. USA,* 82:4274–4276.
149. Struble, R. G., Price, D. L., Jr., Cork, L. A., and Price, D. L. (1985): Senile plaques in cortex of aged normal monkeys. *Brain Res.,* 361:267–275.
150. Torack, R. M., and Lynch, R. G. (1981): Cytochemistry of brain amyloid in adult dementia. *Acta Neuropathol. (Berl.),* 53:189–196.
151. Troncoso, J. C., Sternberger, N. G., Sternberger, L. A., Hoffman, P. N., and Price, D. L. (1986): Immunocytochemical studies of neurofilament antigens in the neurofibrillary pathology induced by aluminum. *Brain Res.,* 364:295–300.
152. Ulrich, J. (1985): Alzheimer changes in nondemented patients younger than sixty-five: possible early stages of Alzheimer's disease and senile dementia of Alzheimer type. *Ann. Neurol.,* 17:273–277.
153. Wang, G. P., Grundke-Iqbal, I., Kascsak, R. J., Iqbal, K., and Wisniewski, H. M. (1984): Alzheimer neurofibrillary tangles: monoclonal antibodies to inherent antigen(s). *Acta Neuropathol. (Berl.),* 62:268–275.
154. Westaway, D., and Prusiner, S. B. (1986): Conservation of the cellular gene encoding the scrapie prion protein. *Nucleic Acids Res.,* 14:2035–2044.
155. Wischik, C. M., Crowther, R. A., Stewart, M., and Roth, M. (1985): Subunit structure of paired helical filaments in Alzheimer's disease. *J. Cell Biol.,* 100:1905–1912.
158. Wisniewski, H. M., Merz, P. A., and Iqbal, K. (1984): Ultrastructure of paired helical filaments of Alzheimer's neurofibrillary tangle. *J. Neuropathol. Exp. Neurol.,* 43:643–656.
156. Wisniewski, H. M., and Terry, R. D. (1973): Re-examination of the pathogenesis of the senile plaque. *Prog. Neuropathol.,* 2:1–26.
157. Wisniewski, H. M., and Wen, G. Y. (1985): Substructures of paired helical filaments from Alzheimer's disease neurofibrillary tangles. *Acta Neuropathol. (Berl.),* 66:173–176.
159. Wong, C. W., Quaranta, V., and Glenner, G. G. (1985): Neuritic plaques and cerebrovascular amyloid in Alzheimer disease are antigenically related. *Proc. Natl. Acad. Sci. USA,* 82:8729–8732.
160. Wood, J. G., Mirra, S. S., Pollock, N. J., and Binder, L. I. (1986): Neurofibrillary tangles of Alzheimer's disease share antigenic determinants with the axonal microtubule-associated protein tau ($\tau$). *Proc. Natl. Acad. Sci. USA,* 83:4040–4043.
161. Wood, J. N., Lathangue, W. B., McLachlan, D. R., Smith, B. J., Anderton, B. H., and Dowding, A. J. (1985): Chromatin proteins share antigenic determinants with neurofilaments. *J. Neurochem.,* 44:149–154.
162. Yen, S-H., and Kress, Y. (1983): The effect of chemical reagents or proteases on the ultrastructure of paired helical filaments. In: *Biological Aspects of Alzheimer's Disease,* edited by R. Katzman, Banbury Report 15, pp. 155–165. Cold Spring Harbor Laboratory, New York.
163. Yen, S-H., Gaskin, F., and Fu, S. M. (1983): Neurofibrillary tangles in senile dementia of the Alzheimer type share an antigenic determinant with intermediate filaments of the vimentin class. *Am. J. Pathol.,* 113:373–381.
164. Yen, S-H., Gaskin, F., and Terry, R. D. (1981): Immunocytochemical studies of neurofibrillary tangles. *Am. J. Pathol.,* 104:77–89.
165. Yen, S-H., Horoupian, D. S., and Terry, R. D. (1983): Immunocytochemical comparison of neurofibrillary tangles in senile dementia of Alzheimer type, progressive supranuclear palsy, and postencephalitic parkinsonism. *Ann. Neurol.,* 13:172–175.

Aging and the Brain, edited by R. D. Terry.
Raven Press, New York © 1988.

# Neurofilaments, Axonal Caliber, and Perikaryal Size

Paul N. Hoffman, John W. Griffin, Edward H. Koo,
Nancy A. Muma, and Donald L. Price

*Departments of Ophthalmology, Neurology, Neuroscience, and Pathology,
The Johns Hopkins School of Medicine, Baltimore, Maryland 21205*

This review of the role of neurofilaments (NFs) in the control of axonal caliber and the size of neuronal perikarya examines evidence supporting the hypotheses that NF gene expression is a primary determinant of caliber in large myelinated nerve fibers and that the level of NF gene expression is closely correlated with perikaryal size. Because fiber caliber is the principal determinant of conduction velocity in myelinated fibers (13,27,35), the control of caliber has important implications for the functional properties of neurons, e.g., the latency (duration) of the monosynaptic reflex changes when caliber is altered (10). Moreover, conduction velocity decreases in neurological diseases associated with reductions in axonal caliber (e.g., Charcot-Marie-Tooth disease) (37). Conduction velocity (46,48), axonal caliber (29), and perikaryal size (R. D. Terry and L. A. Hansen, *this volume*) decrease in older individuals. We propose that such reductions in axonal caliber and perikaryal size could result from decreased expression of NF genes.

## NF AND AXONAL CALIBER

### Morphological Correlates of Axonal Caliber

Several observations support the hypothesis that NFs are major intrinsic determinants of axonal caliber in large myelinated nerve fibers (3,22). The density of NFs, the most numerous cytoskeletal organelles in these fibers, remains relatively constant over a wide range of calibers; the number of NFs correlates closely with axonal cross-sectional area (3,12,22,50) (Fig. 1).

Studies of the radial growth of developing nerve fibers are also consistent with the concept that NFs are principal intrinsic determinants of axonal caliber. Prior to undergoing myelination, embryonic axons are thin (less than 1 $\mu$m in diameter) and principally contain microtubules (MTs) and relatively few NFs (3,40,43). Radial growth correlates with a dramatic increase in

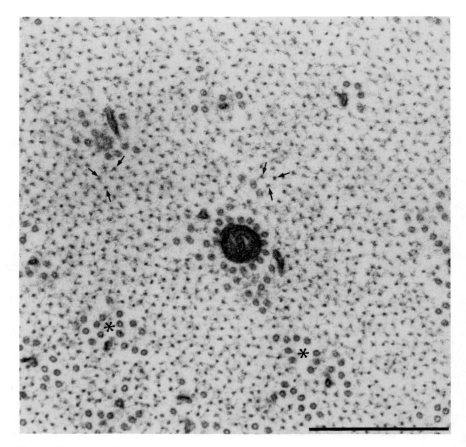

**FIG. 1.** High-resolution electron micrograph of organelles in axoplasm of a large myelinated nerve fiber. NFs (*small arrows*) greatly outnumber MTs (*asterisks*) in this cross-sectional view. Bar = 0.5 μm.

axonal NF content. Although the number of MTs in developing nerve fibers increases during radial growth, the increase in NFs is greater (3). In large myelinated nerve fibers, NFs outnumber MTs by more than 10:1 (12). It should be noted that NF content is not as closely correlated with axonal caliber in small myelinated central nervous system (CNS) fibers, where NF density may vary considerably along the length of the axon, e.g., in optic nerve (39) or in mature unmyelinated fibers, which contain relatively few NFs (3,43). Also, it is clear from morphological observations that NF density in large myelinated nerve fibers can be altered with disease. Marked increases in NF density accompany NF accumulation in giant axonal neuropathy (2), in hexacarbon (45), IDPN (7), and aluminum intoxication (47), and in inter-

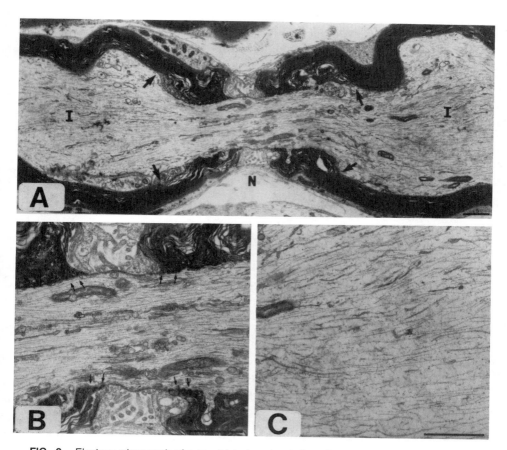

**FIG. 2.** Electron micrograph of a constricted segment viewed in the longitudinal plane of an axon. **A:** Low-power micrograph demonstrates that the caliber of the constricted segment is significantly less than that of the internodes (*I*) in a rat motor fiber. The constricted segment, comprised of the node of Ranvier (*N*) and the paranodal regions, is delineated by *large arrows*. **B:** Myelin attachment sites (*small arrows*) are present in the paranodal regions. **C:** High-power view of the internode demonstrates numerous NFs. Bars = 1 μm. (From ref. 25, with permission.)

nodes that have undergone segmental demyelination (38). These observations indicate that NF spacing can be altered in a variety of pathological settings.

Myelination of axons is closely correlated with the radial growth of developing nerve fibers (3,11,49). Myelinated fibers show distinct regional differences in the composition of their cytoskeletons. These fibers are made up of a series of myelinated segments (internodes) that are relatively long (up to 2,000 μm in the rat) and equal in length. Internodes are separated from one another by short (1–2 μm) unmyelinated regions (the nodes of Ranvier) (3) (Fig. 2). Axonal cross-sectional areas are as much as 10-fold greater at internodes than at nodes (3). Although NF density may be slightly greater at nodes than internodes, total NF content is substantially greater at internodes (3). In contrast, the MT number is comparable in both regions; i.e., MT density is significantly higher at nodes than at internodes (3).

### Role of NF Gene Expression in the Control of Axonal Caliber

The expression of NF genes is the primary step in the sequence of events leading to the appearance of NFs in axons. Each of the three NF subunit polypeptides [200, 145, and 68 kilodaltons (KD)] (20,21) is encoded by a separate gene (34). Transcription of these genes yields NF mRNAs, which are translated exclusively in perikarya and proximal dendrites. Shortly after they are synthesized, these proteins are assembled into stable heteropolymers. This assembly also appears to occur exclusively in perikarya (4). Because axons do not contain ribosomes (33) NFs must be delivered to axons, where they undergo somatofugal translocation via slow axonal transport (21). The absence of unassembled NF subunits in axons precludes local assembly (36) (i.e., NF proteins are transported in the form of NF organelles). Normally, there is relatively little turnover of axonal NFs, except at the axon terminals (31,32). NFs are degraded as they enter the axon terminals, presumably through the action of calcium-activated proteases (32,42).

The axotomy model has been used to investigate the role of NF gene expression in the control of axonal caliber. Previous studies have shown that axonal caliber is reduced in the proximal stumps of transected nerve fibers (1,8,17,19,28). In this setting the axonal cross-sectional area is selectively reduced; myelin sheath thickness, axonal perimeter, and internodal length are relatively unaffected (13). Reductions in caliber correlate with decreases in conduction velocity in the proximal stump (8,13,30), providing a clear demonstration of the relative importance of axonal cross-sectional area as a determinant of conduction velocity (13,35).

In these atrophic axons, the density of NFs is unchanged, but numbers of NFs are reduced in proportion to the diminution in axonal cross-sectional area (9,22) (Fig. 3). In contrast, the MT content of atrophic nerve fibers either remains constant or increases slightly; MT density increases in proportion to the reduction in axonal cross-sectional area (22). The reduction in axonal NF content correlates with a decrease in the relative amount of NF protein (com-

---

→

**FIG. 3.** **A:** NF content is reduced in the atrophic proximal stump of a hypoglossal motor fiber 2 weeks after axotomy. Loss of circularity and an inappropriately thick myelin sheath (for axonal area) indicate that this axon has undergone a reduction in cross-sectional area. MT number is relatively unchanged; MT density is increased in proportion to the decrease in axonal cross-sectional area. **B:** Control motor fiber (with axonal perimeter and myelin sheath thickness comparable to that of the atrophic fiber) is circular and contains many NFs. Bars = 0.5 μm.

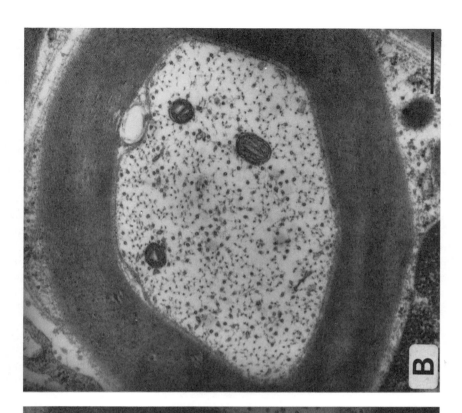

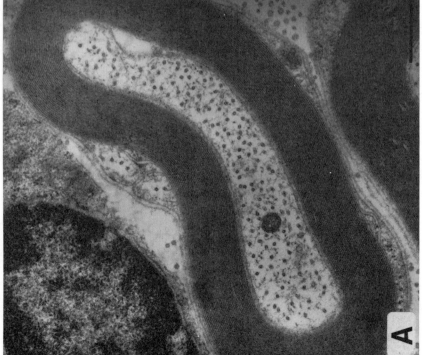

pared to actin and tubulin) undergoing axonal transport in these nerve fibers (26). This axonal atrophy begins near the cell body (soma) and proceeds anterogradely at the rate of slow axonal transport (22); we have termed this process somatofugal atrophy (Fig. 4).

We have demonstrated that the reduction in NF transport in axotomized neurons is related to a selective decrease in NF gene expression. In sensory neurons in dorsal root ganglia (DRG) of normal and axotomized rats, we used cDNA probes to measure levels of mRNA encoding the 68-KD NF protein (NF68), β-tubulin, and actin. RNA blots show that levels of NF68 mRNA in DRG decrease between 4 and 42 days after axotomy (24). *In situ* hybridization studies demonstrate that levels of NF mRNAs are reduced two- to three-fold within individual neurons of axotomized ganglia. This reduction in NF mRNA is selective; in the same ganglia there is a corresponding elevation in levels of mRNAs for actin and tubulin, the other major proteins of the axonal cytoskeleton (24). Because the incorporation of labeled amino acids into NF protein by DRG *in vitro* is also selectively reduced after axotomy with a time course similar to that of the reductions in mRNA levels (16), we infer that specific alterations in NF mRNA levels are mirrored by concomitant changes in the rates of NF synthesis. The decrease in NF mRNA levels correlates temporally with the appearance of axonal atrophy in axotomized sensory fibers; recovery of caliber coincides with the return of NF mRNA levels to

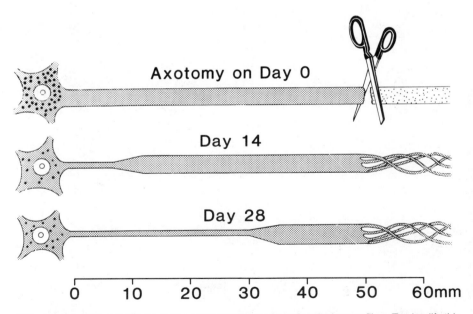

**FIG. 4.** Somatofugal atrophy in the proximal stump of a transected motor fiber. To simplify this diagram, myelin sheaths and nodes of Ranvier are not shown. (From ref. 22, with permission.)

control values (24). Thus NF gene expression is a primary intrinsic determinant of axonal NF content.

## Axonal Caliber and Alterations in NF Transport Kinetics

Axonal NF content depends on both the level of NF gene expression (which determines the amount of NF protein undergoing axonal transport) and the kinetics of NF transport. The interrelation between these parameters is illustrated by the changes in axonal caliber (and NF content) induced by intoxication with $\beta,\beta'$-iminodipropionitrile (IDPN), an agent that impairs the axonal transport of NFs (18). In this model newly synthesized NFs continue to enter the axon but fail to move distally; the result is a massive accumulation of NFs and a dramatic enlargement of the proximal portion of the axon (7). The pathological changes produced by IDPN comprise an example of how a mismatch between the amounts of transported NFs entering and leaving a region of the axon leads to a net accumulation of NFs and an abnormal increase in axonal caliber. Our hypothesis predicts that the rate at which NFs accumulate after IDPN intoxication should correlate with the level of NF gene expression. This prediction is consistent with the observation that NFs accumulate more slowly in neurons in which NF gene expression is reduced (i.e., by axotomy 2 weeks prior to intoxication) than in normal (intact) neurons (J. W. Griffin, P. N. Hoffman, and K. Fahnestock, *unpublished observations*). Thus given the same degree of transport impairment, the rate of NF accumulation correlates with the level of NF gene expression (i.e., NFs accumulate faster in neurons having higher levels of NF gene expression).

## Radical Growth of Developing Nerve Fibers

Neurofilament gene expression and alterations in the kinetics of NF transport play important roles in the radial growth of developing nerve fibers. NF velocity decreases continuously with increasing distance along nerve fibers (25). As a result, NFs enter every region of the axon slightly faster than they leave, leading to a continuous increase in local NF content. If the rate of this accumulation exceeds the local rate of NF turnover (which is normally quite low, except at the axon terminals), axonal NF content should increase, resulting in an increase in axonal caliber. Such a mechanism is consistent with the synchronous pattern of radial growth observed in developing nerve fibers; i.e., growth occurs simultaneously at proximal and distal levels of the fiber without significant tapering of axonal caliber (25). Confining this velocity-dependent accumulation of NFs to the internodal segments of maturing fibers could account for the greater NF content of internodal as compared to nodal segments in mature fibers (23).

As in the case of IDPN intoxication, the rate at which the NF content of developing nerve fibers increases in response to alterations in transport kinetics is related to the level of NF gene expression. Axonal caliber correlates with the level of NF gene expression. For example, in rat DRG the largest fibers arise from the neurons with the highest levels of NF gene expression; the smallest (unmyelinated) fibers arise from neurons with the lowest levels of NF expression (24). In addition, the rate at which NFs accumulate in developing nerve fibers correlates with axonal caliber (i.e., NFs accumulate fastest in the largest-caliber fibers) (25). Therefore the rate at which NF content increases in developing nerve fibers correlates with the level of NF gene expression.

Once the level of NF gene expression has been established in developing neurons, nerve fibers undergo maturational growth without concomitant changes in NF gene expression. For example, after the induction of increased NF gene expression at 10 days of age, levels of NF mRNA in rat DRG reach plateau values over a period of several days and remain constant for the next several months (i.e., during the period of sustained radial growth in these nerve fibers) (N. A. Muma, E. H. Koo, and P. N. Hoffman, *unpublished observations*). Thus the level of NF gene expression remains relatively constant during the radical growth of developing nerve fibers.

### Aging and Axonal Atrophy

Axonal calibers are maintained within narrow limits in mature nerve fibers (5). Relatively little is known about the mechanisms responsible for the cessation of radial growth in mature nerve fibers. As in developing nerve fibers, the velocity of NF transport decreases with increasing distance along nongrowing fibers in mature rats (D. Watson, *unpublished observations*). The level of NF gene expression determines the rate at which NFs accumulate in mature nerve fibers (i.e., in response to the decrease in transport velocity). Therefore one way to stop radial growth is by reducing NF gene expression to the level at which the rate of accumulation equals the local rate of NF turnover. Under these conditions the net rate of accumulation would be zero; i.e., axonal NF content (and axonal caliber) would remain constant. Further reductions in NF gene expression (or increases in the rate of NF turnover) would lead to a net loss of axonal NF, resulting in axonal atrophy. Thus, decreases in NF gene expression could account for the cessation of radial growth in mature nerve fibers and for the axonal atrophy that occurs in these fibers during aging (29) (Fig. 5).

### NF GENE EXPRESSION AND PERIKARYAL SIZE

The level of NF gene expression also appears to correlate with perikaryal size. In rat DRG reduced NF expression after axotomy correlates with the

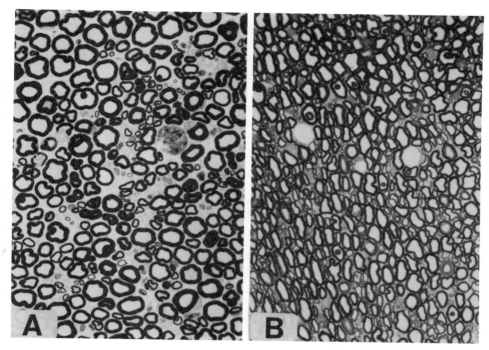

**FIG. 5.** Light micrographs comparing axonal caliber at 12 (**A**) and 20 (**B**) months of age in the sciatic nerve (**A**) and lumbar ventral root (**B**) of the rat. The calibers of axons were comparable in the sciatic nerve and ventral root at both ages (data not shown). Clearly, axonal caliber is greater at 12 than at 20 months of age, indicating that a significant degree of axonal atrophy has occurred between 12 and 20 months. Magnification is identical in the two micrographs.

reduction in the size of perikarya (6,24). Conversely, during postnatal development increased NF gene expression in some DRG neurons correlates with the onset of perikaryal growth (N. A. Muma et al., *unpublished observations*). Furthermore, *in situ* hybridization studies in these sensory neurons demonstrate that the size of perikarya correlates with the level of NF gene expression (24), a finding consistent with the observation that large perikarya in DRG show significant immunoreactivity with NF antibodies, whereas small perikarya show little or no immunoreactivity (41). It has been suggested that neurons in human cerebral cortex undergo age-related reductions in perikaryal size (R. D. Terry and L. A. Hansen, *this volume*). Reductions in axonal caliber and perikaryal size are the morphological correlates of decreased NF gene expression in axotomized neurons (24). Therefore age-related reductions in NF gene expression would be expected to lead to decreases in both the size of perikarya and axonal caliber (29).

## FACTORS REGULATING NF GENE EXPRESSION

The factors that regulate the level of NF gene expression play a primary role in determining axonal caliber. For example, somatofugal atrophy, the morphological correlate of decreased NF gene expression, is initiated when a neuron is disconnected from its targets. If the sciatic nerve is cut and regeneration prevented, the proximal stumps of axons remain atrophic throughout the life of the animal (9). On the other hand, if the nerve is crushed and effective regeneration allowed, caliber recovers in the proximal stump. The time of initial restoration of normal caliber in the proximal axon coincides in a general fashion with that of the reinnervation of target tissues (22,30). This recovery of caliber correlates with the return of NF mRNA levels to normal values (24).

This change in caliber after axotomy does not depend on degeneration of the distal axon. For example, all sensory axons undergo somatofugal atrophy early in the course of exposure to acrylamide (14), a neurotoxin that, after more prolonged exposure, induces distal axonal degeneration in long, large-caliber fibers. In addition, somatofugal atrophy occurs in motor fibers after intramuscular injection of botulinum toxin (15), which blocks muscle activity by inhibiting release of quanta of the neurotransmitter acetylcholine from motor nerve terminals (44). These observations suggest that interactions between neurons and their targets play an important role in maintaining NF gene expression.

We propose that the signal(s) generated by neuron–target interactions travels, by retrograde transport, from the axon terminals to its site of action in neuronal perikarya. This signal could be either a molecule produced by target cells and transferred transsynaptically to axon terminals or a molecule produced in neurons that is modified upon entering the axon terminals and returns to the cell body as a signal. In either case, the continued production of this signal would depend on maintaining normal axon–target cell interactions.

Although the available evidence indicates that the level of NF gene expression is a major determinant of axonal caliber in large myelinated nerve fibers, an unresolved issue is the role of target cells in regulating NF gene expression. Each class of target cells is innervated by axons of a specific caliber. For example, extrafusal muscle fibers and encapsulated sensory receptors are innervated by large myelinated axons, intrafusal muscle fibers are innervated by small myelinated axons, and free nerve endings that lack specific receptors arise from small unmyelinated sensory fibers (5). This relation between the physiological function of targets and axonal caliber raises the possibility that target cells help to specify the level of NF gene expression. According to this hypothesis, the quantity or quality of target-induced signal would determine the rate of NF gene expression, and each class of target cells would specify characteristic levels of signal. The levels of these signals could decrease with aging, resulting in a decrease of NF gene expression. Initially, this decrease in

NF gene expression could result in the cessation of radial growth; further reductions in expression could lead to axonal atrophy and reduction in perikaryal size.

## CONCLUSION

Neurofilament gene expression plays primary roles in the control of axonal caliber and the size of neuronal perikarya. Because axonal caliber is the principal determinant of conduction velocity in large myelinated fibers, the maintenance of caliber is necessary for the preservation of normal function. We propose the NF gene expression, which may be regulated by trophic interactions between neurons and their targets, is impaired during aging. Decreased expression of NF genes would be expected to lead to the reductions in axonal caliber and perikaryal size observed in older individuals.

## ACKNOWLEDGMENT

We thank Kenneth Fahnestock for preparation of the figures.

## REFERENCES

1. Aitkin, J. T., and Thomas, P. K. (1962): Retrograde changes in fibre size following nerve section. *J. Anat.*, 96:121–129.
2. Asbury, A. K., Gale, M. K., Cox, S. C., Baringer, J. R., and Berg, B. O. (1972): Giant axonal neuropathy—a unique case with segmental neurofilamentous masses. *Acta Neuropathol. (Berl.)*, 20:237–247.
3. Berthold, C. H. (1978): Morphology of normal peripheral axons. In: *Physiology and Pathobiology of Axons*, edited by S. G. Waxman, pp. 3–63. Raven Press, New York.
4. Black, M. M. (1987): Spatial relationships between the synthesis and assembly of cytoskeletal proteins in cultured neurons. In: *Intrinsic Determinants of Neuronal Form*, edited by R. J. Lasek. Alan R. Liss, New York (*in press*).
5. Brodal, A. (1981): *Neurological Anatomy in Relation to Clinical Medicine*. Oxford University Press, New York.
6. Cavanaugh, M. W. (1951): Quantitative effects of the peripheral innervation area on nerves and spinal ganglion cells. *J. Comp. Neurol.*, 94:181–219.
7. Clark, A. W., Griffin, J. W., and Price, D. L. (1980): The axonal pathology of chronic IDPN intoxication. *J. Neuropathol. Exp. Neurol.*, 39:42–55.
8. Cragg, B. G., and Thomas, P. K. (1961): Changes in conduction velocity and fibre size proximal to peripheral nerve lesions. *J. Physiol. (Lond.)*, 157:315–327.
9. Dyck, P. J., Nukada, H., Lais, A. C., and Karnes, J. L. (1984): Permanent axotomy: a model of chronic neuronal degeneration preceded by axonal atrophy, myelin remodeling, and degeneration. In: *Peripheral Neuropathy*, edited by P. J. Dyck, P. K. Thomas, E. H. Lambert, and R. Bunge, pp. 666–690. Saunders, Philadelphia.
10. Farel, P. B. (1978): Reflex activity of regenerating frog spinal motoneurons. *Brain Res.*, 158:331–341.
11. Friede, R. L. (1972): Control of myelin formation by axonal caliber (with a model of the control mechanism). *J. Comp. Neurol.*, 144:233–252.
12. Friede, R. L., and Samorajski, T. (1970): Axon caliber related to neurofilaments and microtubules in sciatic nerve fibers of rats and mice. *Anat. Rec.*, 167:379–387.

13. Gillespi, M. J., and Stein, R. B. (1983): The relationship between axon diameter, myelin thickness and conduction velocity during atrophy of mammalian peripheral nerves. *Brain Res.*, 259:41–56.

14. Gold, B. G., Griffin, J. W., and Price, D. L. (1985): Slow axonal transport in acrylamide neuropathy: different abnormalities produced by single-dose and continuous administration. *J. Neurosci.*, 5:1755–1768.

15. Gold, B. G., Griffin, J. W., Pestronk, A., Hoffman, P. N., Stanley, E. F., and Price, D. L. (1987): Axonal atrophy induced by intramuscular injection of botulinum toxin. *Submitted.*

16. Greenberg, S. G. (1986): Changes in cytoskeletal protein synthesis during axonal regeneration. Ph.D. thesis, Case Western Reserve University, Cleveland.

17. Greenman, M. J. (1913): Studies on the regeneration of the peroneal nerve of the albino rat: number and sectional area of fibers: area relation of axis to sheath. *J. Comp. Neurol.*, 23:479–513.

18. Griffin, J. W., Hoffman, P. N., Clark, A. W., Carroll, P. T., and Price, D. L. (1978): Slow axonal transport of neurofilament proteins: impairment by $\beta,\beta'$-iminodipropionitrile administration. *Science,* 202:633–635.

19. Gutmann, E., and Sanders, F. K. (1943): Recovery of fibre numbers and diameters in the regeneration of peripheral nerves. *J. Physiol. (Lond.)*, 101:489–518.

20. Hirokawa, N., Glicksman, M. A., and Willard, M. B. (1984): Organization of mammalian neurofilament polypeptides within the neuronal cytoskeleton. *J. Cell Biol.*, 98:1523–1536.

21. Hoffman,, P. N., and Lasek, R. J. (1975): The slow component of axonal transport: identification of the major structural polypeptides of the axon and their generality among mammalian neurons. *J. Cell Biol.*, 66:351–366.

22. Hoffman, P. N., Griffin, J. W., and Price, D. L. (1984): Control of axonal caliber by neurofilament transport. *J. Cell Biol.*, 99:705–714.

23. Hofman, P. N., Griffin, J. W., and Price, D. L. (1984): Neurofilament transport in axonal regeneration: implications for the control of axonal caliber. In: *Advances in Neurochemistry, Axonal Transport in Neuronal Growth and Regeneration,* edited by J. S. Elam and P. Cancalon, pp. 243–260. Plenum Press, New York.

24. Hoffman, P. N., Cleveland, D. W., Griffin, J. W., Landes, P. W., Cowan, N. J., and Price, D. L. (1987): Neurofilament gene expression: a major determinant of axonal caliber. *Proc. Natl. Acad. Sci. USA,* 84:3472–3476.

25. Hoffman, P. N., Griffin, J. W., Gold, B. G., and Price, D. L. (1985): Slowing of neurofilament transport and the radial growth of developing nerve fibers. *J. Neurosci.* 5:2920–2929.

26. Hoffman, P. N., Thompson, G. W., Griffin, J. W., and Price, D. L. (1985): Changes in neurofilament transport coincide temporally with alterations in the caliber of axons in regenerating motor fibers. *J. Cell Biol.,* 101:1332–1340.

27. Hursh, J. B. (1939): Conduction velocity and diameter of nerve fibers. *Am. J. Physiol.,* 127:131–139.

28. Kreutzberg, G. W., and Schubert, P. (1971): Volume changes in the axon during regeneration. *Acta Neuropathol. (Berl.)*, 17:220–226.

29. Krinke, G., Suter, J., and Hess, R. (1981): Radicular myelinopathy in aging rats. *Vet. Pathol.,* 18:335–341.

30. Kuno, M., Miyata, Y., and Munoz-Martinez, E. J. (1974): Properties of fast and slow alpha motoneurones following motor reinnervation. *J. Physiol. (Lond.)*, 242:273–288.

31. Lasek, R. J., and Black, M. M. (1977): How do axons stop growing? Some clues from the metabolism of the proteins in the slow component of axonal transport. In: *Mechanisms, Regulation and Special Functions of Protein Synthesis in the Brain,* edited by E. Roberts, pp. 161–169. Elsevier/North Holland, New York.

32. Lasek, R. J., and Hoffman, P. N. (1976): The neuronal cytoskeleton, axonal transport and axonal growth. *Cold Spring Harbor Conf. Cell Prolif.*, 3:1021–1049.

33. Lasek, R. J., Dabrowski, C., and Nordlander, R. (1973): Analysis of axoplasmic RNA from invertebrate giant axons. *Nature [New Biol.],* 244:162–165.

34. Lewis, S. A., and Cowan, N. J. (1985): Genetics, evolution and expression of the 68,00-molwt neurofilament protein: isolation of a cloned cDNA probe. *J. Cell Biol.,* 100:843–850.

35. Minwegen, P., and Friede, R. L. (1984): Conduction velocity varies with osmotically induced changes of the area of the axon's profile. *Brain Res.,* 297:105–113.

36. Morris, J. R., and Lasek, R. J. (1982): Stable polymers of the axonal cytoskeleton: the axoplasmic ghost. *J. Cell Biol.*, 92:192–198.

37. Nukada, H., and Dyck, P. J. (1984): Decreased axonal caliber and neurofilaments in hereditary motor and sensory neuropathy, type I. *Ann. Neurol.*, 16:238–241.

38. Parhad, I. M., and Swedberg, E. A. (1986): Neurofilament content in the demyelinated segments of the peripheral nerve. In: *Peripheral Neuropathy Association of America, Abstracts*, p. 44.

39. Parhad, I. M., Griffin, J. W., Hoffman, P. N., and Koves, J. F. (1986): Selective interruption of axonal transport of neurofilament proteins in the visual system by beta, beta'-iminodipropionitrile (IDPN) intoxication. *Brain Res.*, 363:315–324.

40. Peters, A., and Vaughn, J. E. (1967): Microtubules and filaments in the axons and astrocytes of early postnatal optic nerves. *J. Cell Biol.*, 32:113–119.

41. Price, J. (1985): An immunohistochemical and quantitative examination of dorsal root ganglion neuronal subpopulations. *J. Neurosci.*, 5:2051–2059.

42. Roots, B. I. (1983): Neurofilament accumulation induced in synapses by leupeptin. *Science*, 221:971–972.

43. Sasaki-Sherrington, S. E., Jacobs, J. R., and Stevens, J. K. (1984): Intracellular control of axial shape in non-uniform neurites: a serial electron microscopic analysis of organelles and microtubules in AI and AII retinal amacrine cells. *J. Cell Biol.*, 98:1279–1290.

44. Simpson, L. L. (1981): The origin, structure and pharmacological activity of botulinum toxin. *Pharmacol. Rev.*, 33:155–188.

45. Spencer, P. S., and Schaumberg, H. H. (1977): Ultrastructural studies of the dying-back process. III. The evolution of experimental peripheral giant axonal degeneration. *J. Neuropathol. Exp. Neurol.*, 36:276–299.

46. Swallow, J. S., and Griffiths, I. R. (1977): Age related changes in the motor nerve conduction velocity in dogs. *Res. Vet. Sci.*, 23:29–32.

47. Troncoso, J. C., Price, D. L., Griffin, J. W., and Parhad, I. M. (1982): Neurofibrillary axonal pathology in aluminum intoxication. *Ann. Neurol.*, 12:278–283.

48. Wagman, I. H., and Lesse, H. (1952): Maximum conduction velocities of motor fibers of ulnar nerve in human subjects of various ages and sizes, *J. Neurophysiol.*, 15:235–244.

49. Webster, H. DeF., and Favilla, J. T. (1984): Development of peripheral nerve fibers. In: *Peripheral Neuropathy*, edited by P. J. Dyck, P. K. Thomas, E. H. Lambert, and R. Bunge, pp. 329–359: Saunders, Philadelphia.

50. Weiss, P. A., and Mayr, R. (1971): Organelles of neuroplasmic ("axonal") flow: neurofilaments. *Proc. Natl. Acad. Sci. USA*, 68:846–850.

*Aging and the Brain,* edited by R. D. Terry.
Raven Press, New York © 1988.

# Prion Diseases and Brain Dysfunction

## Stanley B. Prusiner

*Departments of Neurology and of Biochemistry and Biophysics, University of
California, San Francisco, California 94143*

In 1920 Creutzfeldt described a progressive dementing illness in a 22-year-old woman (23). The following year, Jakob described four older patients with a clinically similar presentation and course (57). During the ensuing four decades, numerous cases of Creutzfeldt-Jakob disease (CJD) were described clinically and pathologically.

In 1954 Sigurdsson introduced the concept of slow infections. He characterized slow infections as having four cardinal features: (a) a prolonged incubation period ranging from several months to decades; (b) a brief, progressive clinical course leading to death; (c) pathology confined to a single organ; and (d) a natural host usually confined to a single species (115). It appears that slow infections are caused by at least two classes of infectious agent: viruses and prions.

In 1959 Klatzo et al. noted the neuropathologic similarities between CJD and kuru, a degenerative cerebellar disorder of New Guinea natives (65). That same year, Hadlow described the neuropathologic similarities between kuru and scrapie and suggested that kuru might be transmissible to laboratory animals after a prolonged incubation period (53). During the next decade kuru and CJD were transmitted to apes and monkeys (44,46,47). Kuru, CJD, and scrapie are all slow infections.

## PRION DISEASES

The unusual properties of the infectious pathogens causing CJD as well as the animal disease scrapie prompted introduction of the term "prion" to distinguish this class of particles from viruses and viroids (95). Six diseases, three of animals and three of humans, are probably caused by prions (Table 1). The slow infectious agents causing transmissible mink encephalopathy (TME), chronic wasting disease (CWD), kuru, and Gerstmann-Sträussler syndrome (GSS) are not well characterized; thus further knowledge about the properties of these infectious agents must be obtained before they can be firmly classified as prions. For ease of discussion, all the diseases listed in Table 1 are referred to as prion diseases even though a prion etiology must be

TABLE 1. *Prion diseases*[a]

| Disease | Natural host |
|---------|--------------|
| Scrapie[b] | Sheep, goats |
| Transmissible mink encephalopathy (TME) | Mink |
| Chronic wasting disease (CWD) | Mule deer, elk |
| Kuru | Humans—Fore |
| Creutzfeldt-Jakob disease (CJD)[b] | Humans |
| Gerstmann-Sträussler syndrome (GSS) | Humans |

[a]Alternative terminologies include subacute transmissible spongiform encephalopathies and unconventional slow virus diseases (43).

[b]Prions have been shown to cause scrapie and CJD; they are presumed to cause the other diseases listed.

considered tentative until the molecular properties of each slow infectious agent are well defined (96).

Prion diseases share many features; all known prion diseases are confined to the central nervous system (CNS). Prolonged incubation periods ranging from 2 months to more than three decades have been observed. The clinical course in these diseases is usually rather stereotyped and progresses to death. The clinical phase of prion illnesses may last for periods ranging from a few weeks to a few years. A reactive astrocytosis is found throughout the CNS in all these diseases (6,131). Neuronal vacuolation is also found, but it is not a constant or obligatory feature. The infectious agents or prions causing these diseases possess unusual molecular properties that appear to distinguish them from both viruses and viroids (32,95).

The three human prion diseases (kuru, CJD, and GSS) are likely to be variants of the same disorder. By analogy with studies on experimental scrapie, it seems likely that all three of these human diseases require the appearance of an abnormal isoform of the prion protein. The prion protein is encoded by a single copy gene in hamsters and mice (5,91,118). Both chromosomal localization (118) and Southern analyses of human DNA (K. Hsiao, D. Westaway, S. J. DeArmond, and S. B. Prusiner, *in preparation*) suggest that the human PrP gene is single copy.

The human prion diseases illustrate three mechanisms by which this degenerative CNS disorder might arise: (a) slow infection; (b) sporadic degeneration; and (c) genetic transmission. That the three human prion diseases can be transmitted by inoculation to experimental animals is well documented (44,47,75). Kuru is thought to have been spread exclusively through the slow infectious mechanism by ritualistic cannibalism (1,43).

Although a few CJD cases can be traced to inoculation with prions, i.e., human growth hormone (48,66,121,127), cornea transplantation (35), and cerebral electrode implantation (9), the vast majority appear to be sporadic despite considerable effort to implicate scrapie-infected sheep as an exogenous source of prions (25,26). Certainly, sporadic CJD could be explained by prions being ubiquitous in our food chain, with their efficiency of infection being low. We have shown that scrapie prion infection in hamsters by the oral route is $10^9$ times less efficient than intracerebral inoculation in hamsters (100). Whether CJD can arise endogenously without any molecules being contributed from exogenous prions remains to be established. If it is possible for prions to arise endogenously, it is important to identify the macromolecule or events that initiate their production.

Gerstmann-Sträussler syndrome seems to represent the genetic form of prion disease, although 10 to 15% of CJD may also have a genetic basis (75,77). The genetic mechanism whereby patients develop GSS during their fifth decade of life is unknown. One possibility is that a genetic locus renders these individuals susceptible to infection by exogenous prions. Genetic control of the scrapie and CJD incubation periods in mice after inoculation with prions is well documented (19,30,63). Alternatively, GSS might be due to a gene that activates the synthesis of the abnormal isoform of the prion protein as well as any other components of the prion, if they exist. Whether the PrP gene in GSS patients is different from that in unaffected family members is unknown.

Certainly, all of the considerations raised by these three forms of prion disease are equally compatible with a prion structure that either is devoid of any nucleic acid or includes one. Much evidence has been accumulated showing that the abnormal isoform of the prion protein is a component of the infectious particle. No other components of the prion have been identified to date, yet many investigators continue to believe that a small nucleic acid is buried within the interior of the prion. Current data are insufficient to allow us to state that prions are devoid of nucleic acid; however, arguments in support of this hypothesis are growing.

## PURIFICATION AND MOLECULAR STRUCTURE OF PRIONS

Progress in the purification of the hamster scrapie prion (13,99) led to the discovery of a unique protein PrP 27-30, which was shown to be a major component of the infectious particle (14,80). PrP 27-30 is a sialoglycoprotein (15) and was found to polymerize into rods possessing the ultrastructural and histochemical characteristics of amyloid (108). The development of a large-scale purification protocol provided sufficient immunogen for the production of antiserum to PrP 27-30 (7). The availability of this antiserum has provided a means for the molecular comparison in rodents of the infectious particles causing scrapie with those causing CJD (8). We have also used this antiserum to show that amyloid plaques in the brains of scrapie-infected hamsters are composed of paracrystalline arrays of prion proteins (7,28).

Direct evidence for the presence of protease-resistant prion proteins isolated from the brains of patients dying of CJD has been obtained (11). Purified fractions from the brains of two patients with CJD were found to contain protease-resistant proteins ranging in apparent molecular weight ($M_r$) from 10,000 to 50,000. These proteins reacted with antibodies raised against the scrapie prion protein PrP 27-30. Rod-shaped particles were found in sucrose gradient fractions prepared from the brains of these patients that were similar to those isolated from rodents with either scrapie or experimental CJD (8,108). After being stained with Congo red dye, the protein polymers from patients with CJD exhibited green birefringence when examined under polarized light. The findings suggested that the amyloid plaques found in the brains of patients with CJD might be composed of paracrystalline arrays of prions similar to those in prion diseases in laboratory animals; studies show that this situation is the case not only in CJD but also in GSS and kuru (64).

**Purification of Prions**

Development of an incubation time interval assay (99,104) facilitated purification of the infectious particles (33,101,108,109). Partial purification of the scrapie agent led to experiments that provided convincing evidence for a protein within the prion that is required for scrapie infectivity (83,109). Subsequently, a concerted effort was made to identify the protein (13,99). Using both purification steps derived from earlier protocols (102,104–107,109) and centrifugation through a discontinuous sucrose gradient formed in a reorienting vertical rotor, highly purified preparations of scrapie prions were obtained (99).

Considerable evidence indicates that the major protein found in purified prion preparations, PrP 27–30, is a component of the infectious particle (Table 2) (80,108). The concentration of PrP 27-30 was found to be proportional to the prion titer. Many attempts to separate native PrP 27-30 from scrapie prion infectivity were unsuccessful. Indeed, scrapie PrP 27-30 seems to be required for and inseparable from prion infectivity. Furthermore, the murine PrP gene has been shown to be linked to the scrapie incubation time gene (19); the PrP gene has been mapped to murine chromosome 2 (118).

In view of many of the foregoing results, PrP 27-30 was further purified and subjected to gas phase amino acid sequencing (103,108). Once the N-terminal sequence was determined, an isocoding mixture of oligonucleotides corresponding to a portion of this sequence was synthesized and used as a probe to select a clone encoding PrP 27-30 from a scrapie-infected hamster brain cDNA library (91). The identification of the PrP cDNA was confirmed by sequencing additional peptides from PrP 27-30 generated by CNBr cleavage

TABLE 2. *Glossary of prion terminology*

| | |
|---|---|
| **Prion** | Small *proteinaceous infectious* particle that resists inactivation by procedures that modify nucleic acids. It causes scrapie and CJD. Scrapie agent is a synonym. |
| **PrP 27-30** | This protein is the only identifiable macromolecule in purified preparations of hamster scrapie prions. Digestion of PrP 33-35[Sc] with proteinase K generates PrP 27-30. |
| **PrP[Sc]** | Scrapie isoform of the prion protein (PrP 33-35[Sc]). |
| **PrP[c]** | Cellular isoform of the prion protein (PrP 33-35[c]). |
| **Prn-p** | PrP gene in mice located on chromosome 2. |
| **PRNP** | PrP gene in humans located on chromosome 20. |
| **Pid-1** | Gene in mice on chromosome 17 controlling CJD and probably scrapie incubation times. |
| **Prn-i** | Gene in mice on chromosome 2 controlling scrapie and CJD incubation times. *Prn-i* and *Prn-p* form the prion gene complex (*Prn*). |
| **Sinc** | Genetic locus in mice controlling scrapie incubation times, location unknown. |
| **Prion rod** | An aggregate of prions composed largely, if not entirely, of PrP[Sc] or PrP 27-30 molecules. Created by detergent extraction of membranes. Morphologically and histochemically indistinguishable from many amyloids. |

and showing that all were found within the translated sequence of the cloned cDNA insert. Southern blotting with PrP cDNA revealed a single gene with the same restriction patterns in normal and scrapie-infected hamster brain DNA. A single PrP gene was also detected in murine (21,91) and human (91) DNA. PrP mRNA was found at similar levels in both normal and scrapie-infected hamster brain, as well as at lower levels in many other normal tissues. Using antisera raised against PrP 27-30, PrP proteins were detected in crude extracts of infected and normal brains (91); these isoforms were designated PrP 33-35[Sc] and PrP 33-35[c], respectively (4,88). Proteinase K digestion yielded PrP 27-30 in the case of infected brain extract, but it completely degraded PrP 33-35[c]. No PrP-related nucleic acids were found in purified preparations of scrapie prions, indicating that PrP 33-35[Sc] is not encoded by a nucleic acid carried within the infectious particles (91). Studies show that both the scrapie and cellular isoforms of PrP are present in scrapie-infected brains (88).

## Sialoglycoprotein in Scrapie Prions

Purification led to the first identification of a putative macromolecule within the scrapie prion (7,13–15,81,103,108). This molecule (PrP 27-30) is a sialoglycoprotein with an apparent $M_r$ of 27,000 to 30,000 (Table 2) (15). The development of a large-scale purification protocol has allowed determination of the N-terminal sequence of PrP 27-30 and production of antibodies against the protein (7,8,103). Other investigators using purification steps similar to those developed by us seem to have demonstrated the presence of this protein in their preparations (34,55).

That PrP 27-30, which is derived from PrP 33-35[Sc], is a component of the infectious scrapie prion is supported by five major lines of evidence: (a) PrP 27-30 and scrapie prions copurify (99); PrP 27-30 is the most abundant macromolecule in purified preparations of prions (108). (b) PrP 27-30 concentration is proportional to the prion titer (13,80). (c) Procedures that denature, hydrolyze, or selectively modify PrP 27-30 also diminish the prion titer (14,80). (d) The PrP gene (*Prn-p*) in mice is linked to a gene controlling scrapie incubation times (*Prn-i*) (19). (e) PrP 27-30 and scrapie prion infectivity partition together into many forms: membranes, rods, spheres, detergent–lipid–protein complexes, and liposomes (42,81,88,108). These drastically different physical forms all contain PrP 27-30 and high prion titers. These experiments argue for the essential role of PrP 27-30 in the transmission of scrapie infection. To date, all attempts to separate the scrapie isoform of the prion protein (PrP[Sc] or PrP 33-35[Sc]) from infectivity have been unsuccessful.

Some investigators have suggested that the scrapie prion protein (PrP 27-30 or PrP 33-35[Sc]) is unrelated to scrapie infectivity (16,21,111,116,126). They seem not to have considered the differences between the cellular and scrapie isoforms of the prion protein (Table 3). Furthermore, no macromolecule other than PrP 27-30 has been associated with scrapie infectivity.

Considerable evidence suggests that the infectious particles or prions causing scrapie and CJD are composed largely, if not entirely, of protein. The possibility that prions contain a small nucleic acid molecule, though unlikely, cannot be excluded by currently available experimental data. How prions multiply is unknown for they do not contain a gene encoding the prion protein—that gene is found in cellular DNA.

In healthy cells only one isoform of the prion protein is synthesized, and it is designated PrP[C] or PrP 33-35[C] (4,88,91). This protein has an $M_r$ of 33,000 to

TABLE 3. *Cellular and scrapie prion protein isoforms in hamsters*

| Properties | PrP 33-35[C] | PrP 33-35[Sc] |
|---|---|---|
| Uninfected brain | Present | Absent |
| Scrapie brain | Level unchanged | Accumulates |
| Concentration[a] | $< 1 \mu g/g$ | $\sim 10 \mu g/g$ |
| Purified prions | Absent | $10^4$ Molecules/ID$_{50}$ |
| Genetic origin | One cellular gene | One cellular gene |
| mRNA | 2.1 kb | 2.1 kb |
| Localization | | |
| Intracellular | Membrane-bound | Membrane-bound |
| Extracellular | None | Amyloid filaments within plaques |
| Detergent extraction | Soluble | Amyloid rods formed |
| Protease digestion | Degraded | Converted to PrP 27-30[b] |

[a]Expressed as micrograms of prion protein per gram of brain tissue.
[b]PrP 27-30 is derived from PrP 33-35[Sc] during proteinase K digestion in the absence or presence of detergent.

35,000, is sensitive to proteases, and does not polymerize upon exposure to detergents (88,91). The counterpart of PrP$^C$ found only in scrapie-infected animals, PrP$^{Sc}$, is resistant to proteases and does polymerize into amyloid rods and filaments.

## Structure of the Prion Protein Deduced from PrP cDNA Sequence

Studies (5) have shown that initiation of translation at an ATG codon begins 42 nucleotides upstream from the ATG near the 5' of the cDNA clone initially reported (91). The initiation methionine is the first of 22 amino acid residues that comprise a signal peptide (5,111) (Fig. 1). The signal peptide is cleaved by cellular proteases as the native prion protein is synthesized. The first 67 amino acids of PrP 33-35 are not found in PrP 27-30; these amino acids are hydrolyzed during purification, which utilizes proteinase K digestion. Western blot analysis shows that homogenates of scrapie-infected brain contain two immunoreactive proteins of apparent $M_r$ 33,000 to 35,000 (88). One protein, PrP 33-35$^C$, is degraded on digestion with proteinase K, and the other, PrP 33-35$^{Sc}$, is converted to PrP 27-30 during proteinase K digestion (Table 3). The region of the protein that is proteolytically digested contains an interesting set of repeated sequences. Two small repeats of GG(N/S)RYP are followed by a longer set of five repeats of P(H/Q)GGG(__/T)WGQ. Although these repeats possess a high degree of beta structure, they are unnecessary for the amyloid properties exhibited by PrP polymers (108). The significance of these repeats is unknown, but it is of interest that they are highly conserved in the hamster, mouse, and human proteins (21,71,73,91). Because these repeats are hydrolyzed when PrP 27-30 is generated and there is no loss of scrapie infectivity, we surmise that they may be important for the cellular function of the prion protein.

Analysis of the deduced prion protein sequence shows that it has a hydrophobic C-terminus and a hydrophobic domain near the N-terminus (91). The sequence between the hydrophobic regions presumably exhibits considerable beta structure, and there is a segment that probably folds into an amphipathic helix (40). The hydrophobic domains as well as the amphipathic helix are probably buried within cellular membranes, as studies have shown that the prion protein is an integral membrane protein that spans the membrane bilayer at least twice (54a). Multiple forms of scrapie prions have been attributed to their hydrophobicity (107), and numerous studies have documented the association of scrapie infectivity with membranes (56).

The difference between predicted and observed molecular weights of PrP 27-30 [~19 kilodaltons (KD) and 27-30 KD, respectively) appears to be due largely, if not entirely, to glycosylation (15). Chemical deglycosylation of PrP 27-30 with hydrogen fluoride or trifluoromethane sulfonic acid followed by

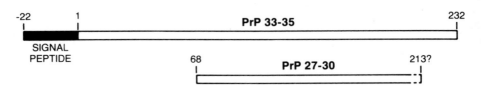

**FIG. 1.** Structure of the hamster prion protein (PrP). The open reading frame encodes a protein of 254 amino acids. The first 22 amino acids comprise a signal peptide that is cleaved during synthesis of PrP 33-35. Digestion of the scrapie isoform of PrP 33-35$^{Sc}$ with proteinase K generates a smaller protease-resistant polypeptide designated PrP 27-30.

sodium dodecyl sulfate polyacrylamide gel electrophoresis (SDS-PAGE) had yielded a protein of about $M_r$ 20,000 (T. Haraguchi-Hiraoka, R. A. Barry, and S. B. Prusiner, *in preparation*). There are two potential N-glycosylation sites of type Asn-X-Thr, at codons 181 to 183 and 197 to 199, respectively (5,91).

Attempts to find meaningful sequence homologies for the PrP cDNA or its translated protein sequence with other macromolecules in computerized data bases (45,94) have been unsuccessful to date. The amino acid and cDNA sequences of the prion protein were also compared to that for known amyloids, and no homology was found. One study suggested that PrP shares significant homology with a portion of the reverse transcriptase and its gene of the AIDS and visna viruses (54). The proposed alignment of small fragments of these sequences employing numerous gaps does not seem to be more significant than that obtained when PrP is compared with many other proteins and their genes.

## PRION PROTEIN GENES

### Hamster PrP Gene

Once correspondence between the cDNA and the amino acid sequence of PrP 27-30 was established, the cDNA was used to probe the genome of the hamster. Both normal and scrapie-infected animals exhibit the same restriction nuclease patterns on Southern blot analysis. A single restriction fragment of 2.6 kb was observed after Eco RI digestion (117). It suggested that the gene for the prion protein might be compact. Other studies show that the entire open reading frame is contained within a single exon (Fig. 2) (5). The 5' end of the PrP gene contains multiple initiation sites, located between 82 and 50

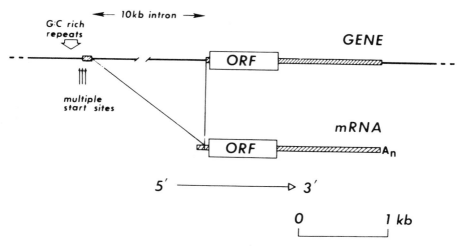

**FIG. 2.** Structure of the hamster PrP gene and mRNA. The features presented were deduced from the nucleotide sequences of PrP genomic and cDNA clones. Untranslated regions of the mRNA are represented by *hatched boxes*. An open reading frame is represented by an *open box*. A splicing event that joins the 5' leader sequences to the remainder of the coding sequences is shown by a vertical and a diagonal line.

nucleotides upstream of a splice donor site. These start sites have been defined by $S_1$ nuclease and primer extension analysis of brain RNA, as well as by *in vitro* transcription of cloned DNA. (Because of a cloning artifact, the 33-terminal nucleotides of the cDNA clone HaPrPcDNA-s11 are an inverted version of the genomic sequences.) The transcription start sites are preceded by G + C rich region that contains three direct repeats of the nonanucleotide GCCCCGCCC. This tandem array strikingly resembles the consensus binding site of the Sp1 protein (36,37,58) and GC motifs found in several viral and cellular promoters (41,84,110,122). This promoter structure, which lacks a "TATA" box, is reminiscent of several housekeeping genes. A 10-kb intron follows the splice donor site. A splice acceptor precedes an uninterrupted block of coding sequences that define the remainder of the PrP mRNA. An ATG codon possessing the features of an initiation site (68,69) is located 11 nucleotides downstream of this splice site. It corresponds to the ATG at nucleotide positions 91 to 93 of the HaPrPcDNA-s11 sequence (5).

Hamster chromosomal DNA was cleaved with individual restriction enzymes, electrophoresed through an agarose gel, and analyzed by Southern blotting (117) using the radiolabeled PrP gene probes. We have constructed three probes corresponding to (a) the first exon, (b) the intron (5), and (c) the second exon (91); both normal and scrapie-infected animals (75 days after inoculation) gave the same restriction patterns with these probes. From these results, we concluded that PrP 27-30 is encoded by a cellular gene, and that rearrangements of this gene are unlikely to figure in the pathogenesis of scrapie. These and other experimental results demonstrate that the PrP gene is single copy.

The degree of sequence conservation observed between hamster and human PrP is consistent with filter hybridization experiments that revealed that mouse, rat, sheep, goat, nematode, *Drosophila,* and possibly yeast harbor candidate PrP gene sequences (128). It is therefore likely that all mammals susceptible to scrapie contain PrP genes. These results are compatible with the preeminent role assigned to PrP 27-30 in scrapie pathogenesis (80). Our results suggest that all mammals may have PrP-related sequences and raise the question of how many other prion diseases may exist.

### CJD Prions and the Human PrP Gene

Hybridization (91) and immunochemical studies on CJD prion proteins (11) have implied that the human genome contains a PrP gene. A single RNA species of ~2.5 kb was observed in human polyadenylated RNA samples on a Northern transfer (71).

A human retinal cDNA library was screened using a hamster PrP cDNA probe under conditions of reduced stringency (91), and nine positive clones were identified and selected. Using the established hamster PrP cDNA sequence as a guide for computer arrangement (23) of the human cDNA fragments, a PrP-related open reading frame was established in the human cDNA (71). The predicted amino acid sequence of this human PrP protein has been aligned with the hamster PrP sequence in Fig. 3 (5,91). These protein sequences differ in length by one amino acid (253 versus 254). Twenty-seven amino acid residues differ between the hamster and human sequence; this sequence divergence (10.67%) is paralleled by 96/759 (12.65%) variation at the nucleotide sequence level.

The amino terminus of the human PrP protein displays a segment of 22 residues that is typical of signal peptides (125). They include a hydrophobic core (MLVLFV) and a small uncharged residue (C) at the putative signal sequence cleavage site; we predict that the mature protein commences at the lysine residue 23; and prior to posttranslational modification human PrP has an $M_r$ of 25,239 daltons. Seven of 22 of the putative signal peptide residues differ from the hamster PrP sequence (Fig. 3). Signal peptide sequence variation is well documented (114,124).

Biochemical similarities have been established between the prions causing scrapie and CJD because antibodies raised against hamster scrapie PrP 27-30 or PrP synthetic peptides cross-react with human CJD prion proteins (11) as well as CJD and GSS amyloid plaques (64). Subsequently other investigators also demonstrated cross-reactivity between rodent and human prion proteins

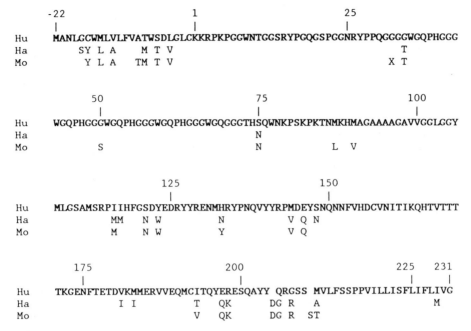

**FIG. 3.** Comparison of the human PrP sequence (Hu) (71) with the hamster (Ha) (7,91,111) and the mouse equivalents (Mo) (21,73). Identical amino acids are not shown. Only amino acid replacements are presented. A deletion in the mouse sequence (residue 32 of Hu and HaPrP) is represented by an X.

(12,18,48,74). Molecular cloning studies demonstrate that this cross-immuno-reactivity results from the highly conserved sequences among PrP molecules. Furthermore, like scrapie prion proteins, CJD prion proteins polymerize into amyloid rods and exhibit green birefringence after staining with Congo red dye.

### Human and Mouse PrP Gene Chromosomal Localizations

Studies with somatic cell hybrids have localized the human PrP gene (PRNP) to chromosome 20 and the mouse PrP gene (*Prn-p*) to chromosome 2 (118). These assignments of the human and mouse PrP genes to homologous chromosomes provide additional evidence for the hypothesis that a common ancestor of man and mouse possessed a PrP gene. *In situ* hybridization studies have confirmed the assignment of the human PrP gene (PRNP) to chromosome 20 and have localized it to band 20p12→pter. Linkage analysis of the mouse PrP gene (*Prn-p*) has located it within 10 cM of the agouti locus on chromosome 2

(20). Additional studies described below have shown that *Prn-p* is tightly linked to a gene controlling the scrapie incubation time (*Prn-i*) (19). *Prn-p* and *Prn-i* have been designated the prion gene complex (*Prn*) in mice.

## Scrapie and CJD Incubation Time Genes

A fascinating question in studies on prions concerns the mechanism controlling the prolonged incubation periods in scrapie and CJD. Early studies with sheep showed that the genetic background of the host could influence both their incubation times and their susceptibility to scrapie (92). Dickinson and co-workers, using specific inbred strains of mice and "strains" of scrapie prions, defined a genetic locus in mice they labeled *Sinc* (29,31). They were unable to link *Sinc* to any known genetic markers or determine its chromosomal location. Neither the strains of mice nor prions have been made available to other investigators, and little progress in understanding *Sinc* has been made (62).

Two genes that influence the prion incubation periods in mice have been identified and their chromosomal assignments determined. *Pid-1* is located on chromosome 17 within the D-subregion of the H-2 complex (63). This gene has been shown to modulate the incubation period of experimental CJD using congenic mice. Of greater influence in both experimental scrapie and CJD is the *Prn-i* gene. The dominant allele of *Prn-i* codes for longer incubation times. Using a restriction fragment length polymorphism, *Prn-i* has been shown to be linked to the gene encoding the prion protein (*Prn-p*) (19). The relation of *Sinc* to *Pid-1* and *Prn-i* remains to be established.

Defining the precise nucleotide sequences responsible for short and long incubation times is of paramount importance. Such studies should, for the first time, begin to elucidate the molecular mechanisms controlling incubation times in prion diseases. In CJD and kuru incubation times of 30 years appear to be common (43). Perhaps these studies will help us understand why many degenerative diseases manifest late in life. It is tempting to speculate that the prion clock gene (*Prn-i*) might have a more general influence and possibly even play a role in the timing of senescence (98).

## EXPRESSION OF PrP mRNA

Polyadenylated RNA prepared from brains of normal and scrapie-infected hamsters at different times after inoculation with prions was analyzed by Northern blotting (120) using a PrP cDNA (91). There was no significant difference between the samples obtained from infected and control animals. Using a mouse PrP cDNA probe, Chesebro and co-workers (21) obtained similar results.

*In situ* hybridization of normal and scrapie-infected hamster brains showed that neurons contain the highest levels of PrP mRNA (equivalent to 50 copies per cell). In contrast, glial cells contain less than three mRNA copies per cell (70). These findings are in accord with the well established observation that CNS neurons are probably the only cell type that undergoes degeneration in prion diseases. (131).

Although PrP mRNA levels were unchanged throughout the course of scrapie infection, we have found that the expression of the PrP gene is developmentally regulated (82). During the first 20 days after birth, PrP mRNA increases in the neonatal hamster brain as measured by Northern blot analysis of polyadenylated RNA and cell-free translation of total brain RNA (82). By 20 days of age, PrP mRNA levels reach a maximum. Apparently the levels of PrP mRNA remain constant throughout the adult life of the hamster.

## IMMUNOLOGIC AND MORPHOLOGIC STUDIES OF PRIONS

### Immunologic Studies of Prion Proteins

One of the most perplexing questions in scrapie and CJD research is now beginning to yield. The lack of an immune response to a lethal "slow infection" has posed a biologic puzzle that is unprecedented. Our discovery of PrP 33-35[C] may explain why animals and humans do not mount immune response to PrP 33-35[Sc] during scrapie or CJD infection (91). This tolerance to PrP 33-35[C], which is induced by PrP 33-35[C], may also explain why antibodies to PrP 33-35[Sc] were so difficult to raise (7,59). We have succeeded in producing monoclonal antibodies (MAb) to PrP 27-30 (3); these PrP MAb recognize both PrP 33-35[C] and PrP 33-35[Sc] (Table 3). Studies with PrP MAb as well as antisera raised against PrP synthetic peptides have unequivocally established a relation between PrP 33-35[C] and PrP 33-35[Sc] (4).

### Ultrastructural Studies of Scrapie and CJD Prions

Many investigations have used the electron microscope to search for a scrapie-specific particle. Spheres, rods, fibrils, and tubules have been described in scrapie, kuru, and CJD-infected brain tissue (2,10,27,38,39,72, 90,123). Notable among the early studies are reports of filamentous virus-like particles in human CJD brain measuring 15 nm in diameter (123) and rod-shaped particles in sheep, rat, and mouse scrapie brain measuring 15 to 26 nm in diameter and 60 to 75 nm in length (38,90). Studies with ruthenium red and lanthanum nitrate suggested that the rod-shaped particles possessed polysaccharides on their surface; these findings are of special interest, as PrP 27-30 has been shown to be a sialoglycoprotein (15).

In purified fractions prepared from scrapie-infected brains, rod-shaped particles were found measuring 10 to 20 nm in diameter and 100 to 200 nm in length (99,108). Although no unit morphologic structure could be identified, most of the rods exhibited a relatively uniform diameter and appeared as flattened cylinders. Some of the rods had a twisted structure suggesting that they might be composed of protofilaments. In the fractions containing rods, one major protein (PrP 27-30) and $\sim 10^{9.5}$ $ID_{50}$ units of prions per milliliter were found. The high degree of purity of our preparations demonstrated by radiolabeling and SDS-PAGE allowed us to establish that the rods are composed of PrP 27-30 molecules. Because PrP 27-30 had already been shown to be required for and inseparable from infectivity (80), we concluded that the rods must be a form of the prion (108). Immunoelectron microscopic studies using antibodies raised against PrP 27-30 have confirmed that the rods are composed of PrP 27-30 molecules (4).

Studies have shown that the rod-shaped particles in purified preparations of prions are created upon detergent extraction of membranes containing PrP 33-35$^{Sc}$ (Fig. 4A,B) (88). Detergent extraction of membranes containing only PrP 33-35$^{C}$ did not produce rods (Table 3). These observations support our hypothesis that the rods are aggregates of prions (99,108).

Sonication of the prion rods reduced their mean length to 60 nm and generated many spherical particles without altering infectivity titers (Fig. 4C) (81). In contrast, fragmentation of M-13 filamentous bacteriophage by brief sonication reduced infectivity significantly. These studies demonstrate that the scrapie agent is not a filamentous animal virus as some investigators have suggested (85).

### Scrapie and CJD Prion Proteins Forming Amyloids

The ultrastructure of the prion rods is indistinguishable from many purified amyloids (108). Histochemical studies with Congo red dye have extended this analogy to purified preparations of prions (108) as well as to scrapie-infected brain where amyloid plaques have been shown to stain with antibodies to PrP 27-30 (7). In addition, PrP 27-30 has been found to stain with periodic acid-Schiff reagent (15); amyloid plaques in tissue sections readily bind this reagent.

Immunocytochemical studies with antibodies to PrP 27-30 have shown that filaments measuring approximately 16 nm in diameter and up to 1,500 nm in length within amyloid plaques of scrapie-infected hamster brain are composed of prion proteins (28). The antibodies to PrP 27-30 did not react with neurofilaments, glial filaments, microtubules, and microfilaments in brain tissue. The prion filaments have a relatively uniform diameter, rarely show narrowings, and possess all the morphologic features of amyloid. Except for their length, the prion filaments appear to be identical ultrastructurally with the rods found in purified fractions of prions (Fig. 4B).

In extracts of scrapie-infected rodent brains, abnormal structures were found by electron microscopy and labeled scrapie-associated fibrils (86).

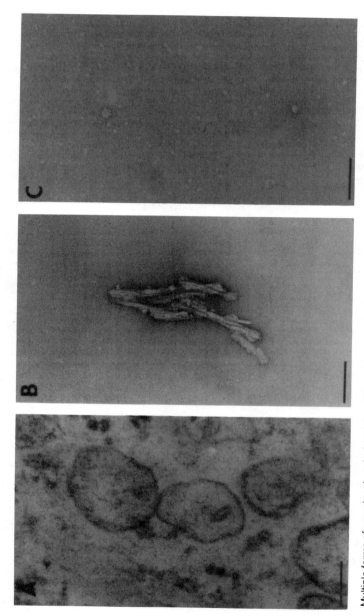

**FIG. 4.** Multiple forms of scrapie prions isolated from infected hamster brain. **A:** Microsomal membranes containing prions. **B:** Purified prion rods that are generated upon detergent extraction of membranes from scrapie-infected brain. **C:** Prion spheres generated from extensive sonication of rods and isolated by sucrose gradient sedimentation. All three forms contain high levels of prion infectivity ( $>10^7$ ID$_{50}$/ml). Bars = 100 nm.

These abnormal fibrils were distinguished from other filamentous structures including amyloids by their characteristic and well defined morphology (85–87). Some investigators have equated these fibrils with the prion rods (33) even though the rods are both ultrastructurally and histochemically identical to many amyloids (108). Although the rods are composed largely, if not entirely, of scrapie or CJD prion proteins, the composition of the fibrils remains to be established.

## ALZHEIMER DISEASE AND PRIONS

In addition to demonstrating that prions are unique biologic particles and fundamentally different from viruses, our studies have also shown that cerebral amyloids may not be inert waste products as most investigators have assumed for nearly a century (7,28,108). Indeed, scrapie prions fulfill all of the criteria required for their classification as a form of cerebral amyloid. This discovery has intensified interest in the possible etiologic role of amyloids in Alzheimer disease (AD) (97). For nearly a century, the accumulation of amyloid filaments with senile plaques and neurofibrillary tangles (NFTs) was appreciated, but their significance in the causation of AD has been a subject of continuing controversy (61).

Studies have shown that the major protein of vascular amyloid in AD and probably in AD senile plaques is unrelated to the prion protein; this conclusion is based on both amino acid sequencing (49,50,79,113,129) and immunostaining studies (17,64,112). The proteins comprising paired helical filaments (PHFs) of the NFTs are less well characterized (24,52,67,78,89,93,119,130). Interestingly, some antisera raised against partially purified PHFs from AD brains do stain amyloid plaques in CJD, GSS, and kuru; the molecular basis for this cross-reactivity remains to be established (60).

The lack of AD transmissibility to experimental animals was the first evidence suggesting that the etiologic molecules in AD were not CJD prions even though the two diseases share many clinical and pathologic features (51). On the other hand, learning about the molecular changes that differentiate the cellular prion protein from its CJD isoform may be informative about the pathogenesis of AD. Of interest are familial pedigrees that contain multiple cases of both AD and CJD (76). Whether these pedigrees demonstrate a significant relation between these two dementing CNS degenerative disorders or AD is simply an incidental finding in familial CJD is unknown.

It will be important to define the human prion gene complex and learn if any gene within the complex or nearby plays a role in the pathogenesis of AD. Presumably, a human prion incubation time gene controls the timing of CJD, GSS, and kuru. Perhaps this same clock gene regulates the age-dependent susceptibility observed in one or more of some common CNS degenerative diseases such as AD, Parkinson disease, and amyotrophic lateral sclerosis.

## PRIONS AND HUMAN DEGENERATIVE NEUROLOGIC DISEASES

The studies described here have clearly demonstrated that knowledge about scrapie prions is relevant to understanding CJD in humans. The approaches developed first for the investigation of experimental scrapie in rodents have proved to be directly applicable to the study of CNS degeneration in humans caused by CJD prions.

Perhaps most important, the current study of prions may represent a point of departure for future investigations of other degenerative diseases. Many disorders may eventually be shown to be caused by prion-like macromolecules. The genetic origin of prions and the slow amplification mechanisms that account for their replication make these unique macromolecules interesting candidates to explore with respect to many diseases that occur later in life.

Due largely to the chemical studies described above, any clinical description of prion diseases in humans must be considered provisional and incomplete. Research on human prions is in its infancy, but the availability of both antibodies and cDNA probes should lead to an explosion of new information about the classification, etiology, clinical course, pathogenesis, and intervention during the next decade.

### ACKNOWLEDGMENTS

Portions of this chapter were adapted from Prusiner, S. B. (1987): Prions causing degenerative neurological diseases. *Annu. Rev. Med.*, 38:381–398, 1987.

Important contributions from Drs. R. Barry, C. Bellinger-Kawahara, J. Bockman, S. DeArmond, R. Gabizon, K. Gilles, M. McKinley, R. Meyer, M. Scott, and D. Westaway are gratefully acknowledged. Collaborative studies with Drs. G. Carlson, J. Cleavor, T. Diener, W. Hadlow, L. Hood, S. Kent, D. Kingsbury, B. Oesch, D. Riesner, and C. Weissmann have been important to the progress of these studies and are greatly appreciated. The author thanks K. Bowman, D. Groth, M. Vincent, and M. Wälchli for technical assistance as well as L. Gallagher for manuscript production assistance.

This work was supported by research grants from the National Institutes of Health (AG02132 and NS14069) and a Senator Jacob Javits Center of Excellence in Neuroscience (NS22786), as well as by gifts from RJR-Nabisco, Inc. and Sherman Fairchild Foundation.

### REFERENCES

1. Alpers, M. P. (1979): Epidemiology and ecology of kuru. In: *Slow Transmissible Diseases of the Nervous System*, Vol. 1, edited by S. B. Prusiner and W. J. Hadlow, pp. 67–92. Academic Press, New York.

2. Baringer, J. R., and Prusiner, S. B. (1978): Experimental scrapie in mice—ultrastructural observations. *Ann. Neurol.*, 4:205–211.
3. Barry, R. A., and Prusiner, S. B. (1986): Monoclonal antibodies to the cellular and scrapie prion proteins. *J. Infect. Dis.*, 154:518–521.
4. Barry, R. A., Kent, S. B., McKinley, M. P., Meyer, R. K., DeArmond, S. J., Hood, L. E., and Prusiner, S. B. (1986): Scrapie and cellular prion proteins share polypeptide epitopes. *J. Infect. Dis.*, 153:848–854.
5. Basler, K., Oesch, B., Scott, M., Westaway, D., Wälchli, M., Groth, D. F., McKinley, M. P., Prusiner, S. B., and Weissmann, C. (1986): Scrapie and cellular PrP isoforms are encoded by the same chromosomal gene. *Cell*, 46:417–428.
6. Beck, E., Daniel, P. M., and Parry, H. B. (1964): Degeneration of the cerebellar and hypothalamoneurohypophysial systems in sheep with scrapie; and its relationship to human system degenerations. *Brain*, 87:153–176.
7. Bendheim, P. E., Barry, R. A., DeArmond, S. J., Stites, D. P., and Prusiner, S. B. (1984): Antibodies to a scrapie prion protein. *Nature*, 310:418–421.
8. Bendheim, P. E., Bockman, J. M., McKinley, M. P., Kingsbury, D. T., and Prusiner, S. B. (1985): Scrapie and Creutzfeldt-Jakob disease prion proteins share physical properties and antigenic determinants. *Proc. Natl. Acad. Sci. USA*, 82:997–1001.
9. Bernoulli, C., Siegfried, J., Baumgartner, G., Regli, F., Rabinowicz, T., Gajdusek, D. C., and Gibbs, C. J., Jr. (1977): Danger of accidental person to person transmission of Creutzfeldt-Jakob disease by surgery. *Lancet*, 1:478–479.
10. Bignami, A., and Parry, H. B. (1971): Aggregations of 35-nanometer particles associated with neuronal cytopathic changes in natural scrapie. *Science*, 171:389–399.
11. Bockman, J. M., Kingsbury, D. T., McKinley, M. P., Bendheim, P. E., and Prusiner, S. B. (1985): Creutzfeldt-Jakob disease proteins in human brains. *N. Engl. J. Med.*, 312:73–78.
12. Bode, L., Pocchiari, M., Gelderblom, H., and Diringer, H. (1985): Characterization of antisera against scrapie-associated fibrils (SAF) from affected hamster and cross-reactivity with SAF from scrapie-affected mice and from patients with Creutzfeldt-Jakob disease. *J. Gen. Virol.*, 66:2471–2478.
13. Bolton, D. C., McKinley, M. P., and Prusiner, S. B. (1982): Identification of a protein that purifies with the scrapie prion. *Science*, 218:1309–1311.
14. Bolton, D. C., McKinley, M. P., and Prusiner, S. B. (1984): Molecular characteristics of the major scrapie prion protein. *Biochemistry*, 23:5898–5905.
15. Bolton, D. C., Meyer, R. K., and Prusiner, S. B. (1985): Scrapie PrP 27-30 is a sialoglycoprotein. *J. Virol.*, 53:596–606.
16. Braig, H., and Diringer, H. (1985): Scrapie: concept of a virus-induced amyloidosis of the brain. *EMBO J.*, 4:2309–2312.
17. Brown, P., Coker-Vann, M., Pomeroy, K., Franko, M., Asher, D. M., Gibbs, C. J., Jr., and Gajdusek, D. C. (1986): Diagnosis of Creutzfeldt-Jakob disease by Western blot identification of marker protein in human brain tissue. *N. Engl. J. Med.*, 314:547–551.
18. Brown, P., Gajdusek, D. C., Gibbs, C. J., Jr., and Asher, D. M. (1985): Potential epidemic of Creutzfeldt-Jakob disease from human growth hormone therapy. *N. Engl. J. Med.*, 313:728–731.
19. Carlson, G. A., Kingsbury, D. T., Goodman, P., Coleman, S., Marshall, S. T., DeArmond, S. J., Westaway, D., and Prusiner, S. B. (1986): Prion protein and scrapie incubation time genes are linked. *Cell*, 46:503–511.
20. Carlson, G. A., Lovett, M., Epstein, C. J., Westaway, D., Goodman, P. A., Marshall, S. T., and Prusiner, S. B. (1986): The prion gene complex: polymorphism of Prn-p and its linkage with agouti. Presented at the XIVth Molecular and Biochemical Genetics Workshop, Bar Harbor, Maine (abstract).
21. Chesebro, B., Race, R., Wehrly, K., Nishio, J., Bloom, M., Lechner, D., Bergstrom, S., Robbins, K., Mayer, L., Keith, J. M., Garon, C., and Haase, A. (1985): Identification of scrapie prion protein-specific mRNA in scrapie-infected and uninfected brain. *Nature*, 315:331–333.
22. Conrad, B., and Mount, D. W. (1982): Microcomputer programs for DNA sequence analysis. *Nucleic Acids Res.*, 10:31–38.
23. Creutzfeldt, H. G. (1920): Über eine eigenartige herdförmige Erkrankung des Zentralnervensystems. *Z. Ges. Neurol. Psychiatr.*, 57:1–18.

24. Crowther, R. A., and Wischik, C. M. (1985): Image reconstruction of the Alzheimer paired helical filament. *EMBO J.*, 4:3661–3665.
25. Davanipour, Z., Alter, M., and Sobel, E. (1986): Creutzfeldt-Jakob disease. *Neurol. Clin.*, 4:341–353.
26. Davanipour, Z., Goodman, L., Alter, M., Sobel, E., Asher, D., and Gajdusek, D. C. (1984): Possible modes of transmission of Creutzfeldt-Jakob disease. *N. Engl. J. Med.*, 311:1582–1583.
27. David-Ferreira, J. F., David-Ferreira, K. L., Gibbs, C. J., Jr., and Morris, J. A. (1968): Scrapie in mice: ultrastructural observations in the cerebral cortex. *Proc. Soc. Exp. Biol. Med.*, 127:313–320.
28. DeArmond, S. J., McKinley, M. P., Barry, R. A., Braunfeld, M. B., McColloch, J. R., and Prusiner, S. B. (1985): Identification of prion amyloid filaments in scrapie-infected brain. *Cell*, 41:221–235.
29. Dickinson, A. G., and Meikle, V. M. (1971): Host-genotype and agent effects in scrapie incubation: change in allelic interaction with different strains of agent. *Mol. Gen. Genet.*, 112:73–79.
30. Dickinson, A. G., and Outram, G. W. (1979): The scrapie replication-site hypothesis and its implications for pathogenesis. In: *Slow Transmissible Diseases of the Nervous System*, Vol. 2, edited by S. B. Prusiner and W. J. Hadlow, pp. 13–31. Academic Press, New York.
31. Dickinson, A. G., Bruce, M. E., Outram, G. W., and Kimberlin, R. H. (1984): Scrapie strain differences: the implications of stability and mutation. In: *Proceedings of Workshop on Slow Transmissible Diseases*, edited by J. Tateishi, pp. 105–118. Japanese Ministry of Health and Welfare, Tokyo.
32. Diener, T. O., McKinley, M. P., and Prusiner, S. B. (1982): Viroids and prions. *Proc. Natl. Acad. Sci. USA*, 79:5220–5224.
33. Diringer, H., Gelderblom, H., Hilmert, H., Ozel, M., Edelbluth, C., and Kimberlin, R. H. (1983): Scrapie infectivity, fibrils and low molecular weight protein. *Nature*, 306:476–478.
34. Diringer, H., Hilmert, H., Simon, D., Werner, E., and Ehlers, B. (1983): Towards purification of the scrapie agent. *Eur. J. Biochem.*, 134:555–560.
35. Duffy, P., Wolf, J., Collins, G., Devoe, A., Streeten, B., and Cowen, D. (1974): Possible person to person transmission of Creutzfeldt-Jakob disease. *N. Engl. J. Med.*, 290:692–693.
36. Dynan, W. S., and Tijian, R. (1983): Isolation of transcription factors that discriminate between different promoters recognized by RNA polymerase II. *Cell*, 32:669–680.
37. Dynan, W. S., Sazer, S., Tijian, R., and Schimke, R. T. (1986): Transcription factor Spl recognizes a DNA sequence in the mouse dihydrofolate reductase promoter. *Nature*, 319:246–248.
38. Field, E. J., and Narang, H. K. (1972): An electron-microscopic study of scrapie in the rat: further observations on "inclusion bodies" and virus-like particles. *J. Neurol. Sci.*, 17:347–364.
39. Field, E. J., Mathews, J. D., and Raine, C. S. (1969): Electron microscopic observations on the cerebellar cortex in kuru. *J. Neurol. Sci.*, 8:209–224.
40. Finer-Moore, J., and Stroud, R. M. (1984): Amphipathic analysis and possible formation of the ion channel in an acetylcholine receptor. *Proc. Natl. Acad. Sci. USA*, 81:155–159.
41. Fromm, M., and Berg, P. (1982): Deletion mapping of DNA regions required for SV40 early region promoter function in vivo. *J. Mol. Appl. Genet.* 1:457–481.
42. Gabizon, R., McKinley, M. P., and Prusiner, S. B. (1986): Reconstitution of scrapie prion proteins into liposomes. *J. Cell Biol.* (abstract), 103:337a.
43. Gajdusek, D. C. (1977): Unconventional viruses and the origin and disappearance of kuru. *Science*, 197:943–960.
44. Gajdusek, D. C., Gibbs, C. J., Jr., and Alpers, M. (1966): Experimental transmission of a kuru-like syndrome to chimpanzees. *Nature*, 209:794–796.
45. GenBank Genetic Sequence Data Bank (1986): GenBank (R) Release 44.0, August 4, 1986. 8823 loci, 8442357 bases, from 11413 reported sequences.
46. Gibbs, C. J., Jr., and Gajdusek, D. C. (1969): Infection as the etiology of spongiform encephalopathy. *Science*, 165:1023–1025.
47. Gibbs, C. J., Jr., Gajdusek, D. C., Asher, D. M., Alpers, M. P., Beck, E., Daniel, P. M., and Matthews, W. B. (1968): Creutzfeldt-Jakob disease (spongiform encephalopathy): transmission to the chimpanzee. *Science*, 161:388–389.

48. Gibbs, C. J., Jr., Joy, A., Heffner, R., Franko, M., Miyazaki, M., Asher, D. M., Parisi, J. E., Brown, P. W., and Gajdusek, D. C. (1985): Clinical and pathological features and laboratory confirmation of Creutzfeldt-Jakob disease in a recipient of pituitary-derived human growth hormone. *N. Engl. J. Med.*, 313:734–738.

49. Glenner, G. G., and Wong, C. W. (1984): Alzheimer's disease and Down's syndrome: sharing of a unique cerebrovascular amyloid fibril protein. *Biochem. Biophys. Res. Commun.*, 122:1131–1135.

50. Glenner, G. G., and Wong, C. W. (1984): Alzheimer's disease: initial report of the purification and characterization of a novel cerebrovascular amyloid protein. *Biochem. Biophys. Res. Commun.*, 120:885–890.

51. Goudsmit, J., Morrow, C. H., Asher, D. M., Yanagihara, R. T., Masters, C. L., Gibbs, C. J., Jr., and Gajdusek, D. C. (1980): Evidence for and against the transmissibility of Alzheimer's disease. *Neurology*, 30:945–950.

52. Grundke-Iqbal, I., Iqbal, K., Tung, Y., Quinlan, M., Wisniewski, H. M., and Binder, L. I. (1986): Abnormal phosphorylation of the microtubule-associated protein $\tau$ (tau) in Alzheimer cytoskeletal pathology. *Proc. Natl. Acad. Sci. USA*, 83:4913–4917.

53. Hadlow, W. J. (1959): Scrapie and kuru. *Lancet*, 2:289–290.

54. Haseltine, W. A., and Patarca, R. (1986): AIDS virus and scrapie agent share protein. *Nature*, 323:115–116.

54a. Hay, B., Barry, R. A., Lieberburg, I., Prusiner, S. B., and Ligappa, V. R. (1987): Biogenesis and transmembrane orientation of the cellular isoform of the scrapie prion protein. *Mol. Cell. Biol.*, 7:914–920.

55. Hilmert, H., and Diringer, H. (1984): A rapid and efficient method to enrich SAF-protein from scrapie brains of hamsters. *Biosci. Rep.*, 4:165–170.

56. Hunter, G. D. (1979): The enigma of the scrapie agent: biochemical approaches and the involvement of membranes and nucleic acids. In: *Slow Transmissible Diseases of the Nervous System*, Vol. 2, edited by S. B. Prusiner and W. J. Hadlow, pp. 365–385. Academic Press, New York.

57. Jakob, A. (1921): Über eigenartige Erkrankungen des Zentralnervensystems mit bemerkenswertem anatomischen Befunde (spatische Pseudosclerose-encephalomyelopathie mit disseminierten Degenerationsherden) [preliminary communication]. *Dtsch. Z. Nervenheilk.*, 70:132–146.

58. Kadonaga, J. T., Jones, K. A., and Tjian, R. (1986): Promoter-specific activation of RNA polymerase II transcription by Sp1. *Trends Biochem. Sci.*, 11:20–23.

59. Kasper, K. C., Bowman, K., Stites, D. P., and Prusiner, S. B. (1981): Toward development of assays for scrapie-specific antibodies. In: *Hamster Immune Responses in Infectious and Oncologic Diseases*, edited by J. W. Streilein, D. A. Hart, J. Stein-Streilein, W. R. Duncan, and R. E. Billingham, pp. 401–413. Plenum Press, New York.

60. Kates, J., DeArmond, S. J., Borcich, J., Barry, R. A., and Prusiner, S. B. (1986): Paired helical filament antisera stain cerebral amyloid plaques in prion diseases. *Neurology*, 36(Suppl. 1):224 (abstract).

61. Katzman, R. (1986): Medical progress: Alzheimer's disease. *N. Engl. J. Med.*, 314:964–973.

62. Kimberlin, R. H. (1986): Scrapie: how much do we really understand? *Neuropathol. Appl. Neurobiol.*, 12:131–147.

63. Kingsbury, D. T., Kasper, K. C., Stites, D. P., Watson, J. C., Hogan, R. N., and Prusiner, S. B. (1983): Genetic control of scrapie and Creutzfeldt-Jakob disease in mice. *J. Immunol.*, 131:491–496.

64. Kitamoto, T., Tateishi, J., Tashima, T., Takeshita, I., Barry, R. A., DeArmond, S. J., and Prusiner, S. B. (1986): Amyloid plaques in Creutzfeldt-Jakob disease stain with prion protein antibodies. *Ann. Neurol.*, 20:204–208.

65. Klatzo, I., Gajdusek, D. C., and Zigas, V. (1959): Pathology of kuru. *Lab. Invest.*, 8:799–847.

66. Koch, T. K., Berg, B. O., DeArmond, S. J., and Gravina, R. F. (1985): Creutzfeldt-Jakob disease in a young adult with idiopathic hypopituitarism: possible relation to the administration of cadaveric human growth hormone. *N. Engl. J. Med.*, 313:731–733.

67. Kosik, K. S., Joachim, C. L., and Selkoe, D. J. (1986): Microtubule-associated protein tau ($\tau$) is a major antigenic component of paired helical filaments in Alzheimer disease. *Proc. Natl. Acad. Sci. USA*, 83:4044–4048.

68. Kozak, M. (1984): Compilation and analysis of sequences upstream from the translational start site in eukaryotic mRNAs. *Nucleic Acids Res.*, 12:857–872.

69. Kozak, M. (1984): Point mutations close to the AUG initiator codon affect the efficiency of translation of rat preproinsulin in vivo. *Nature*, 308:241–246.

70. Kretzschmar, H. A., Prusiner, S. B., Stowring, L. E., and DeArmond, S. J. (1986): Scrapie prion proteins are synthesized in neurons. *Am. J. Pathol.*, 122:1–5.

71. Kretzschmar, H. A., Stowring, L. E. Westaway, D., Stubblebine, W. H., Prusiner, S. B., and DeArmond, S. J. (1986): Molecular cloning of a human prion protein cDNA. *DNA*, 5:315–324.

72. Lampert, P. W., Gajdusek, D. C., and Gibbs, C. J., Jr. (1971): Experimental spongiform encephalopathy (Creutzfeldt-Jakob disease) in chimpanzees. *J. Neuropathol. Exp. Neurol.*, 30:20–32.

73. Locht, C., Chesebro, B., Race, R., and Keith, J. M. (1986): Molecular cloning and complete sequence of prion protein cDNA from mouse brain infected with the scrapie agent. *Proc. Natl. Acad. Sci. USA*, 83:6372–6376.

74. Manuelidis, L., Valley, S., and Manuelidis, E. E. (1985): Specific proteins associated with Creutzfeldt-Jakob disease and scrapie share antigenic and carbohydraate determinants. *Proc. Natl. Acad. Sci. USA*, 82:4263–4267.

75. Masters, C. L., Gajdusek, D. C., and Gibbs, C. J., Jr. (1981): Creutzfeldt-Jakob disease virus isolations from the Gerstmann-Straussler syndrome. *Brain*, 104:559–588.

76. Masters, C. L., Gajdusek, D. C., and Gibbs, C. J., Jr. (1981): The familial occurrence of Creutzfeldt-Jakob disease and Alzheimer's disease. *Brain*, 104:535–558.

77. Masters, C. L., Gajdusek, D. C., Gibbs, C. J., Jr., Bernoulli, C., and Asher, D. M. (1979): Familial Creutzfeldt-Jakob disease and other familial dementias: an inquiry into possible modes of virus-induced familial diseases. In: *Slow Transmissible Diseases of the Nervous System*, Vol. 1, edited by S. B. Prusiner and W. J. Hadlow, pp. 143–194. Academic Press, New York.

78. Masters, C. L., Multhaup, G., Simms, G., Pottgiesser, J., Martins, R. N., and Beyreuther, K. (1985): Neuronal origin of a cerebral amyloid: neurofibrillary tangles of Alzheimer's disease contain the same protein as the amyloid of plaque cores and blood vessels. *EMBO J.*, 4:2757–2763.

79. Masters, C. L., Simms, G., Weinman, N. A., Multhaup, G., McDonald, B. L., and Beyreuther, K. (1985): Amyloid plaque core protein in Alzheimer disease and Down syndrome. *Proc. Natl. Acad. Sci. USA*, 82:4254–4249.

80. McKinley, M. P., Bolton, D. C., and Prusiner, S. B. (1983): A protease-resistant protein is a structural component of the scrapie prion. *Cell*, 35:57–62.

81. McKinley, M. P., Braunfeld, M. B., Bellinger, C. G., and Prusiner, S. B. (1986): Molecular characteristics of prion rods purified from scrapie-infected hamster brains. *J. Infect. Dis.*, 154:110–120.

82. McKinley, M. P., Hay, B., Lingappa, V. R., Lieberburg, I., and Prusiner, S. B. (1986): Developmental expression of prion protein gene in brain. *Dev. Biol.*, 121:105–110.

83. McKinley, M. P., Masiarz, F. R., and Prusiner, S. B. (1981): Reversible chemical modification of the scrapie agent. *Science*, 214:1259–1261.

84. McKnight, S. L., and Kingsbury, R. (1982): Transcriptional control signals of a eukaryotic protein coding gene. *Science*, 217:316–325.

85. Merz, P. A., Rohwer, R. G., Kascsak, R., Wisniewski, H. M., Somerville, R. A., Gibbs, C. J., Jr., and Gajdusek, D. C. (1984): Infection-specific particle from the unconventional slow virus diseases. *Science*, 225:437–440.

86. Merz, P. A., Somerville, R. A., Wisniewski, H. M., and Iqbal, K. (1981): Abnormal fibrils from scrapie-infected brain. *Acta Neuropathol. (Berl.)*, 54:63–74.

87. Merz, P. A., Wisniewski, H. M., Somerville, R. A., Bobin, S. A., Masters, C. L., and Iqbal, K. (1983): Ultrastructural morphology of amyloid fibrils from neuritic and amyloid plaques. *Acta Neuropathol. (Berl.)*, 60:113–124.

88. Meyer, R. K., McKinley, M. P., Bowman, K. A., Barry, R. A., and Prusiner, S. B. (1986): Separation and properties of cellular and scrapie prion proteins. *Proc. Natl. Acad. Sci. USA*, 83:2310–2314.

89. Miller, C. J., Brion, J-P., Calvert, R., Chin, T. K., Eagles, P. A. M., Downes, M. J., Flament-Durand, J., Haugh, M., Kahn, J., Probst, A., Ulrich, J., and Anderton, B. H.

(1986): Alzheimer's paired helical filaments share epitopes with neurofilament side arms. *EMBO J.*, 5:269–276.

90. Narang, H. K. (1974): An electron microscopic study of natural scrapie sheep brain: further observations on virus-like particles and paramyxovirus-like tubules. *Acta Neuropathol. (Berl.)*, 28:317–329.

91. Oesch, B., Westaway, D., Wälchli, M., McKinley, M. P., Kent, S. B. H., Aebersold, R., Barry, R. A., Tempst, P., Teplow, D. B., Hood, L. E., Prusiner, S. B., and Weissmann, C. (1985): A cellular gene encodes scrapie PrP 27-30 protein. *Cell*, 40:735–746.

92. Parry, H. B., editor (1983): *Scrapie Disease in Sheep*. Academic Press, New York.

93. Perry, G., Rizzuto, N., Autilio-Gambetti, A., and Gambetti, P. (1985): Paired helical filaments from Alzheimer's disease patients contain cytoskeletal components. *Proc. Natl. Acad. Sci. USA*, 82:3916–3920.

94. Protein Sequence Database of the Protein Identification Resource (PIR) (1986): Supported by the Division of Research Resources of the National Institutes of Health. Release 10.0, August 13, 1986. W. C. Barker, L. T. Hunt, D. G. George, L. S. Yeh, H. R. Chen, M. C. Blomquist, E. I. Seibel-Ross, A. Elzanowski, M. K. Hong, D. A. Ferrick, J. K. Bair, S. L. Chen, and R. S. Ledley. National Biomedical Research Foundation, Georgetown University Medical Center, Washington, D. C. 3800 sequences, 890703 residues.

95. Prusiner, S. B. (1982): Novel proteinaceous infectious particles cause scrapie. *Science*, 216:136–144.

96. Prusiner, S. B. (1984): Prions—novel infectious pathogens. *Adv. Virus Res.*, 29:1–56.

97. Prusiner, S. B. (1984): Some speculations about prions, amyloid and Alzheimer's disease. *N. Engl. J. Med.*, 310:661–663.

98. Prusiner, S. B. (1987): Degenerative neurologic diseases, biological clocks and aging—an epilogue. In: *Prions—Novel Infectious Pathogens Causing Scrapie and Creutzfeldt-Jakob Disease*, edited by S. B. Prusiner and M. P. McKinley, pp. 523–534. Academic Press, Orlando.

99. Prusiner, S. B., Bolton, D. C., Groth, D. F., Bowman, K. A., Cochran, S. P., and McKinley, M. P. (1982): Further purification and characterization of scrapie prions. *Biochemistry*, 21:6942–6950.

100. Prusiner, S. B., Cochran, S. P., and Alpers, M. P. (1985): Transmission of scrapie in hamsters. *J. Infect. Dis.*, 152:971–978.

101. Prusiner, S. B., Cochran, S. P., Groth, D. F., Downey, D. E., Bowman, K. A., and Martinez, H. M. (1982): Measurement of the scrapie agent using an incubation time interval assay. *Ann. Neurol.*, 11:353–358.

102. Prusiner, S. B., Garfin, D. E., Cochran, S. P., McKinley, M. P., and Groth, D. F. (1980): Experimental scrapie in the mouse: electrophoretic and sedimentation properties of the partially purified agent. *J. Neurochem.*, 35:574–582.

103. Prusiner, S. B., Groth, D. F., Bolton, D. C., Kent, S. B., and Hood, L. E. (1984): Purification and structural studies of a major scrapie prion protein. *Cell*, 38:127-134.

104. Prusiner, S. B., Groth, D. F., Cochran, S. P., Masiarz, F. R., McKinley, M. P., and Martinez, H. M. (1980): Molecular properties, partial purification and assay by incubation period measurements of the hamster scrapie agent. *Biochemistry*, 19:4883–4891.

105. Prusiner, S. B., Groth, D. F., Cochran, S. P., McKinley, M. P., and Masiarz, F. R. (1980): Gel electrophoresis and glass permeation chromatography of the hamster scrapie agent after enzymic digestion and detergent extraction. *Biochemistry*, 19:4892–4898.

106. Prusiner, S. B., Hadlow, W. J., Eklund, C. M., Race, R. E., and Cochran, S. P. (1978): Sedimentation characteristics of the scrapie agent from murine spleen and brain. *Biochemistry*, 17:4987–4992.

107. Prusiner, S. B., Hadlow, W. J., Garfin, D. E., Cochran, S. P., Baringer, J. R., Race, R. E., and Eklund, C. M. (1978): Partial purification and evidence for multiple molecular forms of the scrapie agent. *Biochemistry*, 17:4993–4997.

108. Prusiner, S. B., McKinley, M. P., Bowman, K. A., Bolton, D. C., Bendheim, P. E., Groth, D. F., and Glenner, G. G. (1983): Scrapie prions aggregate to form amyloid-like birefringent rods. *Cell*, 35:349–358.

109. Prusiner, S. B., McKinley, M. P., Groth, D. F., Bowman, K. A., Mock, N. I., Cochran, S. P., and Masiarz, F. R. (1981): Scrapie agent contains a hydrophobic protein. *Proc. Natl Acad. Sci. USA*, 78:6675–6679.

110. Reynolds, G. A., Basu, S. K., Osborne, T. F., Chin, D. J., Gil, G., Brown, M. S., Goldstein, J. L., and Luskey, K. L. (1984): HMG CoA reductase: a negatively regulated gene with unusual promoter and 5′ untranslated regions. *Cell*, 38:275–285.
111. Robakis, N. K., Sawh, P. R., Wolfe, G. C., Rubenstein, R., Carp, R. I., and Innis, M. A. (1986): Isolation of a cDNA clone encoding the leader peptide of prion protein and expression of the homologous gene in various tissues. *Proc. Natl. Acad. Sci. USA*, 83:6377–6381.
112. Roberts, G. W., Lofthouse, R., Brown, R., Crow, T. J., Barry, R. A., and Prusiner, S. B. (1986): Prion protein immunoreactivity in human transmissible dementias. *N. Engl. J. Med.*, 315:1231–1233.
113. Roher, A., Wolfe, D., Paultke, M., and Kukuruga, D. (1986): Purification, ultrastructure and chemical analysis of Alzheimer disease amyloid plaque core protein. *Proc. Natl. Acad. Sci. USA*, 83:2662–2666.
114. Sabatini, D. D., Kreibich, G., Morimoto, T., and Adesnik, M. (1982): Mechanisms for the incorporation of proteins in membranes and organelles. *J. Cell Biol.*, 92:1–22.
115. Sigurdsson, B. (1954): Rida, a chronic encephalitis of sheep with general remarks on infections which develop slowly and some of their special characteristics. *Br. Vet. J.*, 110:341–354.
116. Sklaviadis, T., Manuelidis, L., and Manuelidis, E. E. (1986): Characterization of major peptides in Creutzfeldt-Jakob disease and scrapie. *Proc. Natl. Acad. Sci. USA*, 83:6146–6150.
117. Southern, E. M. (1975): Detection of specific sequences among DNA fragments separated by gel electrophoresis. *J. Mol. Biol.*, 98:503–517.
118. Sparkes, R. S., Simon, M., Cohn, V. H., Fournier, R. E. K., Lem, J., Klisak, I., Heinzman, C., Blatt, C., Lucero, M., Mohandas, T., DeArmond, S. J., Westaway, D., Prusiner, S. B., and Weiner, L. P. (1986): Assignment of the human and mouse prion protein genes to homologous chromosomes. *Proc. Natl. Acad. Sci. USA*, 83:7358–7362.
119. Sternberger, N. H., Sternberger, L. A., and Ulrich, J. (1985): Aberrant neurofilament phosphorylation in Alzheimer disease. *Proc. Natl. Acad. Sci. USA*, 82:4274–4276.
120. Thomas, P. S. (1980): Hybridization of denatured RNA and small DNA fragments to nitrocellulose. *Proc. Natl. Acad. Sci. USA*, 77:5201–5205.
121. Tintner, R., Brown, P., Hedley-Whyte, E. T., Rappaport, E. B., Piccardo, C. P., and Gajdusek, D. C. (1986): Neuropathologic verification of Creutzfeldt-Jakob disease in the exhumed American recipient of human pituitary growth hormone: epidemiologic and pathogenic implications. *Neurology*, 36:932–936.
122. Valerio, D., Duyvesteyn, M. G., Dekker, B. M., Weeda, G., Berkvens, T. M., van der Voorn, L., van Ormondt, H., and van der Eb, A. J. (1985): Adenosine deaminase: characterization and expression of a gene with a remarkable promoter. *EMBO J.*, 4:437–443.
123. Vernon, M. L., Horta-Barbosa, L., Fuccillo, D. A., Server, J. L., Baringer, J. R., and Birnbaum, G. (1970): Virus-like particles and nucleoprotein-type filaments in brain tissue from two patients with Creutzfeldt-Jakob disease. *Lancet*, 1:964–966.
124. Von Heijne, G. (1983): Patterns of amino acids near signal-sequence cleavage sites. *Eur. J. Biochem.*, 133:17–21.
125. Von Heijne, G. (1985): Signal sequences, the limits of variation. *J. Mol. Biol.*, 184:99–105.
126. Weitgrefe, S., Zupancic, M., Haase, A., Chesebro, B., Race, R., Frey, W., II, Rustan, T., and Friedman, R. L. (1985): Cloning of a gene whose expression is increased in scrapie and in senile plaques. *Science*, 230:1177–1181.
127. Weller, R. O., Steart, P. V., and Powell-Jackson, J. D. (1986): Pathology of Creutzfeldt-Jakob disease associated with pituitary-derived human growth hormone administration. *Neuropathol. Appl. Neurobiol.*, 12:117–129.
128. Westaway, D., and Prusiner, S. B. (1986): Conservation of the cellular gene encoding the scrapie prion protein PrP 27-30. *Nucleic Acids Res.*, 14:2035–2044.
129. Wong, C. W., Quaranta, V., and Glenner, G. G. (1985): Neuritic plaques and cerebrovascular amyloid in Alzheimer disease. *Proc. Natl. Acad. Sci. USA*, 82:8729–8732.
130. Wood, J. G., Mirra, S. S., Pollock, N. J., and Binder, L. I. (1986): Neurofibrillary tangles of Alzheimer disease share antigenic determinants with axonal microtubule-associated protein tau ($\tau$). *Proc. Natl. Acad. Sci. USA*, 83:4040–4043.
131. Zlotnik, I. (1962): The pathology of scrapie: a comparative study of lesions in the brain of sheep and goats. *Acta Neuropathol. [Suppl.] (Berl.)*, 1:61–70.

Aging and the Brain, edited by R. D. Terry.
Raven Press, New York © 1988.

# Grafts of Fetal Cholinergic Neurons in Rat Models of Aging and Dementia

Anders Björklund and *Fred H. Gage

*Department of Histology, University of Lund, Lund, Sweden; and *Department of Neurosciences, School of Medicine, University of California, San Diego, La Jolla, California 92093*

The role of the basal forebrain cholinergic system in learning and memory processes has attracted considerable attention. Pharmacological manipulation of central cholinergic transmission has been shown to have profound effects on learning and memory in both human subjects and experimental animals (3,22,23). Moreover, neuropathological and neurochemical studies on autopsy material from patients with Alzheimer disease have demonstrated substantial degeneration or atrophy of the cholinergic neurons in the basal forebrain, including the nucleus basalis, substantia innominata, and the septal-diagonal band area (1,20,50,63). This degeneration is associated with a loss of the acetylcholine synthetic enzyme choline acetyltransferase (ChAT) in wide areas of the neo- and allocortex (14,21,51). Moreover, the magnitude of the cortical ChAT reduction, as assessed in postmortem tissue analyses, has been reported to correlate with the severity of the dementia in Alzheimer patients (51).

In aged rodents as well, impairments in learning and memory have been associated with an age-dependent decline in parameters of forebrain cholinergic transmission (24,36,42,55,58). Data have demonstrated significant shrinkage, with or without actual cell loss, in all parts of the basal forebrain cholinergic system in aged rats or mice (4,30,38,44). Thus as in Alzheimer-type dementia in man, it seems possible that functional deterioration of the limbic and cortical cholinergic projection systems may also contribute to the age-related cognitive impairments in rodent species. This suggestion is consistent with experiments in young rats showing that surgical or excitotoxic damage to either of the two major components of the basal forebrain cholinergic system, i.e., the septohippocampal or basalocortical projections, causes severe impairment in a variety of learning and memory tasks (25,37,48,62).

In this chapter we review a series of studies on the ability of grafts of fetal basal forebrain cholinergic neurons to substitute, structurally and functionally, for a lost or age-impaired cholinergic afferent input to the hippocampal formation or the neocortex in aged rats or in young rats with lesions of the septohippocampal or the basalocortical projection systems. The results show that intrahippocampal or intracortical grafts of tissue rich in developing cholinergic neurons can compensate at least partly for lesion-induced or age-dependent cognitive impairments in rats, and that this effect may be due to the restoration of cholinergic neurotransmission in the deafferented or dysfunctioning host target.

## TECHNICAL ASPECTS OF INTRACEREBRAL NEURAL GRAFTING

Two principal techniques have been used in our laboratory to graft fetal central nervous system (CNS) tissue. The first involves the transplantation of solid pieces of tissue to a surgically prepared transplantation cavity in which the graft is placed (with or without a delay period) in direct contact with the denervated hippocampus. In this procedure good graft survival is ensured by preparing the cavity in such a way that the graft can be placed on a richly vascularized surface (e.g., the pia in the choroidal fissure) that can serve as a "culturing bed" for the graft (57). The vessel-rich ventral surface of the aspirative fimbria-fornix lesion, used to transect the septohippocampal pathway in the present experiments, provides such a culturing bed. This cavity is in direct communication with the lateral ventricle, which may allow the cerebrospinal fluid (CSF) to circulate through the graft cavity and thus probably help the graft to survive, particularly during the early postoperative period.

The second technique involves injection of dissociated cell suspensions into the depth of the brain (13). In this technique pieces of fetal CNS tissue are trypsinized and mechanically dissociated into a milky cell suspension. Small volumes of the suspension can then be stereotactically injected into the desired site using a microsyringe. A major advantage of this technique is that it allows precise and multiple placements of the cells. The technique also makes possible accurate monitoring of the number of cells injected by estimation of the density of cells in the suspension. For the remainder of this chapter the first technique is referred to as the "solid graft" and the second technique as the "cell suspension."

Central nervous tissue survives grafting only if it is taken from fetal or neonatal donors, and optimum survival for a CNS region seems to coincide with the period when the neurons are undergoing their last cell divisions but before they have established extensive axonal projections. For grafting of basal forebrain cholinergic neurons in the rat, we have found the optimal donor age to be between days 14 and 17 of gestation.

## GRAFT SURVIVAL AND FIBER OUTGROWTH

The ability of cholinergic-rich grafts of fetal basal forebrain tissue to ameliorate lesion-induced learning and memory deficits has been studied in rats with aspirative fimbria-fornix lesions (transecting the septohippocampal cholinergic pathway) or excitotoxic lesions of the nucleus basalis region, which provides the major cholinergic afferent input to the fronto/parietal neocortical areas. Intrahippocampal grafts of basal forebrain tissue have also been studied in aged rats without any preceding denervating lesions.

## Intrahippocampal Grafts in Young or Aged Rats

Solid pieces of the embryonic septal-diagonal band area have been found to be capable of providing a new cholinergic innervation of the cholinergically denervated hippocampal formation in fimbria-fornix-lesioned young rats (5). With such solid grafts the reinnervation process is protracted over several months. With cell suspension grafts of the septal-diagonal band region, injected directly into the denervated hippocampus, we have been able to increase the rate of reinnervation of the denervated hippocampus as well as to increase the total area of the denervated hippocampus that is reinnervated by the acetylcholine esterase (AChE)-positive fibers growing out from the grafted cells (9).

The septal cell suspension grafts are found as several cellular aggregates or tissue masses within the hippocampal or choroidal fissures, within the overlying ventricle, or embedded in the host hippocampal tissue. It has been estimated that the implanted tissue grows to about twice its initial volume and that approximately 60% of the potential number of cholinergic neurons survive, provided the implants are made into a cholinergically denervated (i.e., fimbria-fornix-lesioned) hippocampus (32).

A new AChE-positive innervation is established from the grafts, starting between 1 and 3 weeks after implantation. By 3 months the entire hippocampal formation was reached by the ingrowing fibers, with a terminal density approaching that of the normal hippocampus (9).

The laminar pattern established by the newly formed AChE-positive terminal networks was remarkably similar to that of the normal AChE-positive innervation, even with respect to finer details. This finding suggests that the distribution of the ingrowing fibers from the graft was highly specific. Other experiments, using grafts of various types of monoaminergic neurons, have shown that the patterning of the ingrowing axons is characteristic for each neuron type, and that it is greatly dependent on both graft placement and the presence or absence of the intrinsic cholinergic innervation (6,10–12).

In aged rats grafting has been performed into the intact hippocampal formation using the cell suspension technique (33,34). Graft survival assessed 3 to 4 months after grafting was comparable to that seen in our previous studies in young adult recipients. Fiber outgrowth into the host brain was evaluated in animals that had had their intrinsic septohippocampal pathway removed (by a fimbria-fornix lesion) 6 to 10 days before killing. Dense outgrowth of AChE-positive fibers occurred up to about 2 mm away from the septal implants. The overall magnitude of fiber outgrowth was less than that generally seen in the previously denervated hippocampus in young adult recipients, but it appeared to be as extensive as in young recipients when the grafts are placed in the nondenervated hippocampal formation. In addition, the distribution of the AChE-positive fibers from the septal implants in the host hippocampus suggested that the pattern formed in the nondenervated target tissue of the aged recipients was more diffuse and somewhat different from normal.

Electron microscopy, using ChAT immunocytochemistry, has shown that the ingrowing cholinergic axons from the grafts form abundant synaptic contacts with neuronal elements in the host dentate gyrus in both the fimbria-fornix-lesioned young rats and the nondenervated aged rats (17,18). Although the graft-derived synapses in the aged rats were remarkably similar to normal synapses qualitatively and quantitatively, some abnormalities were found in the fimbria-fornix-lesioned young rats with respect to the relative distribution of contacts on dentrites and neuronal perikarya.

### Intracortical Grafts in Rats with Lesions of the Nucleus Basalis

Grafts of basal forebrain cholinergic neurons implanted as a cell suspension into the frontoparietal neocortex have been studied in rats with ibotenic acid lesions of the nucleus basalis (27–29). Similar to the grafts placed in the hippocampal formation, the intracortical grafts produced a new AChE-positive terminal network in an approximately 2 mm wide area around each cell deposit, and the outgrowing fibers showed a clear tendency to organize themselves in an appropriate laminar pattern within the host cortex (29). Electron microscopy using ChAT immunocytochemistry has shown that the ingrowing cholinergic fibers form abundant synaptic contacts with perikarya and dentrites of cortical neurons in the host (16). By 1 month after transplantation the ChAT activity levels in the graft-reinnervated frontoparietal cortical region was increased from about 40% of control in the animals with lesions alone to about 60% of control in the grafted animals (29).

### BIOCHEMICAL MEASURES OF GRAFT FUNCTION

The activity of the cholinergic innervation of the denervated hippocampus, derived from solid or suspension grafts of the septal-diagonal band area, has been monitored biochemically by measurements of the acetylcholine-synthesizing enzyme ChAT and of acetylcholine synthesis rates *in vitro* (5,8). Although AChE is a useful anatomical marker in the septohippocampal cholinergic projection system, the AChE enzyme is not a specific marker for cholinergic neurons. The synthetic enzyme ChAT, by contrast, is an enzyme specifically localized in cholinergic neurons and is a better marker of cholinergic neurotransmission. ChAT enzyme activity has therefore been used to measure the time course and magnitude of fiber outgrowth from both solid and suspended septal grafts. Graft-derived ChAT activity was barely detectable by 10 days after the implantation of cell suspension grafts, but it sharply increased between 10 days and 1 month in the region of the host hippocampus close to the graft. By 6 months ChAT activity was restored to near-normal levels in all segments of the previously denervated hippocampal formation. When comparing the total ChAT activity derived from the solid grafts and the cell suspension grafts, the cell suspension grafts appeared to be about twice as effective as the solid grafts, although the amount of tissue grafted was about the same in each case.

The functional activity of the septal grafts was further assessed by measurements of [14C]acetylcholine synthesis from [14C]glucose *in vitro* in fimbria-fornix-lesioned rats with septal suspensions implanted into the depth of the denervated hippocampus (8). The overall hippocampal [14C]acetylcholine synthesis was restored to normal levels in the grafted animals, and estimates of acetylcholine turnover rate suggested that the transmitter machinery of the newly established septohippocampal connections operated at a rate similar to that of the intrinsic septohippocampal pathway. Thus these septal cell suspensions seem capable of maintaining function at a relatively "physiological" level despite their abnormal position.

In a subsequent study, Kelly et al. (40) investigated the magnitude of lesion-induced functional alterations in different regions of the hippocampal formation, as reflected in the local rates of [14C]2-deoxyglucose (2-DG) utilization, and the degree to which this index of functional activity could be normalized following reinnervation by solid septal grafts. Transection of the septohippocampal pathway by a unilateral fimbria-fornix lesion resulted in a 30 to 50% reduction in 2-DG utilization throughout the ipsilateral hippocampal formation, and this depressed metabolism persisted 6 months after the lesion. Interestingly, the areas of depressed 2-DG utilization within the lesioned hemisphere were largely coextensive with the areas of the cingulate cortex and the hippocampal formation that had been substantially cholinergically denervated as a consequence of the fimbria-fornix transection. Fimbria-fornix-lesioned rats that had received solid septal grafts displayed a significant recovery in hippocampal 2-DG use compared to the rats with lesion alone. The graft-induced recovery in 2-DG utilization was significantly correlated with the graft-induced recovery in AChE staining density in adjacent sections from the same brains ($r=0.84$; $p<0.01$), thus suggesting a relation between the cholinergic reinnervation from the septal grafts and the restoration of functional glucose utilization. Indeed, the area of the host hippocampus and dentate gyrus that showed a complete restoration of AChE-positive innervation in these grafted animals was normalized with respect to 2-DG utilization rate, whereas the area with only partial AChE-positive reinnervation showed a partial but incomplete recovery of 2-DG use. Together with the biochemical data cited above, these results strongly suggest that the cholinergic component of the grafts is functional at the biochemical level and influencing, or normalizing, the overall functional performance of the deafferented hippocampal formation.

## ELECTROPHYSIOLOGICAL STUDIES

A series of studies have applied *in vivo* or *in vitro* electrophysiological techniques to analyze the functional properties of the graft–host connections in the septum-grafted animals, as well as the degree of functional integration of the septal grafts with the host brain. In the first of these studies (43), stimulation of solid septal grafts evoked characteristic field potentials in the dentate gyrus, and the depth profile revealed diffuse innervation characteristics of the normal septal afferents. Prepulse stimulation of the septal grafts was found to potentiate the field potentials evoked by perforant path stimulation. The latter effect, which is also a characteristic response of the granule cells to septal stimulation in the intact dentate gyrus, can probably be related to a synaptic cholinergic action, either directly onto the dentate granule cells or indirectly via local interneurons. The electron microscopic immunocytochemical demonstration of such synapses from the septal grafts (17) is consistent with this interpretation.

Segal et al. (53) analyzed the connections of septal suspension implants in fimbria-fornix-lesioned rats using intracellular recordings in hippocampal slices 4 to 8 weeks after grafting. Stimulation of the septal graft contained within the slice produced a slow and long-lasting, voltage-dependent depolarization in some host CA1 neurons located up to about 2 mm away from the graft. This depolarization was associated with an increase in spontaneous action potential discharges and spontaneous postsynaptic potentials. These responses were similar to those seen after topical application of acetylcholine. Because topical application of atropine attenuated, and physostigmine potentiated, the graft-induced depolarizing responses, these results are consistent with the formation of functional excitatory cholinergic synapses by the grafted septal neurons onto the host pyramidal neurons.

In another study (15), electroencephalograms (EEGs), evoked field responses, and cellular activity were recorded from animals with and without cholinergic grafts. Prior to the electrophysiological experiment the rats were trained to run in a wheel for water reward. In animals without transplants no recovery of rhythmic slow activity (RSA, or theta) occurred up to 9 months after the lesion. RSA is a characteristic EEG correlate of exploratory behavior in normal rats and is lost in animals with fimbria-fornix lesions (59). Instead, large-amplitude sharp waves and fast activity were present. In all rats with solid septal grafts, but in none of the rats with septal suspension grafts, behavior-dependent RSA reappeared several months after transplantation. The recovered RSA showed a strict and constant covariation with behavior: It was present during running in the wheel and absent while the animal was drinking or sitting still. Interestingly, the RSA recorded from the graft-reinnervated hippocampus and the RSA recorded from the contralateral hippocampus occurred in synchrony. In addition, granule cells and interneurons were found to fire rhythmically and phase-locked to the RSA. The rats with septal suspension grafts displayed only short-duration bursts of RSA (not present in the lesioned rats without transplants) and mainly during immobility.

These findings suggest that at least a portion of the RSA pacemaker cells of the host septum survives the fimbria-fornix transection, and that a solid graft of septal tissue, implanted into the fimbria-fornix-lesion cavity, may be capable of relaying this pacemaker activity to the host hippocampus. Alternatively, the grafted septal neurons, in the absence of normal connections, could be providing the pacemaker qualities. It would require, however, that the pacemaker cells in the graft be under the same brainstem control as the host septum. In either case, these data provide strong evidence that the grafts can become at least partly integrated with the host brain and that they are capable of influencing the target neuronal population in a near-normal manner.

## GRAFT-INDUCED AMELIORATION OF LEARNING AND MEMORY IMPAIRMENT

### Lesions of the Septohippocampal Pathway

The hippocampus has a special role in learning and memory, and bilateral fimbria-fornix or medial septal lesions in rats are known to result in severe impairment in both working memory (see ref. 48, for review) and spatial memory (see ref. 46, for review). These lesions disrupt several major afferent and efferent connection systems of the hippocampal formation. Nevertheless, because similar (but less pronounced) effects are obtained by pharmacological blockade of cholinergic transmission (48,61,62), it appears that damage to the cholinergic septohippocampal pathway contributes greatly to the memory impairments seen after fimbria-fornix or medial septal lesions.

In the eight-arm radial maze (43) rats with solid septal grafts (7 months after transplantation) showed a positive linear trend in maze performance over days of testing but overall did not differ significantly from nongrafted rats with lesions. However, potentiation of cholinergic transmission by pretreatment with the acetylcholinesterase inhibitor physostigmine produced significant enhancement of maze performance in the grafted group but not in the lesioned control group, and in some cases the grafted rats performed as well as the nonlesioned control animals. In a more recent study on intrahippocampal grafts of septal cell suspensions in rats with medial septal lesions, Pallage et al. (49) have obtained significant graft-induced recovery of radial maze performance also in the absence of acetylcholinesterase inhibition.

In a study using a T-maze forced-choice alternation test (performed 6 months after transplantation), Dunnett et al. (26) reported that seven of nine rats with solid septal grafts and four of five rats with septal suspension grafts were able to learn the task, some of them up to the level of control rats. The remaining rats with septal grafts and a separate group of rats with control grafts taken from the brainstem locus ceruleus region performed at chance level, similar to the rats that received only the fimbria-fornix lesion. The subsequent microscopic analysis showed a significant correlation between performance of the grafted rats and the amount of graft-derived AChE-positive staining in the previously denervated hippocampus ($r = 0.50; p < 0.02$).

Nilsson et al. (47) tested the ability of septal suspension or solid grafts to improve spatial reference and working memory in the Morris water-maze task (45) in rats with bilateral fimbria-fornix lesions. Sixty to eighty percent of the grafted rats showed significant recovery of spatial memory. This observation was seen in rats that had been pretrained in the task prior to lesion and grafting and in rats that had not been exposed to the water maze prior to lesion and transplantation. In the pretrained rats the bilateral fimbria-fornix lesion completely abolished the acquired performance. Whereas the lesioned, nongrafted rats could relearn the task partially using nonspatial strategies, the lesioned rats with septal grafts were capable of reacquiring a spatial memory of the platform site. Interestingly, central muscarinic receptor blockade by atropine (50 mg/kg) completely abolished the reacquired spatial memory in the grafted animals. This atropine effect was also seen in the normal control rats but to a lesser extent. Peripheral receptor blockade induced by atropine methylbromide, which passes the blood–brain barrier poorly, had no effect. Segal et al. (54) have reported similar results on intrahippocampal septal suspension grafts in rats with medial septal lesions.

### Nucleus Basalis Lesions

Large bilateral ibotenic acid lesions of the nucleus basalis region induce severe eating and drinking impairment. However, because large unilateral lesions of the nucleus basalis were also found to induce long-lasting learning and memory deficits in both passive avoidance and place-navigation in the Morris water-maze task, the first series of behavioral experiments were made on rats with unilateral lesions and unilateral intracortical grafts (27,28). Grafts of cholinergic-rich basal forebrain tissue, but not control grafts of hippocampal tissue, were found to significantly ameliorate the deficits seen in both passive avoidance and the water-maze task. In the passive avoidance test the grafts had no effects on the acquisition of the initial avoidance, whereas the retention impairments tested 2 days later were completely reversed. Similarly, the grafts had no effect on the acquisition of the water-maze task, whereas the grafted animals showed significant improvement in their ability to locate the platform site after platform removal.

Because the graft-induced effects were seen not only on parameters of learning and memory but also on some aspects of the sensorimotor impairments induced by the nucleus basalis lesion, these results indicate that the cholinergic-rich intracortical grafts may be capable of influencing some more general aspects of cortical function than memory per se (27).

## RECOVERY OF LEARNING AND MEMORY IN AGED RATS

Aged rats are known to display significant impairment in spatial working memory and spatial reference memory (2,33,39,60). In addition, there is evidence from several laboratories of decrements in parameters of cholinergic synaptic function in the hippocampal formation of aged rats, e.g., in muscarinic binding sites (42), acetylcholine synthesis (24,27), and high-affinity choline uptake (55). These age-dependent cholinergic deficits are further supported by observations that pyramidal cells of aged rats have a reduced responsiveness to iontophoretically applied acetylcholine (41,52). More recent reports (4,30,38,44) have provided evidence for a structural deterioration of the basal forebrain cholinergic neurons in aged rodents. Thus Horberger et al. (38) reported significant atrophy, without any major cell loss, in aged mice, whereas we observed both atrophy and a 40 to 60% cell loss throughout the basal forebrain cholinergic system in aged rats (30).

Taken together, these data provide support for the idea that decreases in memory function observed in aged animals may be dependent at least partly on impaired cholinergic function in the hippocampal formation and its associated limbic and cortical structures, and that the age-dependent decrease in function of the basal forebrain cholinergic system may contribute to decreased cognitive function in aged rodents. Analogous with the graft-induced effects seen in young rats with lesions of the septohippocampal or basalocortical pathway, therefore, grafts of cholinergic-rich septal tissue might be capable of compensating for at least some aspects of the learning and memory deficits seen in the aged rats.

Age-dependent learning and memory deficits were assessed in the Morris water-maze task prior to transplantation (31,33). This test requires that the rat use spatial cues in the environment to find a platform hidden below the surface of a pool of opaque water. Normal young rats have no trouble learning this task with speed and accuracy. Because our initial studies showed that only a portion (one-fourth to one-third) of our 21- to 23-month-old rats were markedly impaired in this task, a pretransplantation test served to identify the impaired individuals in the aged rat group. Based on the performance of the young controls, we set the criterion for impaired performance in the aged rats such that the mean escape latency (i.e., swim time to find the platform) should be above an upper 99% confidence limit of the escape latencies recorded in the young control group. A subgroup of old rats showed mean escape latencies greater than the criterion and were thus allocated to the "old impaired" group, which was used for subsequent transplantation. The remaining subgroup of aged rats constituted the "old nonimpaired" group. The latter group, together with a young control group, served as reference groups. A portion of the "old impaired" group received bilateral suspension grafts prepared from the septal-diagonal band area obtained from 14- to 16-day-old embryos of the same rat strain. Three implant deposits were made stereotactically into the hippocampal formation on each side. The remaining "old impaired" rats were left unoperated and served as the "old-impaired" control group. On the posttransplantation test 2.5 to 3.0 months after grafting the nongrafted groups remained impaired, whereas the grafted animals, as a group, showed a significant improvement in performance as indicated by their reduced escape latency. This improvement of the grafted group was demonstrated by comparisons to its pretransplantation performance as well as to the performance of the nongrafted old controls in the second test.

The ability of the rats to use spatial cues for the location of the platform in the pool was assessed by analyzing their search behavior after removal of the platform on the fifth day of testing. The pretransplantation test rats and rats in the "old nonimpaired" groups focused their search in the quadrant where the platform had previously been placed, whereas the "old impaired" rats failed to do so. In the posttransplantation test the grafted rats, but not the nongrafted "old impaired" group, showed significantly improved performance. Swim distance in the platform quadrant was increased by 83%, and they swam significantly more in the platform quadrant than in other quadrants of the pool. By contrast, the nongrafted controls showed no significant change over their pretransplantation performance.

In a subsequent study (31) we made some initial attempts to analyze the septal graft effects pharmacologically. In these experiments we used a modified water-maze protocol in which the platform was visible ("cue" trials) and invisible ("place" trials) on alternating trials. In this test it was clear that the "old impaired" rats were severely impaired not only when the platform was hidden (i.e., spatial reference memory) but also in the acquisition of the task when the platform was visible (which can be taken as a measure of nonspatial reference memory). The nongrafted impaired rats remained as impaired on both the "cue" and the "place" tasks when retested 2.5 months after the first test, whereas the impaired rats with septal suspension implants in the hippocampal formation were significantly improved on both components of the task. Moreover, whereas the nongrafted animals showed worse performance during the first 2 days of the second test session, compared to the last days of the first test session, the grafted animals retained their level of performance from the end of the first test session. This finding indicates that the septal grafts can have an effect not only on acquisition but also on retention of the learned performance.

In the pharmacological test, atropine (50 mg/kg i.p.) abolished completely the ability to find the platform in the grafted animals, with both visible and nonvisible platforms. Consistent with this finding, the rats' ability to locate the platform site (after platform removal) was eliminated. By contrast, atropine had no significant effect in the "old impaired" rats without grafts and only a marginal effect in the young control rats. Physostigmine (0.05 mg/kg i.p.) had no significant effect on either grafted or nongrafted animals when administered during a single day of trials. These observations seem consistent with the idea that the graft-mediated improvements, seen in the aged rats on both spatial and nonspatial learning and memory in the water-maze test, are dependent on a cholinergic mechanism.

## CONCLUDING COMMENTS

Grafts of basal forebrain tissue rich in cholinergic neurons—but not control grafts from the hippocampus or the locus ceruleus region—can significantly ameliorate (but not completely reverse) the learning and memory deficits seen in rats with lesions of the septohippocampal or basalocortical systems and those with age-dependent cognitive deficits. The combined morphological, biochemical, physiological, and pharmacological data strongly suggest that these graft-induced effects depend, at least in part, on connections established between the graft and the host.

From the studies conducted in young adult rats with lesions of the cholinergic projection systems it appears that implanted embryonic cholinergic neurons in some cases can substitute quite well, morphologically and functionally, for a lost afferent cholinergic input to a denervated brain region. The basal forebrain cholinergic neurons are commonly conceived of as a modulatory or level-setting system that tonically regulates the activity or performance of the hippocampal neuronal machinery. Removal of the cholinergic control mechanisms thus results in inhibition or impairment of hippocampal function. It seems possible therefore that the functional recovery seen after reinstatement of impaired cholinergic transmission by septal grafts could be interpreted as relatively nonspecific reactivation of inhibited, but otherwise intact, hippocampal neuronal machinery.

To what extent the intracerebral implants can be functionally integrated with the host brain is still poorly known, however, and remains therefore an interesting question for further investigation. The chances for extensive integration may be greatest for neuronal suspension grafts implanted as deposits directly into the depth of the brain, but even solid grafts inserted as whole pieces have in several cases been seen to become reinnervated from the host brain, in both adult and developing recipients (see ref. 7, for review). Interestingly, in the above cited study by Buzsaki et al. (15), rats with solid septal grafts showed much better recovery of behavior-related hippocampal theta rhythm, or RSA, than rats with suspension grafts. As discussed above, it may be because of the ability of the solid grafts placed in the fimbria-fornix lesion cavity to act as a "bridge" for axons from the host brain, which could serve to synchronize EEG rhythmicity in the lesioned hippocampus with that on the intact control side.

Whether these observations on grafts in young rats with denerving lesions are valid for the interpretation of the graft-induced functional effects in aged rats (without any preceding experimentally induced brain damage) is unclear. The observations of fiber outgrowth and, ultrastructurally, of synapse formation with neurons in the host hippocampus may support the possibility that even in the nondenervated aged host brain the implanted cholinergic neurons may act via specific efferent connections with the host. We propose the following working hypothesis for both aged rats and young rats with denervating lesions: The functional effects of implanted septal tissue are exerted by a specific action of selective neuronal elements in the graft onto dysfunctioning neuronal elements in the host, and this influence is mediated via the fiber connections established by the implanted neurons. On the assumption that impaired cholinergic neurotransmission contributes to the age-dependent cognitive impairment, we also propose that the ameliorative action of septal grafts in aged rats is at least partly due to a restoration of cholinergic neurotransmission in the area. Our results suggest, however, that although cholinergic reinnervation of the target may be *necessary* for the behavioral effects induced by the implanted basal forebrain tissue it may not be *sufficient* for graft function. Several neuronal cell types may participate, and the presence or absence of specific afferent connections to the grafts may also be important.

## ACKNOWLEDGMENTS

The studies were supported by grants from the Swedish MRC (04X-3874) and the National Institutes of Health (NS-06701 and AG 06088), the Office of Naval Research, and the Margaret and Herbert Horra Jr. Foundation.

## REFERENCES

1. Arendt, T., Bigl, V., Tennstedt, A., and Arendt, A. (1985): Neuronal loss in different parts of the nucleus basalis is related to neuritic plaque formation in cortical target areas in Alzheimer's disease. *Neuroscience*, 14:1–14.
2. Barnes, C. A., Nadel, L., and Honig, W. K. (1980): Spatial memory deficits in senescent rats. *Can. J. Psychol.*, 34:29–39.
3. Bartus, R. T., Dean, R. L., Beer, B., and Lippa, A. S. (1982): The cholinergic hypothesis of geriatric memory dysfunction. *Science*, 217:408–416.
4. Biegon, A., Greenberger, V., and Segal, M. (1986): Quantitative histochemistry of brain acetylcholinesterase and learning rate in the aged rat. *Neurobiol. Aging*, 7:215–217.
5. Björklund, A., and Stenevi, U. (1977): Reformation of the severed septohippocampal

cholinergic pathway in the adult rat by transplanted septal neurons. *Cell Tissue Res.*, 185:289–302.

6. Björklund, A., and Stenevi, U. (1981): In vivo evidence for a hippocampal adrenergic neurotrophic factor specifically released on septal deafferentation. *Brain Res.*, 229:403–428.
7. Björklund, A., and Stenevi, U. (1984): Intracerebral neural implants: neuronal replacement and reconstruction of damaged circuitries. *Annu. Rev. Neurosci.*, 7:279–308.
8. Björklund, A., Gage, F. H., Schmidt, U., Stenevi, U., and Dunnett, S. B. (1983): Intracerebral grafting of neuronal cell suspensions. VII. Recovery of choline acetyltransferase activity and acetylcholine synthesis in the denervated hippocampus reinnervated by septal suspension implants. *Acta Physiol. Scand. [Suppl.]*, 522:59–66.
9. Björklund, A., Gage, F. H., Stenevi, U., and Dunnett, S. B. (1983): Intracerebral grafting of neuronal cell suspensions. VI. Survival and growth of intrahippocampal implants of septal cell suspensions. *Acta Physiol. Scand. [Suppl.]*, 522:49–58.
10. Björklund, A., Kromer, L. F., and Stenevi, U. (1979): Cholinergic reinnervation of the rat hippocampus by septal implants is stimulated by perforant path lesion. *Brain Res.*, 173:57–64.
11. Björklund, A., Segal, M., and Stenevi, U. (1979): Functional reinnervation of rat hippocampus by locus coeruleus implants. *Brain Res.*, 170:409–426.
12. Björklund, A., Stenevi, U., and Svendgaard, N-A. (1976): Growth of transplanted monoaminergic neurons into the adult hippocampus along the perforant path. *Nature*, 262:787–790.
13. Björklund, A., Stenevi, U., Schmidt, R. H., Dunnett, S. B., and Gage, F. H. (1983): Intracerebral grafting of neuronal cell suspensions. I. Introduction and general methods of preparation. *Acta Physiol. Scand. [Suppl.]*, 522:1–7.
14. Bowen, D. M., Smith, C. B., White, P., and Davison, A. N. (1976): Neurotransmitter-related enzymes and indices of hypoxia in senile dementia and other abiotrophies. *Brain*, 99:459–496.
15. Buzsaki, G., Gage, F. H., Czopf, J., and Björklund, A. (1986): Restoration of rhythmic slow activity (theta) in the subcortically denervated hippocampus by fetal CNS transplants. *Brain Res. (in press)*.
16. Clarke, D. J., and Dunnett, S. B. (1986): Ultrastructural organization of choline acetyltransferase immunoreactive fibres innervating the neocortex from embryonic ventral forebrain grafts. *J. Comp. Neurol. (in press)*.
17. Clarke, D. J., Gage, F. H., and Björklund, A. (1986): Formation of cholinergic synapses by intra-hippocampal septal grafts as revealed by choline acetyltransferase immunocytochemistry. *Brain Res.*, 369:151–162.
18. Clarke, D. J., Gage, F. H., Nilsson, O. G., and Björklund, A. (1986): Grafted septal neurons form synaptic connections in the dentate gyrus of behaviorally-impaired aged rats. *J. Comp. Neurol. (submitted)*.
19. Coleman, P. D., Hornberger, J. C., and Buell, S. J. (1985): Stability of number but not size of acetylcholinesterase-positive neurons of basal forebrain in C57B1/6 mice between 7 to 53 months. *Neurosci. Lett.* [Suppl.], 22:S58.
20. Coyle, J. T., Price, D. L., and Delong, M. R. (1983): Alzheimer's disease: a disorder of cortical cholinergic innervation. *Science*, 219:1184–1189.
21. Davies, P., and Maloney, A. J. F. (1976): Selective loss of central cholinergic neurons in Alzheimer's disease. *Lancet*, 2:1403.
22. Deutsch, J. A. (1983): The cholinergic synapse and the site of memory. In: *The Physiological Basis of Memory*, edited by J. A. Deutsch, pp. 367–386. Academic Press, New York.
23. Drachman, D. A., and Sahakian, B. J. (1979): Effects of cholinergic agents on human learning and memory. In: *Nutrition and the Brain*, Vol. 5, edited by A. Barbeau, J.H. Growdon, and R. J. Wurtman, pp. 351–366. Raven Press, New York.
24. Dravid, A. R. (1983): Deficits of cholinergic enzymes and muscarinic receptors in the hippocampus and striatum of senescent rats: effect of chronic hydergine treatment. *Arch. Int. Pharmacodyn.*, 264:195–202.
25. Dunnett, S. B. (1985): Comparative effects of cholinergic drugs and lesions of nucleus basalis or fimbria-fornix on delayed matching in rats. *Psychopharmacology*, 87:357–363.
26. Dunnett, S. B., Low, W. C., Iversen, S. D., Stenevi, U., and Björklund, A. (1982): Septal transplants restore maze learning in rats with fornix-fimbria lesions. *Brain Res.*, 251:335–348.
27. Dunnett, S. B., Toniolo, G., Fine, A., Ryan, C. N., Björklund, A., and Iversen, S. D.

(1985): Transplantation of embryonic ventral forebrain neurons to the neocortex of rats with lesions of nucleus basalis magnocellularis. II. Sensorimotor and memory effects. *Neuroscience*, 16:787–797.

28. Fine, A., Dunnett, S. B., Björklund, A., and Iversen, S. D. (1985): Cholinergic ventral forebrain grafts into the neocortex improve passive avoidance memory in a rat model of Alzheimer disease. *Proc. Natl. Acad. Sci. USA*, 82:5227–5230.

29. Fine, A., Dunnett, S. B., Björklund, A., Clarke, D., and Iversen, S. D. (1985): Transplantation of embryonic ventral forebrain neurons to the neocortex of rats with lesions of nucleus basalis magnocellularis. I. Biochemical and anatomical observations. *Neuroscience*, 16:769–786.

30. Fischer, W., Wictorin, K., and Björklund, A. (1987): Intracerebral infusion of nerve growth factor ameliorates cholinergic neuron atrophy and spatial memory impairments in aged rats. *Nature (submitted)*.

31. Gage, F. H., and Björklund, A. (1986): Cholinergic septal grafts into the hippocampal formation improve spatial learning and memory in aged rats by an atropine sensitive mechanism. *J. Neurosci. (in press)*.

32. Gage, F. H., and Björklund, A. (1986): Enhanced graft survival in the hippocampus following selective denervation. *Neuroscience*, 17:89–98.

33. Gage, F. H., Björklund, A., Stenevi, U., Dunnett, S. B., and Kelly, P. A. T. (1984): Intrahippocampal septal grafts ameliorate learning impairments in aged rats. *Science*, 225:533–536.

34. Gage, F. H., Dunnett, S. B., Stenevi, U., and Björklund, A. (1983): Intracerebral grafting of neuronal cell suspensions. VIII. Survival and growth of implants of nigral and septal cell suspensions in intact brains of aged rats. *Acta Physiol. Scand. [Suppl. ]*, 522:67–75.

35. Gage, F. H., Kelly, P. A. T., and Björklund, A. (1984): Regional changes in brain glucose metabolism reflect cognitive impairments in aged rats. *J. Neurosci.*, 4:2856–2866.

36. Gibson, G. E., Peterson, C., and Jensen, D. J. (1981): Brain acetylcholine synthesis declines with senescence. *Science*, 213:674–676.

37. Hepler, D. J., Olton, D., Wenk, G. L., and Coyle, J. T. (1985): Lesions in nucleus basalis magnocellularis and medial septal area of rats produce qualitatively similar memory impairments. *J. Neurosci.*, 5:866–873.

38. Horberger, J. C., Buell, S. J., Flood, D. G., McNeill, H., and Coleman, P. D. (1985): Stability of numbers but not size of mouse forebrain cholinergic neurons to 53 months. *Neurobiol. Aging*, 6:269–275.

39. Ingram, D. K., London, E. D., and Goodrick, C. L. (1981): Age and neurochemical correlates of radial maze performance in rats. *Neurobiol. Aging*, 2:41–47.

40. Kelly, P. A. T., Gage, F. H., Ingvar, M., Lindvall, O., Stenevi, U., and Björklund, A. (1985): Functional reactivation of the deafferented hippocampus by embryonic septal grafts as assessed by measurements of local glucose utilization. *Exp. Brain Res.*, 58:570–579.

41. Lippa, A. S., Critchett, D. J., Ehlert, F., Yamamura, H. I., Enna, S. J., and Bartus, R. T. (1981): Age-related alterations in neurotransmitter receptors: an electrophysiological and biochemical analysis. *Neurobiol. Aging*, 2:3–8.

42. Lippa, A. S., Pelham, R. W., Beer, B., Critchett, D. J., Dean, R. L., and Bartus, R. I. (1980): Brain cholinergic dysfunction and memory in aged rats. *Neurobiol. Aging*, 1:13–19.

43. Low, W. C., Lewis, P. R., Bunch, S. T., Dunnett, S. B., Thomas, S. R., Iversen, S. D., Björklund, A., and Stenevi, U. (1982): Functional recovery following neural transplantation of embryonic septal nuclei in adult rats with septohippocampal lesions. *Nature*, 300:260–262.

44. Luine, V. N., Renner, K. J., Heady, S., and Jones, K. J. (1986): Age and sex-dependent decreases in ChAT in basal forebrain nuclei. *Neurobiol. Aging*, 7:193–198.

45. Morris, R. G. M. (1981): Spatial localization does not require the presence of local cues. *Learn. Motiv.*, 12:239–260.

46. Morris, R. G. M. (1983): An attempt to dissociate "spatial mapping" and "working memory" theories of hippocampal function. In: *The Neurobiology of the Hippocampus*, edited by W. Seifert. Academic Press, London.

47. Nilsson, O. G., Shapiro, M. L., Gage, F. H., and Björklund, A. (1987): Spatial learning and memory following fimbria-fornix transection and grafting of fetal septal neurons to the hippocampus. *Exp. Brain Res. (in press)*.

48. Olton, D. S., Becker, J. T., and Handelman, G. E. (1979): Hippocampus, space and memory. *Behav. Brain Sci.*, 2:313–365.
49. Pallage, V., Toniolo, G., Will, B., and Hefti, F. (1986): Long-term effects of nerve growth factor and neural transplants on behavior of rats with medial septal lesions. *Brain Res. (in press)*.
50. Pearson, R. C. A., Sofroniew, M. V., Cuello, A. C., Powell, T. P. S., Eckenstein, F., Esiri, M. M., and Wilcock, G. K. (1983): Persistence of cholinergic neurons in the basal nucleus in a brain with senile dementia of the Alzheimer's type demonstrated by immunohistochemical staining for choline acetyltransferase. *Brain Res.*, 289:375–379.
51. Perry, E. K., Tomlinson, B. E., Blessed, G., Bergmann, K., Gibson, P. H., and Perry, R. H. (1978): Correlation of cholinergic abnormalities with senile plaques and mental test scores in senile dementia. *Br. Med. J.*, 2:1457–1459.
52. Segal, M. (1982): Changes in neurotransmitter actions in aged rat hippocampus. *Neurobiol. Aging*, 3:121–124.
53. Segal, M., Björklund, A., and Gage, F. H. (1985): Transplanted septal neurons make viable cholinergic synapses with a host hippocampus. *Brain Res.*, 336:302–307.
54. Segal, M., Greenberger, V., and Milgam, H. W. (1987): A functional analysis of connections between grafted septal neurons and a host hippocampus. *Prog. Brain Res. (in press)*.
55. Sherman, K. A., Kuster, J. E., Dean, R. L., Bartus, R. T., and Friedman, E. (1981): Presynaptic cholinergic mechanisms in brain of aged rats with memory impairments. *Neurobiol. Aging*, 2:99–104.
56. Sims, N. R., Marek, K. L., Bowen, D. M., and Davison, A. N. (1982): Production of ($^{14}$C) acetylcholine and ($^{14}$C) carbon dioxide from (U-$^{14}$C) glucose in tissue prisms from aging rat brain. *J. Neurochem.*, 38:488–492.
57. Stenevi, U., Björklund, A., and Svendgaard, N-Aa. (1976): Transplantation of central and peripheral monoamine neurons to the adult rat brain: techniques and conditions for survival. *Brain Res.*, 114:1–20.
58. Strong, R., Hicks, P., Hsu, L., Bartus, R. T., and Enna, S. J. (1980): Age-related alterations in the rodent brain cholinergic system and behavior. *Neurobiol. Aging*, 1:59–63.
59. Vanderwolf, C. H. (1969): Hippocampal electrical activity and voluntary movement in the rat. *Electroencephalogr. Clin. Neurophysiol.*, 26:407–418.
60. Wallace, J. E., Krauter, E. E., and Campbell, B. A. (1980): Animal models of declining memory in the aged: short term and spatial memory in the aged rat. *J. Gerontol.*, 35:355–363.
61. Whishaw, I. Q. (1985): Cholinergic receptor blockade impairs local but not taxon strategies for place navigation in a swimming pool. *Behav. Neurosci.*, 99:979–1005.
62. Whishaw, I. Q., O'Connor, W. T., and Dunnett, S. B. (1985): Disruption of central cholinergic systems in the rat by basal forebrain lesions of atropine: effects on feeding, sensorimotor behaviour, locomotor activity and spatial navigation. *Behav. Brain Res.*, 17:103–115.
63. Whitehouse, P. J., Price, D. L., Struble, R. G., Clark, A. W., Coyle, J. T., and Delong, M. R. (1982): Alzheimer's disease and senile dementia: loss of neurons in the basal forebrain. *Science*, 215:1237–1239.

*Aging and the Brain,* edited by R. D. Terry.
Raven Press, New York © 1988.

# Neuronotrophic Factors and Their Involvement in the Adult Central Nervous System

*Silvio Varon, *Marston Manthorpe, **Lawrence R. Williams,
and **Fred H. Gage

*Departments of *Biology and **Neurosciences, School of Medicine, University of
California, San Diego, La Jolla, California 92093*

Neuronal populations, in both the central (CNS) and peripheral (PNS) nervous systems, undergo during early development a naturally occurring cell death that reduces the number of embryonic neurons to that found in the adult (11). It has been postulated that developmental neuronal survival is regulated by neuronotrophic factors (NTFs), i.e., special proteins presumably supplied by the innervation territory. The available NTFs would be taken up by the innervating axonal endings and transported retrogradely in the axons to promote survival-supporting activities in the neuronal cell bodies (64). Glial cells, from both PNS and CNS developing tissues, have also been found capable of supplying such NTFs to the neurons (42,66). Glial cells are located around the synapse, along the axons, and in close proximity to the cell body and could therefore present their NTFs to different segments of the associated nerve cells. Identification and investigation of target territory- or glia-derived factors have been made possible by the use of neuronal and glial cell cultures *in vitro* (65).

Much of what is currently known about NTFs comes from the study of developing PNS tissues *in vivo* and of prenatal test neurons *in vitro* (65,69). It has been attractive, however, to speculate that similar if not identical factors play corresponding roles for adult CNS neurons *in vivo;* and such speculations have led to a more comprehensive neuronotrophic hypothesis (2,20,61–63), summarized in Table 1. The hypothesis postulates that adult CNS neurons are not only regulated by CNS endogenous NTFs but are actually dependent on NTF availability. It follows from such a postulated dependence that a reduction or loss of trophic support, i.e., a *trophic deficit,* would cause loss of function, degeneration, and eventual death of the deprived neurons. Trophic deficits could occur at various levels of the trophic chain of events, including: (a) inadequate production or secretion by the source cells (postsynaptic partners, glia); (b) interference with the transfer of NTFs from source to receptors

TABLE 1. *Main elements of the neuronotrophic hypothesis*

1. NTFs regulate adult as well as developing neurons.
2. NTFs also regulate adult CNS neurons *in vivo*.
3. Neuronal performances depend on their NTFs.
4. NTF deficit causes dysfunction and degeneration.
5. NTF deficits may occur at different levels.
6. NTFs may be involved in human CNS pathology.

on the neuronal target membrane; (c) defective axonal transports (antero-grade to deliver receptors to the axonal membrane, retrograde to carry back to the cell body the NTF-occupied receptors); and (d) reduced competence of the target neurons to transduce the NTF message and/or operate the cellular machinery that would benefit from it. Lastly, any such trophic deficit could be the basis for involutive neuronal processes in brain aging, certain neurodegenerative CNS diseases, or even the apparent inability of injured CNS axons to regenerate after traumatic or other lesions.

This chapter first provides a brief survey of NTF investigation techniques and of the few factors already characterized at this time. Next, we evaluate some evidence for the presence of such factors in injured adult neural tissue and their apparent correlation with repair processes in certain PNS and CNS regeneration models. We then review direct evidence for the ability of some such factors to promote both survival and axonal regrowth of adult CNS neurons *in situ*. Lastly, we point out directions in which this research is likely to proceed in future years and speculate about the applicability of these concepts and tools to actual interventions in clinical practice.

## *IN VITRO* ASSAYS FOR NEURONOTROPHIC AND NEURITE-PROMOTING ACTIVITIES

As already mentioned, the most important tool for the recognition and investigation of NTFs is provided by the use of *in vitro* neuronal cell cultures (40,64,65). The neural tissue containing the neurons to be addressed by a putative NTF is dissociated into component cells; the cell suspension is en-riched for its neuronal population; the neurons are seeded at low densities on an appropriate culture substratum and with an appropriate culture medium containing serial dilutions of the NTF source material to be tested; and neuronal survival is determined after a chosen time in culture. The culture conditions are set so that few neurons survive in the absence of the NTF supplement, and maximal survival is achieved at sufficient concentrations of the factor. The NTF dilution providing half-maximal support defines the num-ber of trophic units (TU) per milliliter of original sample. The same type of assay also permits the recognition and quantitative evaluation of inhibitory factors. When the cultured neurons are supplied with a constant and optimal concentration of NTF and with serial dilutions of a material containing the putative inhibitor, neuronal survival is prevented at high inhibitor concentrations and progressively allowed as the inhibitor is diluted out—similarly defining the inhibitory units (IU) per milliliter of test sample from the dilution achieving half-maximal inhibition (40).

A series of studies using test neurons from chick embryo ciliary ganglia has revealed the existence of a second class of factors, designated neurite-promoting factors (NPFs), which regulate the outgrowth of neuronal processes ("neurites") rather than the actual survival by the cultured neurons (1,7). Figure 1 illustrates the relative consequences of NTFs and NPFs. The cultured neurons fail to survive in the absence of both NTF and NPF (o/o), survive but do not grow neurites when only the NTF is present (NTF/o), begin to grow neurites but subsequently die when the NPF but not the NTF is available (o/NPF), and survive and grow profuse neurites when both factors are present (NTF/NPF). It is therefore possible to culture the test neurons in the presence of constant amounts of NTF (to secure their maximal survival) and serial dilutions of an NPF-containing material, determine the percentage of neurons displaying neuritic growth at a selected culture time, and thus define quantitatively the neurite-promoting units (NPU) per milliliter of the original material under study. Similar analyses, using constant and optimal amounts of both NTF and NPF, can be carried out with regard to "neurite-inhibiting" agents.

A standardized *in vitro* assay can then be used to screen various source materials (e.g., extracts of tissues innervated by the test neurons or materials derived from cultures of glial cells), select the most abundant source, and proceed with characterization of the molecule carrying the observed NTF or NPF activity. Usually both types of activity reside with protein molecules, and traditional protein chemistry techniques allow their purification. The factors isolated thus far are active in the picomolar range, and only minute amounts can be obtained in the purified form. Thus extensive work is needed before enough purified factor becomes available to proceed with partial amino acid sequencing, gene cloning, and antibody production, which are the steps required for final characterization and the development of bioengineered production of the factor on a larger scale for potential *in vivo* uses. Eventually *in vivo* models must be developed for the validation and quantitative evaluations of the roles that the purified factor can play in the experimental animal itself.

## KNOWN NEURONOTROPHIC AND NEURITE-PROMOTING FACTORS

### Nerve Growth Factor

The discovery of nerve growth factor (NGF) nearly 40 years ago opened a new era in developmental and cellular neurobiology, with NGF being the first

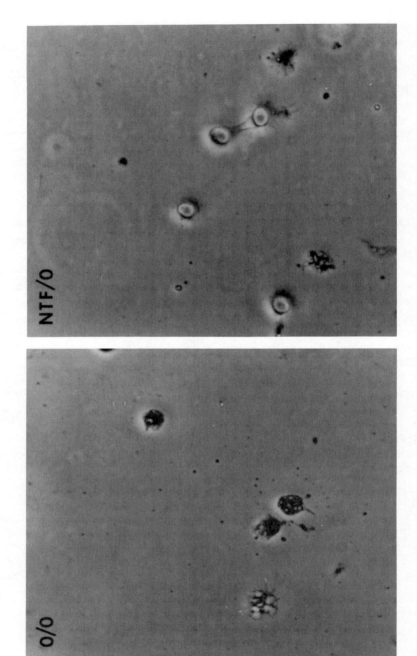

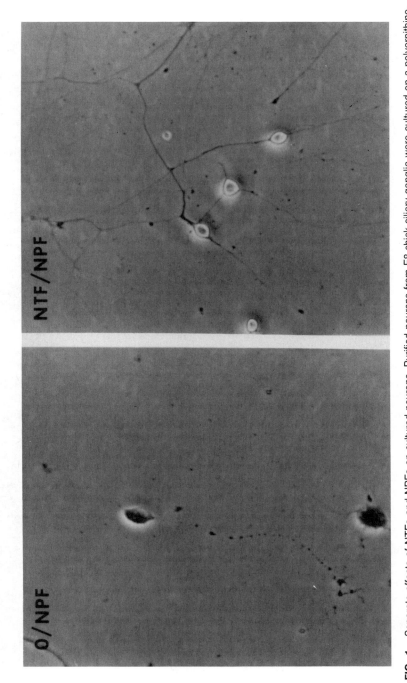

**FIG. 1.** Separate effects of NTFs and NPFs on cultured neurons. Purified neurons from E8 chick ciliary ganglia were cultured on a polyornithine-coated substratum in medium with or without their NTF and/or NPF *(top left corner symbols)*. Survival occurs only in the presence of NTF, and neuritic growth only in the presence of NPF.

identifiable protein factor controlling survival, neurite outgrowth, and transmitter synthesis by selected types of neurons *in vivo* and *in vitro* (for review, see refs. 19,33,59,69). The serendipitous finding that NGF is extraordinarily abundant in the submaxillary gland of adult male mice has permitted the use of this source tissue for the isolation and characterization of the NGF protein (70). The mouse submaxillary NGF occurs as a complex (7S NGF) of three protein subunits and $Zn^{2+}$, in which the NGF activity resides exclusively with the beta subunit (beta, or 2.5S NGF), a highly basic 25-kilodalton (KD) dimer of two identical chains. Identification of the gene for mouse NGF (52) has led to identification of the human NGF gene (60), and the homology between the two genes has demonstrated the highly conserved nature, hence evolutionary stability, of this factor.

Nerve growth factor has been traditionally known to affect two types of PNS neurons: the sensory neurons in dorsal root ganglia (DRG) and the autonomic principal (noradrenergic) neurons in paravertebral and prevertebral sympathetic ganglia. The responses to NGF by these two types of neurons change with their developmental age. Thus neuronal survival no longer appears to strictly require NGF *in vitro* and *in vivo* at late prenatal stages for the DRG and early postnatal stages for the sympathetic ganglia neurons— even though both neurons continue throughout adult life to respond to NGF with, for example, an increase in transmitter synthesizing enzymes. The dependence on NGF for neuronal survival and neurite regrowth, however, may be reinstated in the adult animal upon mechanical or chemical insults to the sympathetic neurons. Further studies revealed the susceptibility to NGF of other PNS ganglionic cells and of adrenochromaffin cells, which all share with DRG and sympathetic ganglia neurons a neutral crest origin.

Of greatest importance has been the discovery that NGF also addresses CNS neurons and, in particular, cholinergic neurons in several CNS locations. Cholinergic neurons in the medial septum and diagonal band innervate the hippocampal formation, and those in the nucleus basalis innervate the neocortex. These two territories for CNS cholinergic innervation contain both NGF and messenger RNA for NGF, revealing a cell ability to actually synthesize NGF (29). Radiolabeled NGF injected into the hippocampus or the neocortex is selectively taken up, retrogradely transported, and accumulated by the innervating neurons of the septum/diagonal band and the nucleus basalis, respectively (53). Transection of the fimbria-fornix tract, which carries the cholinergic axons projecting from septum to hippocampus, causes an increase in the hippocampal content of NGF but not of its mRNA (30)—supporting the view that hippocampal NGF is in fact normally removed from its site of production by the intact cholinergic fibers. Receptors for NGF have been recognized in rat brain tissue (58). The actual ability of NGF to affect directly CNS cholinergic neurons has been demonstrated by an NGF-induced increase in the choline acetyltransferase (ChAT) activity of perinatal rat cortical, septal, and striatal neurons *in vitro* and *in vivo* (23,26,44,45), as well as *in vivo* axotomized adult septal neurons following partial fimbria-fornix transection (22).

Despite the many years of NGF investigation, the molecular mechanisms underlying NGF actions remain to be elucidated. Receptors for NGF have been identified on the surface of the responding neurons, but the nature of the second messages transducing the NGF–receptor complex into regulation of various neuronal machineries is still unclear. A series of *in vitro* studies (55,67), however, has determined that: (a) an adequate performance of the $Na^+,K^+$-pump is essential for the ability of neurons to survive; (b) any NGF-dependent neuron, when deprived of NGF, loses its ability to operate its $Na^+,K^+$-pump several hours before it dies; and (c) NGF controls the maintenance of the neuronal $Na^+, K^+$-pump and/or restores its operation within seconds of its readministration. It appears therefore that one of the early steps in the control by NGF of neuronal viability takes place at the level of the $Na^+,K^+$-pump in the neuronal membrane.

### Ciliary Neuronotrophic Factor

The intrinsic musculature of the eye (in the choroid, ciliary body, and iris) is innervated by the cholinergic neurons of the ciliary ganglion (CG). During development, about half of the CG neurons die at the time they reach the intraocular innervation territories, and their death is increased by prior removal of the target tissue and reduced by preimplantation of an additional eye primordium. This classical example of developmental neuronal death has implied that the intraocular muscle tissue is a source of trophic factors for the CG neurons (38). The hypothesis has been supported by a series of studies leading to the extraction and purification from the chick embryo eye of a ciliary neuronotrophic factor (CNTF), capable of supporting *in vitro* survival and neuritic growth in cultures of CG neurons (3). Subsequent studies revealed a high CNTF activity in extracts of peripheral nerve, and a rat nerve CNTF has also been purified (43). The chick eye CNTF and the rat nerve CNTF proteins share a number of physicochemical properties but differ slightly in charge and size. Unlike NGF, the CNTF protein is acidic and has a monomeric molecular weight of 25 to 28 KD. Amino acid sequences, gene cloning, and anti-CNTF antibodies are being pursued.

In addition to its competence for the cholinergic CG neurons (which NGF does not support), CNTF also supports survival and neuritic growth by DRG and sympathetic ganglia neurons, thereby partially overlapping the neuronal target spectrum of NGF (38). The survival of NGF- and CNTF-dependent neurons has been found to be also supported, in the absence of these trophic proteins, by certain phorbol esters known to activate an intracellular protein kinase C (46). Further studies on the $Na^+,K^+$-pump of DRG neurons have shown that phorbol esters as well as CNTF do, in fact, preserve the competence of the neuronal pump but are unable to restore its losses incurred during early trophic deprivation—unlike NGF, which both protects and restores pump performance (56). One may therefore speculate that a protein phosphorylation step catalyzed by protein kinase C mediates the protection of the neuronal $Na^+,K^+$-pump and, consequently, the viability of these neurons.

## CNS-Addressing Neuronotrophic Factors

Central nervous system tissues comprise a highly heterogeneous neuronal population as well as various types of glial cells. Thus CNS neuronal cell cultures can be readily used for recognition of wide-spectrum neuronotrophic agents, but a search for narrow-spectrum CNS-addressing NTFs (CNS-NTFs) require either purification of the desired neuronal subset or its direct visualization within a mixed neuronal culture by use of specific neuronal markers. Research along these lines is still lagging considerably behind that using PNS neuronal systems.

Low-density neuronal cultures from various prenatal rat and chick CNS tissues have revealed the presence of neuronotrophic agents in media conditioned by glial cell cultures, CNS tissue extracts, and *in vivo* exudates from injured PNS and CNS tissues. The main agent in glia-conditioned media has been found to be pyruvate (54), a critical intermediate in energy metabolism, amino acid (hence protein) synthesis, and lipid anabolism. The finding demonstrated an insufficient capability of the cultured CNS neurons to utilize glucose as their main nutrient and encouraged speculations about a glia–neuron energy coupling that may be critical in the adult CNS under abnormal functional loads and/or pathological circumstances (27,63,71).

Conversely, other studies (40) have revealed that the CNS neuronotrophic activity in PNS and CNS wound fluids, as well as cerebrospinal fluid (CSF) from head trauma human patients (36), resides with protein rather than low-molecular-weight agents. Recognition of a CNS neuronotrophic protein abundantly present in whole blood has led to its purification from human red blood cells and its identification as the enzyme catalase (75). Further investigations led to the demonstration that all the test neurons requiring pyruvate for their *in vitro* survival could be independently supported by catalase or other antioxidants, and to the recognition of a peroxidation-induced block in the utilization of glucose that is either prevented (or corrected) by the antioxidant agents or bypassed by exogenous pyruvate (72). These and other observations draw attention to the role of free radicals in neuronal degeneration and death, as well as brain aging processes, and inspire the speculation that neuronotrophic factors and other agents may promote antioxidant neuronal defenses (72).

Central nervous system neuronotrophic activity has been suggested for a number of "growth" factors purified and characterized for their activities on other test cell systems. A brain-derived growth factor (BDGF), isolated from pig brain, supports *in vitro* survival and neuritic growth by DRG, but not sympathetic or ciliary ganglia neurons (4). Fibroblast growth factor (FGF) designates a family of proteins, extracted from brain and pituitary tissues, that promote proliferation of glial cells as well as fibroblasts. Gene cloning and amino acid sequences have been obtained for both an acidic and a basic FGF. The basic FGF has been reported to promote survival and neurite extension by cultured fetal rat hippocampal neurons (74). Another well-characterized protein from the mouse submaxillary gland, epidermal growth factor (EGF), which promotes growth and differentiation of several nonneural cell types, has also been suggested to play modulatory roles in the nervous system (25). Sera contain promoting as well as inhibitory protein factors for PNS and CNS neurons (13,57). A serum-derived neuronotrophic protein for cultured CNS neurons has been partially purified and characterized (28). The list of and knowledge about CNS-NTFs will undoubtedly be extended over the next few years.

### Anchorage-Dependent NPFs

Early studies with ciliary ganglionic cultures have revealed that several conditioned media contain not only the trophic factor CNTF but also a separate protein factor that binds most effectively to polycationic substrata and confers to them a high neurite-promoting activity, as already illustrated in Fig. 1 (1,7,15). Several additional observations have suggested that such NPFs may be related to extracellular matrix constituents, and *in vitro* assays of several purified extracellular matrix constituents have shown the glycoprotein laminin to be the most potent NPF among them (39). Laminin can be produced by PNS Schwann cells (6) and CNS astroglial cells (51), as well as by other cells. A schwannoma-derived polycation-binding NPF (SW-PNPF) has been characterized in detail and shown to comprise laminin complexed with proteoglycans, another family of extracellular matrix constituents (14,15). The contributions of proteoglycans to the neurite-promoting activity of their complex with laminin remain to be defined and lend themselves to some intriguing speculations (14). Both laminin and SW-PNPF are very active on CNS as well as PNS neuronal cultures.

Extracellular matrix is an abundant component of peripheral nerve, a tissue promoting *in vivo* axonal regeneration from both CNS and PNS neurons, but it is nearly absent in adult CNS parenchyma where axonal regeneration is hampered. If a naturally constructed but cell-free extracellular matrix preparation could be obtained, it should be possible to ascertain if (a) it displays *in vitro* the same neurite-promoting competence as do purified laminin or purified laminin–proteoglycan complexes, and (b) it could be used *in vivo* as a prosthetic terrain for PNS and CNS axonal regeneration, and mimic peripheral nerve tissue despite its lack of living cells. With these goals in mind, we have obtained and tested a human amnion membrane matrix (hAMM) from a readily available source, the human placenta (12,13).

As illustrated in Fig. 2A, the amnion membrane is manually separated from the chorion, and its epithelial cell layer is removed by treatment with ammonium hydroxide and gentle brushing. The resulting cell-free sheet presents a "basement membrane" (BM) layer lined by a "stroma" (ST) layer. Small pieces of it can be laid down and anchored onto nitrocellulose paper with either the BM or the ST surfaces face up. Alternatively, hAMM pieces can be folded or coiled and cross-sections of it similarly laid on nitrocellulose to expose a profile of both layers. A suspension of test neurons can then be seeded on the hAMM preparations with the required neuronotrophic supplements, and the cultures can be fixed after the desired incubation periods to evaluate the neuritic growth (using anti-neurofilament antibody) and its topographical relation to extracellular matrix constituents of the hAMM substratum (e.g., with anti-laminin antibodies) (13). Neurons from both CNS and PNS attach and survive on either the BM or the ST faces of the hAMM but grow neurites only on the basement membrane surface (Fig. 2B). When hAMM cross-sections are used, the neuritic growth is seen to be almost entirely confined to the hAMM layer characterized by the presence of laminin (Fig. 2C). These observations indicate that the laminin-containing extracellular matrix not only promotes regeneration of CNS and PNS axons *in vitro* but can also provide a directional guidance to the regrowing axons.

## *IN VIVO* MODELS FOR NTF AND NPF EVALUATION

### Silicone Chamber Model for PNS Regeneration

Peripheral nerve can regenerate after a complete transection, even in the adult mammal, if the proximal and distal nerve stumps are reapposed and sutured or if a nerve segment from another location is grafted as a bridge between the two stumps. Little is known about the cellular and molecular events triggered by the drastic disruption of the normal microenvironment consequent to the nerve lesion or about the regulatory influences attending success or failure of the nerve regeneration process. In collaboration with Göran Lundborg and co-workers in Sweden, we have developed a nerve regeneration model that allows analyses and manipulations of such events and regulatory influences (68). As shown in Fig. 3A, a sciatic nerve is exposed and resected in the adult rat, and the two nerve stumps are sutured into the opposite end of a silicone tube, generating an interstump gap of 10 mm (the "chamber"). Within 1 month, a new coaxial, fluid-surrounded structure (Fig. 3B) builds up across the chamber gap with all the characteristics of a young regenerated nerve (Fig. 3C): a perineurial outer cell sheath and an endoneurial core comprising blood vessels, Schwann cells, axons, and myelin. Over the next 2 months the regenerating axons grow beyond the chamber confines into the distal nerve segment to reach and functionally connect with their peripheral target tissues.

A spatial-temporal analysis of the events underlying the formation of a nerve regenerate within the chamber has indicated that: (a) the chamber fills with nerve stump exudate within 1 day; (b) an acellular matrix of longitudinally oriented fibrin polymers from chamber fluid precursors forms to bridge the interstump gap within 1 week; (c) perineurial, Schwann, and endothelial cells migrate from both stumps into the fibrin matrix over the next 2 weeks; and (d) axons grow out of the proximal stump following the cell migration and reach the distal end of the chamber over the third and fourth weeks. *In vitro* bioassays have shown that the chamber fluid accumulates, during the first few days, high levels of NTFs for spinal motor neurons, DRG sensory neurons, sympathetic ganglia and autonomic neurons (the three contributors of axons to the sciatic nerve), and that the concentration of these NTFs rapidly decreases to low but sustained levels thereafter (37). Figure 4 shows that this NTF surge precedes by several days the onset of axonal regeneration into the chamber and could therefore play a trophic role in the recovery and maintenance of the axotomized neurons rather than as a trigger for their axonal regrowth. On the other hand, NPFs appear and progressively accumulate in the chamber fluid in approximate coincidence with the later cell immigration and provide a precise temporal correlation with the onset and advance of the axonal outgrowth. Immunohistochemical examinations of the chamber matrix similarly showed the early presence in the acellular matrix of fibronectin (an extracellular matrix glycoprotein known to promote cell migration) and the later appearance of the neurite-promoting extracellular matrix glycoprotein, laminin (35).

## Hippocampal Model for CNS Regeneration

The hippocampal formation (hippocampus plus dentate gyrus) is a relatively simple, highly laminated brain structure that has been extensively investigated in development and regeneration studies. Much of the cholinergic innervation to the hippocampal formation comes from the cholinergic neurons of the medial septum and vertical diagonal band nuclei via the fimbria-fornix tract. Severance of the fimbria-fornix therefore should have at least three major consequences: (a) cholinoceptive sites on hippocampal and dentate gyrus neurons are vacated by their cholinergic presynaptic inputs and become potentially available for reinnervation by new cholinergic (or possibly other) axons; (b) the hippocampal tissue could accumulate trophic factors no longer taken up and removed by the original presynaptic endings or even

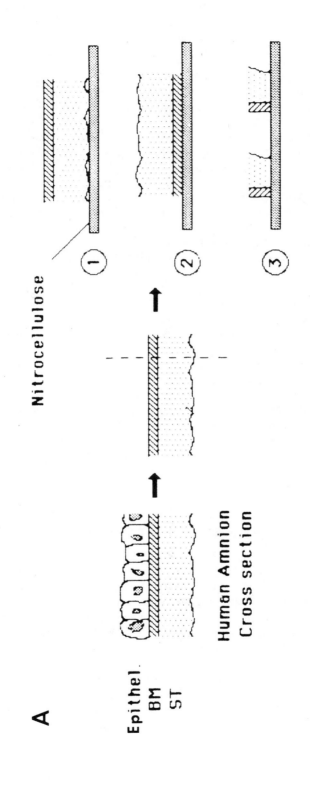

A

Epithel.
BM
ST

Human Amnion
Cross section

Nitrocellulose

① ② ③

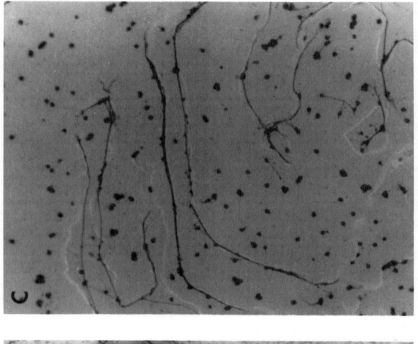

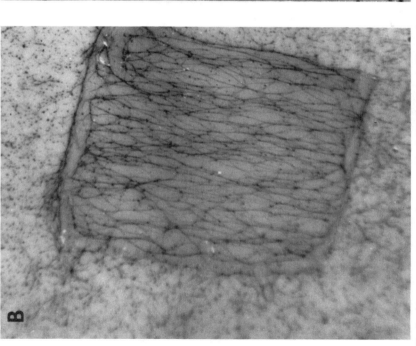

**FIG. 2.** Human amnion membrane matrix (hAMM) as an *in vitro* substratum for neurite regeneration and anchorage on nitrocellulose in different configurations (*1–3*). **B:** Massive and oriented neuritic growth (from E8 chick ciliary ganglionic neurons) is displayed by anti-neurofilament immunostaining on the basement membrane (*BM*) face of the nitrocellulose-anchored hAMM [no neuritic growth occurs on the stroma (*ST*) face—not shown]. **C:** Cross-section of rolled-up hAMM, used as a nitrocellulose-anchored substratum, shows that neuritic growth (*dark lines*) is largely guided along the laminin-immunoreactive regions (*light bands*).

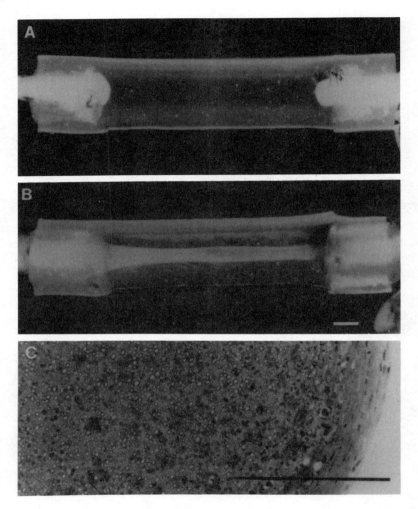

**FIG. 3.** Silicone chamber model for PNS regeneration. The two stumps of a transected sciatic nerve in the adult rat seal a space within a silicone chamber (**A**), across which a nerve structure regenerates within 1 month (**B**). Bar = 1 mm. Cross-sections of the regenerate reveal the typical components of a peripheral nerve (**C**). Bar = 100 $\mu$m.

increase their NTF production in reaction to the lesion; and (c) the axotomized neurons in the septum would be deprived of needed NTFs from their natural supply source, the hippocampal innervation territory, and lose function or die.

Septal or striatal fetal grafts (both of which contain cholinergic neurons), implanted in a cavity made through the retrosplenial cortex, have shown the ability to grow cholinergic fibers into the host rat hippocampus that the entorhinal lesion (in conjunction with a fimbria-fornix lesion) had deprived of

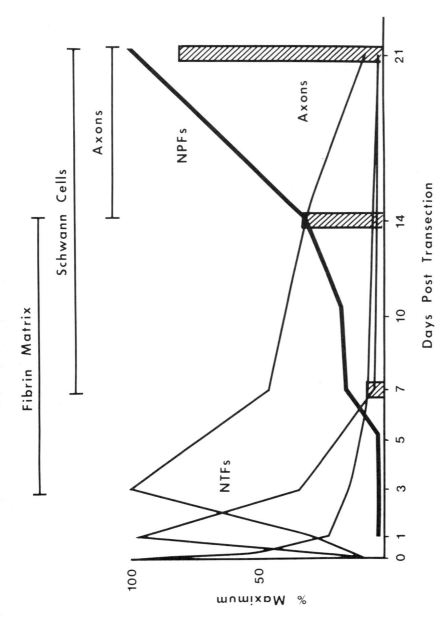

**FIG. 4.** Temporal developments in the silicone chamber model. In the chamber fluid NTFs undergo a transient buildup in the early days, whereas NPFs accumulate later concurrently with the invasion of the chamber matrix by Schwann and other cells. Regenerating axons from the proximal nerve stump advance into the chamber only after the appearance of Schwann cells (and laminin) in the matrix and NPFs in the fluid.

its cholinergic innervation (34). The success of the graft, however, was poor when the fetal tissue was implanted immediately after the lesion and progressively improved with increasingly delayed implantation times. In collaboration with Cotman's group (41,47,48), we were able to show in adult as well as neonatal rats that the entorhinal lesion is followed by a progressive accumulation, in both the injured tissue and its local exudate, of NTFs for a variety of test neurons. The NTF accumulation closely correlated in time with the success of increasingly delayed graft implantation and might therefore account for the latter. Accumulation of NGF in denervated hippocampus has more recently been shown to accompany an ingrowth of sympathetic fibers from adult host or from implanted peripheral sympathetic ganglia (10). Successful survival and axonal outgrowth by several fetal CNS grafts into the adult rat hippocampus may similarly reflect an accumulation in the host tissue of the corresponding NTFs (9,16), although their actual presence and nature have yet to be documented.

**Impact of NGF Septohippocampal Regenerative Processes**

The studies just reviewed of the sciatic nerve chamber model and the hippocampal model have provided clear demonstrations that NTFs and NPFs do occur *in vivo* in both the PNS and CNS of adult animals, and that they do so in the context of and in some correlation with neural regeneration processes. This information, however, does not directly establish that these factors actually engage in the regeneration process itself. Ways to achieve such a demonstration would be to: (a) deprive a selected CNS neuronal population of its innervation territory and thus its putative source of endogenous NTFs; (b) verify a functional deficit or outright death of the axotomized neurons consequent to their presumptive trophic deprivation; and (c) prevent or reduce the neuronal damage by the experimental administration of appropriate exogenous NTFs. The knowledge accumulated on the cholinergic component of the septohippocampal model and the more recent evidence for the ability of NGF to affect septal cholinergic neurons have offered the tools to address this problem. Unequivocal evidence that exogenous NGF can protect septal neurons from axotomy-induced death has now been provided by a detailed collaboration of Gage's, Varon's, and Björklund's groups (17,76,77). Similar evidence has been obtained independently by Hefti (21) and confirmed by Kromer (31).

A complete aspirative lesion of the fimbria-fornix in the adult rat leads to a massive disappearance of cholinergic neurons in the medial septum and vertical diagonal band (MS/VDB), which project their axons to the hippocampus via the fimbria-fornix, but leads to little loss in the horizontal limb of the diagonal band whose axons reach the hippocampus via a more ventral pathway (17). A microcannula device for continuous infusion of exogenous agents into the lateral ventricle (or the parenchyma) in close proximity to the septum (76) was used to administer NGF over 2 weeks following the fimbria-fornix lesion. Examination of the MS/VDB region at 2 weeks provided the following information (77):

1. Coronal sections of the septum stained for acetylcholinesterase (Fig. 5) reveal a conspicuous loss of cholinergic neurons in the MS/VDB regions ipsilateral to the fimbria-fornix lesion (Fig. 5A, B). This loss is no longer apparent in the NGF-treated animals (Fig. 5C). Similar results have been obtained by immunohistochemical staining with anti-choline acetyltransferase antibody. Because the cholinergic neurons can be recognized only by their acetylcholine-related enzymes, it remains conceivable that the apparent loss of stainable cholinergic neurons (which reaches its maximum within the first postoperation week) may reflect an initial loss of "function" followed by later degeneration and death.

2. A numerical analysis of the cell loss in representative septal sections, illustrated in Fig. 6, shows that by 2 weeks 50 to 90% of the medial septal cholinergic neurons would be lost, and that nearly all of them are rescued by exogenous NGF administration. Moreover, Nissl-stained sections reveal that as many as 50% of the total neuronal population are lost as a consequence of the lesion unless exogenous NGF is supplied. Because noncholinergic neurons may outnumber cholinergic ones by about 10-fold, this second finding demonstrates that noncholinergic neurons also (a) undergo massive death as a consequence of the fimbria-fornix lesion and (b) gain protection from the availability of exogenous NGF. The question whether NGF protects these other septal neurons directly or indirectly (by preventing the cholinergic death as a potential secondary source of trophic losses or other damages) remains to be investigated (73). As to the identity of the dying noncholinergic neurons, evidence for a vast participation of GABAergic neurons in the cell death induced by fimbria-fornix transection has been obtained (49), although their potential susceptibility to protection by NGF has not yet been evaluated.

### Axonal Regeneration in the Septohippocampal Model

One additional observation after exogenous NGF administration to the fimbria-fornix-transected adult rat was the appearance of a massive buildup of cholinergic fibers in the dorsal lateral quadrant of the septum (77). As shown in Fig. 7, this NGF-induced cholinergic sprouting is observed only on the side that had undergone the fimbria-fornix transection and faces the region of the lesion. This observation suggests that, in addition to protecting the cholinergic neurons against death, NGF also either protects or promotes new growth of the corresponding cholinergic axons. The intraseptal confinement of these cholinergic fibers further suggests that they may be prevented from growing

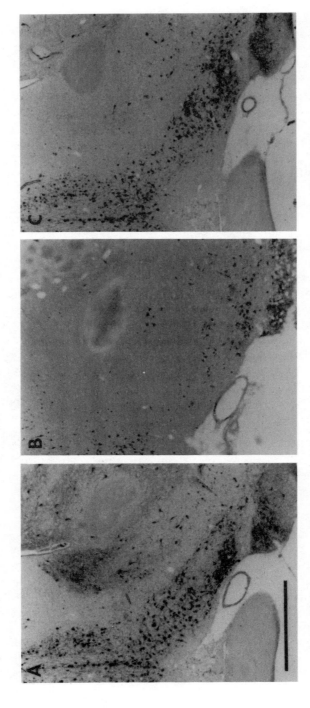

**FIG. 5.** Cholinergic neuronal loss in septum and diagonal band after fimbria-fornix transection and their protection by continuous intraventricular administration of NGF. Coronal sections (only one side shown) of adult rat basal forebrain, stained for AChE to identify cholinergic neurons. **A:** Unoperated animal. **B:** Animal with fimbria-fornix transection but only vehicle infusion. **C:** Animal with fimbria-fornix transection plus NGF administration. Bar = 1 mm.

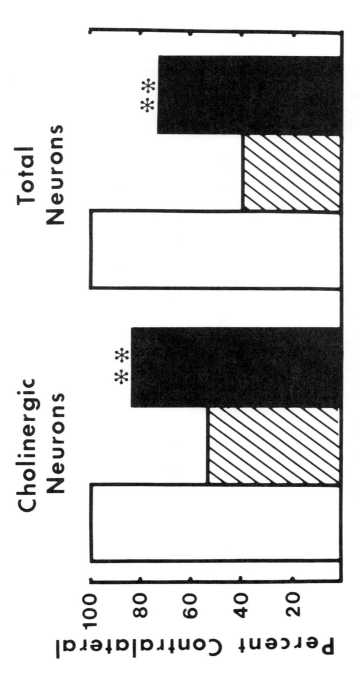

**FIG. 6.** Numerical analyses of cholinergic (AChE) and total (cresyl violet) neurons in the medial septum of fimbria-fornix-transected adult rats. *Open bars:* values contralaterally to the lesion (similar to those of unoperated animals). *Hatched bars:* values ipsilaterally to the lesion, no NGF treatment. *Solid bars:* same, in NGF-treated animals.

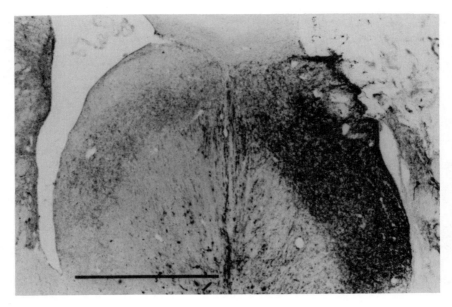

**FIG. 7.** NGF-induced buildup of cholinergic fibers in the dorsal lateral quadrant of the septum after fimbria-fornix transection. *Right side:* AChE staining ipsilateral to the lesion in NGF-infused rats. Bar = 1 mm.

out of the septum by adverse or by nonconducive influences from the lesion microenvironment. If so, the next step for successful regeneration of CNS axons in this model—in addition to the trophic protection of the damaged neurons—would require the presentation of a suitable "neurite-promoting bridge" across the fimbria-fornix lesion.

One such approach was attempted using fetal hippocampal grafts (32), at a time when the axotomy-induced death of septal neurons and their protection by NGF had not yet been defined. Cholinergic fibers, presumably originating from the nonaffected cholinergic cells, did invade the fetal hippocampal graft and extended beyond it into the host hippocampus. The fetal hippocampal graft approach deserves further detailed investigations to evaluate (a) the presumptive benefits of NGF administration and (b) any functional outcome of the invasion of the host hippocampus by the regenerating cholinergic (or other) axons. However, the obvious restriction in the collection and availability of fetal CNS tissue, particularly if the approach would eventually be extended to human subjects, dictates the search for other materials capable of providing neurite-promoting bridges. The human amnion membrane matrix (hAMM), already discussed for its *in vitro* properties, would be an ideal prosthetic material given its human origin, ethical suitability, and relative abundance. We are currently evaluating the effectiveness of hAMM in the septohippocampal system (12).

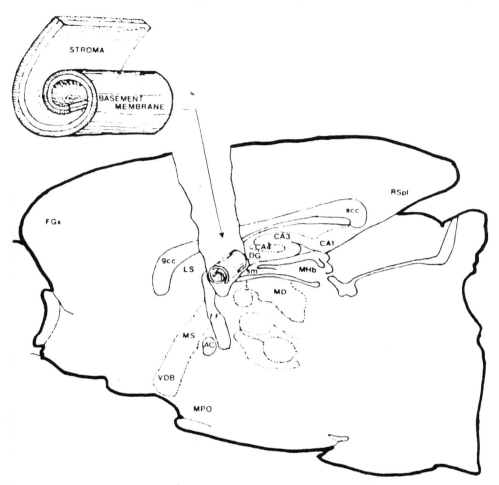

**FIG. 8.** Insertion of a hAMM bridge into the fimbria-fornix aspirative lesion of an adult rat. A sheet of hAMM is rolled into a cylinder (basement membrane face out), and a segment of it is positioned between septal and hippocampal regions of the transected fimbria-fornix. FCx: frontal cortex, gcc: genu corpus calosum, LS: lateral septum nucleus, MS: medial septum nucleus, VDB: nucleus of the vertical limb of the diagonal band, AC: anterior commissure, SM: stria medullaris thalami, DG: dentate gyrus, CA1–4: fields CA1–4 of Ammon's horn, MD: mediodorsal thalamus nucleus, MHb: medial habenular nucleus, scc: splenium corpus callosum, MPO: medial preoptic nucleus, RSpl: retrosplenial cortex, FF: fimbria-fornix.

Figure 8 illustrates the approach. The hAMM was rolled into a tight coil, and a coil segment of the appropriate dimension was inserted into the transected fimbria-fornix lesion so as to appose its cut sections to the septum on one side and the hippocampus on the other. Four weeks later longitudinal sections of the hAMM insert were examined for cholinergic fibers (acetylcholinesterase stain), human laminin (anti-laminin antibodies), and cells (cresyl violet). The hAMM insert was found to be well preserved, with little if any host tissue reaction to it. Figure 9 shows that cholinergic fibers had extended along the hAMM axis between the host septum and hippocampus (Fig. 9A) in general coincidence with laminin immunoreactive regions of the insert (Fig. 9B) and had contributed acetylcholinesterase-positive fibers to hippocampus and dentate gyrus of the host (Fig. 9C). Also present in the insert (not shown) were many nonneuronal cells, including astroglial (GFAP-immunoreactive) cells. In these preliminary experiments, no intraventricular administration of exogenous NGF was provided. The encouraging results warrant future vigorous explorations of several aspects: optimization of the "packaging" and the positioning of the hAMM insert, concurrent intraventricular infusion of NGF, quantitative evaluations of the extent and distribution of the regrowing cholinergic fibers into the host hippocampal formation, potential participation of other NGF-supported septal neurons to the hippocampal reinnervation, and the potential involvement of nonneuronal cells in the insert, among others. Given successful outcomes of such studies, it will become possible to investigate the ability of the regenerating axons to form new synaptic connections with host hippocampal neurons and, possibly, achieve some degree of functional restoration.

## PROJECTIONS AND SPECULATIONS

We have reviewed concepts, information, and test models, *in vivo* and *in vitro*, that establish NTFs and NPFs as important controllers of neuronal maintenance and repair in the CNS as well as the PNS and in the adult as well as the developing mammalian organism. Much of the recent work, although carried out in the context of neural regeneration, provides a clear impetus to the more general neuronotrophic hypothesis (Fig. 1) that at least the NTFs are likely to play considerable roles in other situations where neurons are at risk for involutive or pathological processes. Deficiencies of the basal forebrain cholinergic system are strongly implicated in learning and memory defects (24), e.g., those that accompany brain aging, Alzheimer disease,

**FIG. 9.** *In vivo* regeneration of cholinergic axons across a hAMM bridge and their invasion of the adult rat host hippocampal formation. **A:** AChE-stained fibers along the axis of the hAMM bridge. **B:** Laminin immunoreactive regions of the same section as **A. C:** AChE-positive fibers have left the hAMM insert and invaded the host hippocampus (*HIPP*).

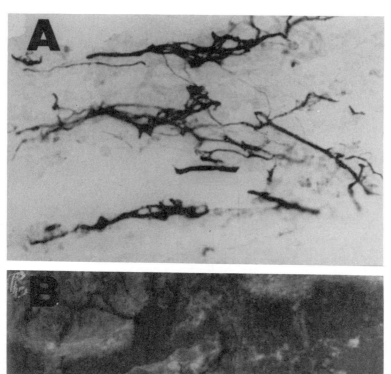

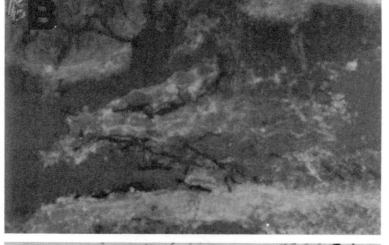

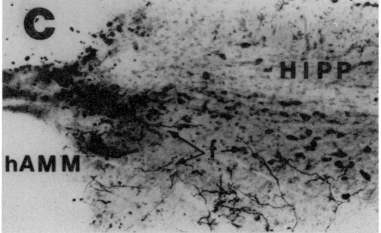

Alzheimer type senile dementia, or Down syndrome dementia (5,8,50). Recent though preliminary work (18) has indicated that continuous infusion of NGF into aged rats selected for learning and memory impairments did in fact result in improved or preserved performances in the Morris water-maze test. We deem it likely that NTFs other than NGF and CNS neuronal subsystems other than the cholinergic ones will eventually be shown to engage in similar neuronotrophic relations.

The task ahead remains formidable: recognition, purification, and bioengineered production of new NTF proteins; quantitative definition of new *in vivo* model systems, and of various experimental insults, susceptible to trophic help; investigation of NTF abnormalities that might occur in suitable neuropathological specimens; extension of NTF interventions to primate models; more efficient or more practical methods for exogenous NTF deliveries; among others. Nevertheless, it no longer appears impossible to conceive that a not too distant future might see the first attempts to use neuronotrophic agents as tools for clinical interventions in the human patient.

## ACKNOWLEDGMENTS

Much of the work reviewed here has been supported by grants from the NINCDS (NS-16349 to S.V.); the National Science Foundation (BNS-81-8847 and BNS-85-01766 to S.V.; BNS-85-02198 to M.M.); and the NIA (AG-03766) and Office of Naval Research to F.H.G.

## REFERENCES

1. Adler, R., Manthorpe, M., Skaper, S. D., and Varon, S. (1981): Polyornithine-attached neurite-promoting factors (PNPFs): culture sources and responsive neurons. *Brain Res.*, 206:129–144.
2. Appel, S. H. (1981): A unifying hypothesis for the cause of amyotrophic lateral sclerosis, parkinsonism, and Alzheimer disease. *Ann. Neurol.*, 10:499–505.
3. Barbin, G., Manthorpe, M. and Varon, S. (1984): Purification of the chick eye ciliary neuronotrophic factor (CNTF). *J. Neurochem.*, 43:1468–1478.
4. Barde, Y.-A., Edgar, D., and Thoenen, H. (1982): Purification of a new neurotrophic factor from mammalian brain. *EMBO J.*, 1:549–553.
5. Bartus, R. T., Dean, R. L., Beer, B., and Lippa, A. S. (1982): The cholinergic hypothesis of geriatric memory dysfunction. *Science*, 217:408–417.
6. Bunge, R. P., and Bunge, M. B. (1983): Interrelationships between Schwann cell function and extracellular matrix production. *Trends Neurosci.*, 6:499–505.
7. Collins, F. (1978): Induction of neuritic outgrowth by a conditioned-medium factor bound to the culture substratum. *Proc. Natl. Acad. Sci. USA*, 75:5210–5213.
8. Coyle, J. T., Price, D. L., and DeLong, M. R. (1983): Alzheimer's disease: a disorder of cortical cholinergic innervation. *Science*, 219:1184–1190.
9. Crutcher, K. A., and Collins, F. (1982): In vitro evidence for two distinct hippocampal growth factors: basis of neuronal plasticity? *Science*, 217:67–68.
10. Crutcher, K. A., and Davis, J. N. (1981): Sympathetic noradrenergic sprouting in response to central cholinergic denervation. *Trends Neurosci.*, 4:70–72.

11. Cunningham, T. J. (1982): Naturally occurring neuron death and its regulation by developing neural pathways. *Int. Rev. Cytol.*, 74:163–186.
12. Davis, G. E., Blaker, S. N., Engvall, E., Varon, S., Manthorpe, M., and Gage, F. H. (1987): Human amnion membrane serves as a substratum for growing axons in vitro and in vivo. *Science*, 236:1106–1109.
13. Davis, G. E., Engvall, E., Varon, S., and Manthorpe, M. (1987): Human amnion membrane as a substratum for cultured peripheral and central nervous system neurons. *Dev. Brain Res.*, 33:1–10.
14. Davis, G. E., Klier, F. G., Engvall, E., Cornbrooks, C., Varon, S., and Manthorpe, M. (1987): Association of laminin with heparan and chondroitin sulfate-bearing proteoglycans in neurite-promoting complexes from rat schwannoma cells. *Submitted.*
15. Davis, G. E., Varon, S., Engvall, E., and Manthorpe, M. (1985): Substratum-binding neurite promoting factors: relationships to laminin. *Trends Neurosci.*, 8:528–532.
16. Gage, F. H., Björklund, A., and Stenevi, U. (1984): Denervation releases a neuronal survival factor in adult rat hippocampus. *Nature,* 308:637–639.
17. Gage, F. H., Wictorin, K., Fischer, W., Williams, L. R., Varon, S., and Björklund, A. (1986): Cell loss and sprouting of cholinergic neurons in medial septum and diagonal band following fimbria-fornix transection: quantitative temporal analysis. *Neuroscience*, 19:241–255.
18. Gage, F. H., Wictorin, K., Fisher, W., Williams, L. R., Varon, S., and Björklund, A. (1986): Chronic intracerebral infusion of nerve growth factor (NGF) improves memory performance in cognitively impaired aged rats. *Soc. Neurosci. Abstr.*, 12:1580.
19. Greene, L. A., and Shooter, E. M. (1980): The nerve growth factor: biochemistry, synthesis, and mechanism of action. *Annu. Rev. Neurosci.*, 3:353–402.
20. Hefti, F. (1983): Alzheimer's disease caused by a lack of nerve growth factor? *Ann. Neurol.*, 13:109–110.
21. Hefti, F. (1986): Nerve growth factor promotes survival of septal cholinergic neurons after fimbrial transections. *J. Neurosci.*, 6:2155–2162.
22. Hefti, F., Dravid, A., and Hartikka, J. (1984): Chronic intraventricular injections of nerve growth factor elevate hippocampal choline acetyltransferase activity in adult rats with partial septo-hippocampal lesions. *Brain Res.*, 293:305–311.
23. Hefti, F., Hartikka, J. J., Eckenstein, R., Gnahn, H., Heumann, R., and Schwab, M. (1985): Nerve growth factor increases choline acetyltransferase but not survival or fiber outgrowth of cultured fetal septal cholinergic neurons. *Neuroscience*, 14:55–68.
24. Hepler, D. J., Wenk, G. L., Cribbs, B. L., Olton, D. S., and Coyle, J. T. (1985): Memory impairments following basal forebrain lesions. *Brain Res.*, 346:8–14.
25. Herschman, H. R., Goodman, R., Chandler, C., Simpson, D., Cawley, D., Cole, R., and DeVellis, J. (1983): Is epidermal growth factor a modulator of nervous system function? *Birth Defects*, 19:79–94.
26. Honegger, P., and Lenoir, D. (1982): Nerve growth factor (NGF) stimulation of cholinergic telencephalic neurons in aggregating cell cultures. *Dev. Brain Res.*, 3:229–238.
27. Hydèn, H. (1967): RNA in brain cells. In: *Neuroscience Study Program*, edited by G. C. Quarton, T. Melnechuk, and F. O. Schmitt, pp. 248–266. University Press, New York.
28. Kaufman, L., and Barrett, J. (1983): Serum factor supporting long-term survival of rat central neurons in culture. *Science*, 220:1394–1396.
29. Korsching, S., Auburger, G., Heumann, R., Scott, J., and Thoenen, H. (1985): Levels of nerve growth factor and its mRNA in the central nervous system of the rat correlate with cholinergic innervation. *EMBO J.*, 4:1389–1393.
30. Korsching, S., Heumann, R., Thoenen, H., and Hefti, F. (1986): Cholinergic denervation of the rat hippocampus by fimbrial transection leads to a transient accumulation of nerve growth factor (NGF) without change in mRNANGF content. *Neurosci. Lett.*, 66:175–180.
31. Kromer, L. F. (1986): Nerve growth factor treatments subsequent to bilateral fornix-fimbria lesions prevent retrograde neuronal death in the rat septum. *Soc. Neurosci. Abstr.*, 12:983.
32. Kromer, L. F., Björklund, A., and Stenevi, U. (1981): Regeneration of the septo-hippocampal pathways in adult rats is promoted by utilizing embryonic hippocampal implants as bridges. *Brain Res.*, 210:173–200.
33. Levi-Montalcini, R. (1982): Developmental neurobiology and the natural history of nerve growth factor. *Annu. Rev. Neurosci.*, 5:341–361.

34. Lewis, E. R., and Cotman, C. W. (1982): Mechanisms of septal lamination in the developing hippocampus analyzed by outgrowth of fibers from septal implants. II. Absence of guidance by degenerative debris. *J. Neurosci.*, 2:66–77.
35. Longo, F. M., Hayman, E. G., Davis, G. E., Ruoslahti, E., Engvall, E., Manthorpe, M., and Varon, S. (1984): Neurite promoting factors and extracellular matrix components accumulating in vivo within nerve regeneration chambers. *Brain Res.*, 309:105–117.
36. Longo, F. M., Selak, I., Zovickian, J., Manthorpe, M., Varon, S., and U, H-S. (1984): Neuronotrophic activities in cerebrospinal fluid of head trauma patients. *Exp. Neurol.*, 84:207–218.
37. Longo, F. M., Skaper, S. D., Manthorpe, M., Williams, L. R., Lundborg, G., and Varon, S. (1983): Temporal changes in neuronotrophic activities accumulating in vivo within nerve regeneration chambers. *Exp. Neurol.*, 81:756–769.
38. Manthorpe, M., and Varon, S. (1985): Regulation of neuronal survival and neuritic growth in the avian ciliary ganglion. In: *Growth and Maturation Factors*, edited by G. Guroff, pp. 77–117. Wiley, New York.
39. Manthorpe, M., Engvall, E., Ruoslahti, E., Longo, F. M., Davis, G. E., and Varon, S. (1983): Laminin promotes neuritic regeneration from cultured peripheral and central neurons. *J. Cell Biol.*, 97:1882–1890.
40. Manthorpe, M., Luyten, W., Longo, F. M., and Varon, S. (1983): Endogenous and exogenous factors support neuronal survival and choline acetyltransferase activity in embryonic spinal cord cultures. *Brain Res.*, 267:57–66.
41. Manthorpe, M., Nieto-Sampedro, M., Skaper, S. D., Lewis, E. R., Barbin, G., Longo, F. M., Cotman, C. W., and Varon, S. (1983): Neuronotrophic activity in brain wounds of the developing rat: correlation with implant survival in the wound cavity. *Brain Res.*, 267:47–56.
42. Manthorpe, M., Rudge, J., and Varon, S. (1986): Astroglial cell contributions to neuronal survival and neuritic growth. In: *Astrocytes*, Vol. 2, edited by S. Fedoroff and A. Vernadakis, pp. 315–376. Academic Press, New York.
43. Manthorpe, M., Skaper, S. D., Williams, L. R., and Varon, S. (1986): Purification of adult rat sciatic nerve ciliary neuronotrophic factor. *Brain Res.*, 367:282–286.
44. Martinez, H. J., Dreyfus, C. F., Jonakait, G. M., and Black, I. B. (1985): Nerve growth factor promotes cholinergic development in brain striatal cultures. *Proc. Natl. Acad. Sci. USA*, 82:7777–7781.
45. Mobley, W. C., Rutkowski, J. L., Tennekoon, G. I., Buchanan, K., and Johnston, M. V. (1985): Nerve growth factor increases choline acetyltransferase activity in the striatum of neonatal rats. *Science*, 229:284–287.
46. Montz, H. P. M., Davis, G. E., Skaper, S. D., Manthorpe, M., and Varon, S. (1985): Tumor-promoting phorbol diester mimics two distinct neuronotrophic factors. *Dev. Brain Res.*, 23:150–154.
47. Nieto-Sampedro, M., Lewis, E. R., Cotman, C. W., Manthorpe, M., Skaper, S. D., Barbin, G., Longo, F. M., and Varon, S. (1982): Brain injury causes a time-dependent increase in neuronotrophic activity at the lesion site. *Science*, 217:860–861.
48. Nieto-Sampedro, M., Manthorpe, M., Barbin, G., Varon, S., and Cotman, C. W. (1983): Injury-induced neuronotrophic activity in adult rat brain: correlation with survival of delayed implants in a wound cavity. *J. Neurosci.*, 3:2219–2229.
49. Peterson, G. M., Williams, L. R., Varon, S., and Gage, F. H. (1987): Loss of GABAergic neurons in medial septum after fimbria-fornix transection. *Submitted.*
50. Price, D. L., Whitehouse, P. J., Struble, R. G., Coyle, J. T., Clark, A. W., DeLong, M. R., Cork, L. C., and Hedreen, J. C. (1982): Alzheimer's disease and Down's syndrome. *Ann. N.Y. Acad. Sci.*, 396:145–164.
51. Rudge, J. S., Manthorpe, M., and Varon, S. (1985): The output of neuronotrophic and neurite-promoting agents from rat brain astroglial cells: a microculture method for screening potential regulatory molecules. *Dev. Brain. Res.*, 19:161–172.
52. Scott, J., Selby, M., Urdea, M., Quiroga, M., Bell, G. I., and Rutter, W. J. (1983): Isolation and nucleotide sequence of cDNA encoding the precursor of mouse nerve growth factor. *Nature*, 302:538–540.
53. Seiler, M., and Schwab, M. E. (1984): Specific retrograde transport of nerve growth factor (NGF) from neocortex to nucleus basalis in the rat. *Brain Res.*, 300:33–39.
54. Selak, I., Skaper, S. D., and Varon, S. (1985): Pyruvate participation in the low molecular weight trophic activity for CNS neurons in glia-conditioned media. *J. Neurosci.*, 5:23–28.

55. Skaper, S. D., and Varon, S. (1983): Control of the Na$^+$, K$^+$-pump by nerve growth factor is essential to neuronal survival. *Brain Res.*, 271:263–271.
56. Skaper, S. D., Montz, H. P. M., and Varon, S. (1986): Control of Na$^+$, K$^+$-pump activity in dorsal root ganglionic neurons by different neuronotrophic agents. *Brain Res. (in press).*
57. Skaper, S. D., Selak, I., and Varon, S. (1983): Serum- and substratum-dependent modulation of neuritic growth. *J. Neurosci. Res.*, 9:359–369.
58. Taniuchi, M., Schweizer, J. B., and Johnson, E. M. (1986): Nerve growth factor receptor molecules in rat brain. *Proc. Natl. Acad. Sci. USA*, 83:1950–1954.
59. Thoenen, H., and Barde, Y-A. (1980): Physiology of nerve growth factor. *Physiol. Rev.*, 60:1284–1335.
60. Ullrich, A., Gray, A., Berman, C., and Dull, T. J. (1983): Human β-nerve growth factor gene sequence highly homologous to that of mouse. *Nature*, 303:821–825.
61. Varon, S. (1975): In vitro approaches to the study of neural tissue aging. In: *Survey of the Aging Nervous System*, edited by G. Maletta, pp. 59–76. DHEW Publ. (NIH) 74–296.
62. Varon, S. (1977): Neural growth and regeneration: a cellular perspective. *Exp. Neurol.*, 54:1–6.
63. Varon, S. (1985): Factors promoting the growth of the nervous system. *Neuroscience*, 2(3): 1–62.
64. Varon, S., and Adler, R. (1980): Nerve growth factors and control of nerve growth. *Curr. Topics Dev. Biol.*, 16:207–252.
65. Varon, S., and Adler, R. (1981): Trophic and specifying factors directed to neuronal cells. *Adv. Cell. Neurobiol.*, 2:115–163.
66. Varon, S., and Manthorpe, M. (1982): Schwann cells: an in vitro perspective. *Adv. Cell. Neurobiol.*, 3:35–95.
67. Varon, S., and Skaper, S. D. (1983): The Na$^+$, K$^+$-pump may mediate the control of nerve cells by nerve growth factor. *Trends Biochem. Sci.*, 8:22–25.
68. Varon, S., and Williams, L. R. (1987): Peripheral nerve regeneration in a silicone model chamber: cellular and molecular aspects. *Peripheral Nerve Repair Regen.*, 1:9–25.
69. Varon, S., Manthorpe, M., Davis, G. E., Williams, L. R., and Skaper, S. D. (1987): Growth factors. In: *Functional Recovery in Neurological Disease*, edited by S. G. Waxman, pp. 493–521. Raven Press, New York.
70. Varon, S., Nomura, J., Perez-Polo, J. R., and Shooter, E. M. (1972): The isolation and assay of the nerve growth factor proteins. In: *Methods and Techniques of Neurosciences*, edited by R. Fried, pp. 203–229. H. Dekker, New York.
71. Varon, S., Rudge, J., Davis, G. E., Manthorpe, M., and Skaper, S. D. (1987): Astroglia production of neuronotrophic and neurite promoting agents. In: *Biochemistry of Glial Cells*, edited by T. Grisar and G. Franck (*in press*).
72. Varon, S., Skaper, S. D., and Manthorpe, M. (1987): Trophic and toxic mechanisms in neuronal survival. In: *Model Systems of Development and Aging in the Nervous System*, edited by A. Vernadakis, pp. 299–317. Nijhoff, Boston.
73. Varon, S., Williams, L. R., and Gage, F. H. (1987): In vivo protection by an exogenous neuronotrophic factor against neuronal death in adult rat CNS. In: *Neuroplasticity: A New Therapeutical Tool in CNS Pathology*, edited by A. Portera-Sanchez and G. Toffano. FIDIA Research Series, Liviana Press, Padua, Italy (*in press*).
74. Walicke, P., Cowan, W. M., Ueno, N., Baird, A., and Guillemin, R. (1986): Fibroblast growth factor promotes survival of dissociated hippocampal neurons and enhances neurite extension. *Proc. Natl. Acad. Sci. USA*, 83:3012–3016.
75. Walicke, P., Varon, S., and Manthorpe, M. (1986): Purification of a human red blood cell protein supporting the survival of cultured CNS neurons, and its identification as catalase. *J. Neurosci.*, 6:1114–1121.
76. Williams, L. R., Vahlsing, H. L., Lindamood, T., Varon, S., Gage, F. H., and Manthorpe, M. (1987): A preformed small gauge cannula device for continuous infusion of exogenous agents into the brain. *Exp. Neurol.*, 95:743–754.
77. Williams, L. R., Varon, S., Peterson, G., Wictorin, K., Fischer, W., Björklund, A., and Gage, F. H. (1986): Continuous infusion of nerve growth factor prevents basal forebrain neuronal death after fimbria-fornix transection. *Proc. Natl. Acad. Sci. USA*, 83:9231–9235.

*Aging and the Brain*, edited by R. D. Terry.
Raven Press, New York © 1988.

# Cholinergic Trophic Factors in Alzheimer Disease

Stanley H. Appel, J. Robert Bostwick, Garrett Crawford, and James L. McManaman

*Department of Neurology, Baylor College of Medicine, Houston, Texas 77030*

Trophic factors influence the survival, growth, and differentiation of neurons in the developing nervous system and appear to play a role in regenerative processes in the adult nervous system. If the function of such factors is disturbed in Alzheimer disease and if they can ameliorate the clinical condition are presently unclear. In the present discussion we review the clinical presentation and the brain pathology in Alzheimer disease to determine if such factors could potentially influence the regenerative process. Our interpretation of the available data is that the cortical pathology consisting in neuritic plaques and cerebrovascular amyloid is primary, and that the subcortical and some of the cortical changes occur by retrograde degeneration. We then review the topic of trophic factors and indicate their retrograde effects in neural tissue. Because such factors act in a retrograde direction, their functional impairment could underlie the retrograde degeneration of ascending subcortical projections in Alzheimer disease, and their administration could be of significant therapeutic value.

## CLINICAL PROBLEM

Alzheimer disease is a disorder of the later decades of life characterized by diffuse deterioration of mental function. It is slowly progressive and presents the picture of gradually increasing forgetfulness in the activities of daily living, an abbreviated attention span, a gradual deterioration in homemaking activities, difficulty in dressing, and an alteration in mood leading to episodes of frustration often associated with delusions, illusions, and even hallucinations. The diagnosis depends on ruling out secondary causes of loss of memory and impaired cognitive function such as depression, multiple infarcts, intracranial mass lesions, infections, or toxic and metabolic disorders (44). However, even when such secondary causes are ruled out, the clinical symptoms of the remaining patients do not comprise a discrete homogeneous entity.

## NEURONAL LOSS IN ALZHEIMER DISEASE

In patients with Alzheimer disease, there is a more significant loss of neurons than in age-matched controls (65). There is an overall weight loss in the brain, attributable to shrinkage of cerebral white matter in hippocampal gyrus and in frontal lobes, and to a lesser extent in the temporoparietal lobes. There is a definite loss of cortical neurons in Alzheimer disease, but the loss is not uniform (64). Fibrous astrocytes are found to be increased (61). Neurons between 40 and 90 $\mu$m were found to be the same or increased as in age-matched controls, whereas neurons greater than 90 $\mu$m were depleted, suggesting a possible shrinkage of large neurons to a smaller size. Almost 50% of cells are also lost from the amygdala, which usually does not show age-related losses (27). Furthermore, in the hippocampus of older Alzheimer patients, a similar percentage of neurons may be lost (7).

Deep subcortical and brainstem nuclei, including the nucleus basalis of Meynert, the periaqueductal region, and the locus ceruleus, also demonstrate significant cell loss. In fact, quantitative studies of cell number and biochemical constituents have demonstrated that cholinergic innervation from the nucleus basalis (70), noradrenergic innervation from the locus ceruleus (17), dopaminergic innervation from ventral tegmentum (40), and serotonergic innervation from the raphe (38) are compromised in Alzheimer disease.

## MICROSCOPIC LESIONS IN ALZHEIMER DISEASE

Four microscopic lesions are pertinent in Alzheimer disease. These lesions include senile or neuritic plaques, neurofibrillary tangles, granulovacuolar degeneration, and Hirano bodies. Senile plaques consist of a spherical mass of degenerating neurites, extracellular fibrils of amyloid, and reactive macrophages and microglia. Some of these degenerating neurites are immunoreactive for neurons definitely known to be affected in Alzheimer disease, e.g., cholinergic (29), noradrenergic (30), and somatostatinergic (6,47), whereas other studies suggest the presence of GABA- (69) and neuropeptide Y-containing (13) terminals. The plaques occur as an age-related change in both animals and man, and may be in proximity to capillaries.

The major distinctive constituent of the classical senile plaque is extracellular amyloid, which has a characteristic $\beta$-pleated sheet structure. The composition of the neuritic plaque has been the subject of considerable controversy. Some authors have suggested that aluminum may comprise 4 to 19% of the plaque core, and that silicone may also represent 6 to 24% of the plaque core (12). Thus inorganic elements may be key constituents of the core and represent either primary or secondary phenomena. Other reports suggest that the amino acid composition of purified amyloid plaque core protein may be identical to that found in cerebrovascular amyloid protein (20).

Neurofibrillary tangles (NFTs) are intraneuronal fibrillary structures whose precise morphological constituents are found only in human brain tissue. These structures are relatively insoluble and may be associated with intraneuronal deposits of aluminum (54). NFTs are not specific for Alzheimer disease but are also found in other conditions, e.g., Down syndrome, parkinsonian–dementia complex of Guam, postencephalitic parkinsonism, subacute sclerosing panencephalitis, tuberous sclerosis, Hallervorden-Spatz syndrome, and dementia pugilistica (74). The composition of the NFT is still a matter of considerable controversy. Data suggest that NFTs are partially made up of modified tau proteins (33) as well as other microtubular-associated antigens (32,55,77), vimentin epitopes (76), and modified neurofilaments (3). However, many constituents of NFTs are still not yet characterized. Such data suggest the association of the NFT with altered components of the cytoskeletal apparatus. Perhaps the most controversial recently described constituent is the amyloid component $(A_4)$ described by Masters et al. (43). Further work is needed to clarify if this constituent is a contaminant of the isolation procedure of NFTs and if such an amyloid constituent is indeed found in the neuritic plaque and cerebrovascular amyloid as well as NFTs.

In Alzheimer disease the lowest density of NFTs is in the primary cortices, and increasing numbers are noted in primary and secondary association cortices, reaching a peak in the multimodal association areas that are reciprocally related to the limbic cortex and the hippocampus (53).

Granulovacuolar degeneration is most commonly noted in Sommer's sector of the hippocampus. It is characterized by an intraneuronal, membrane-bound vesicle with a central electron-dense granule and can be stained with an anti-tubulin antibody (57). It is not unique to Alzheimer disease, as it is also seen with normal aging and other disorders.

Another microscopic finding in aged brains is the Hirano body, which consists of an eosinophilic intracytoplasmic inclusion measuring up to 50 $\mu$m in diameter. Localized predominantly in neurons of Sommer's sector of the hippocampus, it has a crystalline or paracrystalline pattern. It appears with increasing frequency after the sixth decade and has a higher incidence in Alzheimer disease, but it is also seen in other disorders (23). Immunocytochemistry demonstrates the presence of actin (22). Thus the three intracytoplasmic microscopic lesions that are the hallmark of Alzheimer disease are most likely derived from the cytoskeletal apparatus and are not specific for Alzheimer disease.

## BLOOD VESSEL COMPROMISE

The blood vessels in patients with Alzheimer disease may also be compromised by the presence of amyloid. Amyloid usually begins to collect in the middle layer of the brain vasculature; and it may replace all layers, weaken the vessel, and lead to hemorrhage. Glenner (19) has suggested that such cerebrovascular amyloid may be the initial stage in impairing the blood–brain barrier. Increased cerebrospinal fluid (CSF)/serum ratios for immunoglobulin G (IgG) and albumin, together with elevated CSF albumin levels in patients with Alzheimer disease (2,16) are consistent with increased permeability of the blood–brain barrier. The presence of extravasated serum proteins in brain parenchyma as visualized with immunohistological techniques also suggests altered permeability of the brain microvasculature (72,73). Individual capillaries show thickening and reduplication of the basement membrane and covering with astrocytic processes, which stain intensively for serum proteins and immunoglobulins (28,37).

## SITE OF THE PRIMARY LESION IN ALZHEIMER DISEASE

The impairment in several neurotransmitter systems derived from subcortical projections, as well as the impairment of intrinsic cortical and hippocampal somatostatin neurons, clearly implicate both cortical neurons and subcortical projections in the pathogenesis of Alzheimer disease. The key question is if the cortical or the subcortical lesions are primary. If the subcortical changes are primary, anterograde degeneration would be associated with cortical and hippocampal changes. If the cortical changes are primary, the lesions of the cortex or hippocampus at sites where affected neurons converge with projections from subcortical cholinergic, noradrenergic, serotonergic, and dopaminergic neurons may result in retrograde degeneration of these afferent projections. In the latter situation the retrograde effects could be due to an impairment of trophic factors or an impaired action of trophic factors on their specific receptors located on projecting presynaptic axons. Furthermore, senile plaques would be found at the points where the projecting system synapse in cortical association areas. NFTs might then be localized to the projecting axons. With this point of view, the senile plaques may more closely mark the site of initial pathology as cortical and hippocampal, and the cellular loss in nucleus basalis and locus ceruleus may result from retrograde degeneration.

Evidence that the cortical damage is primary and the subcortical damage is secondary is as follows. The subcortical neurons affected in Alzheimer disease are those that project to specific areas of the cortex. Subcortical cells that do not project to the cortex are not affected. For example, cells in locus ceruleus that project to the cortex are significantly compromised, whereas locus ceruleus cells that project to the spinal cord, basal ganglia, and cerebellum are relatively spared (41,42). Furthermore, cells in the locus ceruleus that project to the occipital cortex, which is less involved in Alzheimer disease, are less compromised. In the nucleus basalis the compromise of cells is topographically arranged, and regions of nucleus basalis projecting to the most severely affected cortical areas are themselves most severely compromised (5). Loss of dopaminergic cells follows a similar topographical involvement. Cells from substantia nigra, which project predominantly to the striatum, are far less involved than cells from the ventral tegmentum, which project via the mesocortical and mesolimbic tracts to the cerebral cortex (40).

A second major reason that the lesions are primary in the cortex is related to the loss of intracortical neurons. Somatostatin-containing neurons are primarily located in the cortex and hippocampus and are not derived from subcortical projections. Yet these intracortical cells are also compromised in Alzheimer disease. Furthermore, the loss of cortical choline acetyltransferase activity is far greater than the loss of cells from the nucleus basalis (56), thereby suggesting that not only the subcortical projections but the intracortical cholinergic neurons are also affected. Additionally, animal models have demonstrated that compromise of the cortex can lead to impairment of the structure and function of projecting subcortical cells by retrograde degeneration (63).

Circumstantial evidence for the primacy of the cortical loss is the fact that it would be easier to compromise the numerous cell types as well as the projecting subcortical neurons in the cortex than to assume that a process primarily involves widespread nuclei in various parts of the brainstem and diencephalon and either secondarily or simultaneously involves scattered loci in hippocampus and cortex.

Finally, neuritic plaques in Alzheimer disease are found predominantly in cortical regions, as well as hippocampus and amygdala. The neuritic plaques located elsewhere, e.g., in the nucleus basalis, may be ill-defined in structure. As noted above, there is an apparent correlation between the density of neuritic plaques in the cortex and the extent of cell loss in nucleus basalis (5) or locus ceruleus (29,41) that project to these cortical areas.

## RETROGRADE DEGENERATION

Thus most of the evidence in Alzheimer disease supports the cortex as the localization of the primary process leading to cerebrovascular amyloid and neuritic plaques. Secondarily, the projecting cortical and subcortical cells undergo retrograde degeneration and demonstrate NFTs, Hirano bodies, and granulovacuolar degeneration.

Retrograde transneuronal degeneration has been noted in the limbic system, i.e., in the medial mamillary nucleus or the ventral tegmental nucleus following lesions in the limbic cortex or cerebral cortex (15). It has also been demonstrated in pyramidal cells of precentral cortex following limb amputation or in the inferior olivary nucleus following cerebellar or Purkinje cell damage. Lesions of anterior thalamic nucleus or medial mamillary nucleus result in retrograde transneuronal degeneration in ventral tegmental nucleus. Lesions of the occipital visual cortex have been noted to give rise to changes in retinal ganglion cells, optic nerve, and lateral geniculate body presumably secondary to retrograde transneuronal degeneration. In experimental animals this process may take from 17 days to 2 months, and in the visual system it may take up to 2 years. Within the pathways involved in Alzheimer disease, changes of retrograde transneuronal degeneration may take even longer periods of time and may be associated with altered neurotrophic function.

## TROPHIC FACTORS

In 1981 we suggested that trophic factors may play a role in the pathogenesis of Alzheimer disease (4). Target-derived trophic factors are molecules that exert transynaptic retrograde effects on neuronal survival and differentiation. The discovery of nerve growth factor (NGF) was the first major step in the molecular analysis of neural development (35) and suggested that the effect of the target might be mediated by diffusible molecules (14). NGF can be isolated as an active 26,500-dalton component containing two identical polypeptide chains (11). The gene coding for human NGF has been sequenced (67). NGF can reverse naturally occurring as well as experimentally induced cell death in sympathetic and sensory neurons *in vivo*. Anti-NGF antibodies can block the development of the sympathetic nervous system *in vivo* (34). Thus competition for a limited supply of NGF may determine which neurons live and which die during development. Furthermore, NGF may be required for neuronal maintenance during adulthood (75).

The existence of naturally occurring cell death in most populations of vertebrate neurons (52) and the early realization that only a few neuronal systems are sensitive to NGF led to speculation that NGF may be one of a family of trophic agents. The search for new factors that regulate neuronal growth and development has mostly employed *in vitro* assays similar to those used for NGF. A wide range of activities that stimulate various aspects of neuronal growth and development has been noted in target tissue extracts in cell-conditioned media. However, the significance of such studies is still unclear, as most results have been obtained with impure components and may be dependent on unknown features of the assay. Only complete purification of the trophic factors will permit unambiguous identification. A new factor that stimulates survival of sensory neurons in culture has been purified to homogeneity from pig brain (8). The molecule has a molecular weight of 12,300 daltons, an isoelectric point of 10.1, and a specific activity estimated to be 0.4 mg/ml/unit. It migrates as a single band on sodium dodecyl sulfate (SDS) gel electrophoresis. Its effect is additive to that of NGF, and it is not blocked by antisera to NGF.

Partially purified factors have been documented to have effects on neuronal survival, neurite extension, substrate adhesion and neurite promotion, and development and differentiation. NGF clearly has more than one kind of stimulatory activity, but the degree of multiple activities in other trophic factors is unclear because of the impurity of the preparations employed. Chick ciliary ganglion has been a useful preparation for identifying neuronal survival factors, and such activity has been found in extracts prepared from embryonic eye tissue (1), chick heart, and in CNS wounds in developing and young adult rats (50). Further purification of the eye extract demonstrates activity in a 20,000-dalton component as determined by gel filtration. A similar molecular weight factor has been found in another laboratory to stimulate neuronal growth with no effects on levels of choline acetyltransferase (ChAT). Whether these are identical or merely similar factors is unclear, but they are clearly distinct from pig brain factor. Similar ambiguities surround our understanding of neurite extension factors, substrate adhesion and neurite-promoting factors, and differentiation and development factors (59). Different trophic activities with different specificities and function clearly exist in different target tissues. Whether a single factor can have diverse activities or diverse factors can have a single activity must await both purification and characterization of the specific factors.

The existence of neuronal trophic factors and their release by target tissue is less well clarified in the CNS. Nevertheless, the existence of retrograde transneuronal degeneration within the adult CNS provides circumstantial evidence for the existence of factors which, like NGF, may influence survival, differentiation, and maintenance of innervating neurons (15). In fact, evidence has demonstrated that NGF can act as a neurotrophic factor for central cholinergic neurons. NGF as well as its messenger RNA are present in rat brain, and its levels and anatomical distribution correspond to cholinergic neurons and their target areas (31,62). The NGF mRNA is primarily in hippocampus and cortex, and NGF is present in hippocampus, cortex, as well as septum and nucleus basalis. NGF receptors have been localized to the septum and basal nucleus of the rat brain (58) and are found in a similar distribution in human brain (60). Thus NGF appears to be made in cortex and hippocampus, and to act in a retrograde fashion upon projecting cholinergic processes from septum and nucleus basalis.

Nerve growth factor has been documented to elevate the activity of ChAT when injected into the brain of newborn rats (46) or when applied to cultures of dissociated septal neurons from fetal rat brain (26). Antibodies to NGF reduce the number of cholinergic neurons in tissue culture systems (24). However, NGF antibodies do not reduce ChAT activity when injected *in vivo* (21). Although this latter finding may be related to the fact that antibodies never reach the cholinergic neurons, it is also possible that other trophic factors can compensate for antibody-produced deficiencies in NGF. Because NGF is now known to influence cholinergic neuronal development *in vivo,* it would be important to repeat the *in vivo* antibody experiments and document whether anti-NGF or anti-NGF receptor antibodies do in fact interact with cholinergic neurons.

Nerve growth factor also appears to influence CNS cholinergic neurons in adults. In adult animals with lesions between the septum and hippocampus, cholinergic neurons were reduced approximately 50%; but in similarly lesioned animals treated with NGF, the number of cholinergic neurons was reduced only 10% (25). Thus NGF appears to enhance the survival of damaged cholinergic neurons in adult animals. Similar lesions between the septum and hippocampus can alter behavior, and administration of NGF partially reverses the behavioral deficit (36).

Studies from our own laboratory have documented that factors other than NGF clearly enhance the cholinergic activity of central mammalian neurons. As a model of central cholinergic effects, we selected the septohippocampal system for detailed analysis because it has been extensively studied with respect to its anatomical relations, developmental neurogenesis, neurotransmitter distribution, and capacity for regeneration (10,36,49). In this system extracts of the target rat hippocampus enhance neurite outgrowth as well as cholinergic activity of rat medial septal nucleus cultured in either serum-free defined medium or heat-inactivated horse serum (51).

Medial septal nucleus is obtained from the brains of 16-day-old rat embryos, dissected into 0.3 to 0.4 mm diameter pieces, and explanted onto polylysine-coated dishes. Under these conditions neuronal tissue attaches to the culture dish surface within 1 hr and begins to extend processes within 24 hr after explanation. The processes increase in number and length over at least 6 to 8 days *in vitro*. The major effect of hippocampal extract is an increase in cholinergic activity. Choline acetyltransferase activity is enhanced twofold, choline uptake is enhanced twofold, and acetylcholine synthesis is enhanced more than threefold. Furthermore, the conversion of choline to acetylcholine is increased from 20% to 30% in the presence of hippocampal extract. The effect of hippocampal extract on cholinergic development increases in a linear fashion with protein concentration and saturates at 50 $\mu$g/ml. With further separation techniques employing column chromatography and high-pressure liquid chromatography, we have been able to achieve more than 30,000-fold purification. Characterization of the hippocampal cholinergic activity has demonstrated that it is acid-stable and has an apparent molecular weight less than 1,500 daltons.

Our cholinergic trophic peptide does not appear to be related to NGF, as no small peptide fragment of NGF has been documented to have any trophic effects on sensory neurons, sympathetic neurons, or central cholinergic neurons *in vivo* or *in vitro*. Furthermore, antibodies to NGF do not block the effects of our trophic peptides *in vitro* (51). In our tissue culture systems, NGF has a minimal effect on acetylcholine synthesis, whereas it has a significant stimulatory effect on choline acetyltransferase activity. Conversely, our peptide has maximal effects on acetylcholine synthesis and lesser effects on choline acetyltransferase activity. The effects of NGF and our hippocampal peptide appear to be additive with respect to CAT activity of septal neurons. Our peptide appears to enhance the conversion of choline, which is taken up into the cell into acetylcholine, whereas NGF, which has minimal effects on acetylcholine synthesis, has minimal effects on the conversion of choline to acetylcholine.

Cholinergic-enhancing trophic activity resides in different species, each of which may affect a different aspect of cholinergic metabolism. Clearly, any factor that enhances cell survival apparently stimulates cholinergic activity *in vitro* compared to control cultures. Furthermore, enhancement of choline uptake and the conversion of choline to acetylcholine represent additional mechanisms of enhancing cholinergic activity. Finally, direct enhancement of ChAT activity, either through an increased number of enzyme molecules or an increased activity of each enzyme molecule, represents a potential means of stimulating activity. However, because ChAT activity does not appear to be rate-limiting for acetylcholine synthesis, it is not clear what functional consequence is derived from increasing ChAT activity, compared, for example, to an increase in uptake of choline. Our central factors appear to enhance activity by many of these mechanisms. Further characterization of these trophic moieties should permit us to define the specific mechanism of cholinergic enhancement of each factor, as well as to ascertain the functional consequence of enhancing activity by these different routes.

It is also important to note that basic fibroblast growth factor enhances survival and neurite extension of hippocampal (68) and cortical (48) neurons in dissociated culture. Insulin-like growth factor II also can enhance neuritic extension and thus function as a trophic factor (45). Other defined growth factors may also be found to function as trophic factors in neural tissue.

## IMPLICATIONS FOR ALZHEIMER DISEASE

The data reviewed in the previous section on trophic factors clearly supports the presence of several trophic factors influencing cholinergic neurons within the CNS. However, data are not presently available as to whether NGF of any other cholinergic trophic factors are altered or whether trophic factor receptors are compromised in Alzheimer disease. Nevertheless, the importance of trophic factors in preventing retrograde degeneration in animal models suggests that the loss of projecting nucleus basalis cells may be related to primary cortical pathology, which would result in lack of NGF or central cholinergic trophic factor or a reduced response to such factors owing to compromised receptors for such trophic factors.

If the changes in cerebral cortex in Alzheimer disease are considered to be primary, retrograde degeneration would not only compromise cholinergic ascending projections from nucleus basalis but also noradrenergic projections from locus ceruleus, serotonergic ascending projections from nucleus raphe, and dopaminergic ascending projections from ventral tegmentum. Cholinergic trophic factors per se would not be sufficient to ameliorate the noradrenergic, serotonergic, and dopaminergic cell loss. However, dopaminergic trophic factors have been documented (66); and circumstantial evidence suggests the existence of noradrenergic as well as serotonergic factors. It is possible that trophic function could become compromised as the cortical cells secreting such factors or the trophic factor receptors on ascending projections are engulfed by the cortical pathology. Collateral sprouting of cholinergic and possible glutamatergic terminals has been demonstrated in Alzheimer disease hippocampus (18). Thus the capacity for regeneration is present within the CNS, as it is within the neuromuscular system, and trophic factors may play a significant role in this process. However, as the primary mechanisms of pathogenesis continue, either trophic factors or terminals bearing receptors may become depleted and the regenerative process would be overriden by the degenerative process. The trophic factors may then provide a potential therapeutic intervention that could prevent the retrograde degeneration and possibly ameliorate clinical dysfunction regardless of what initiated the primary process.

## ACKNOWLEDGMENTS

We are grateful to the Harkins Foundation Fund for Alzheimer's Research and the Robert J. Kleberg and Helen C. Kleberg Foundation for support of our research efforts.

## REFERENCES

1. Adler, R., Landa, R. B., Manthorpe, M., et al. (1979): Cholinergic trophic factors: intraocular distribution of trophic activity for ciliary neurons. *Science,* 204:1434–1436.
2. Alafuzoff, I., Adolfsson, R., Bucht, G., et al. (1983): Albumin and immunoglobulin in plasma and cerebrospinal fluid and blood-cerebrospinal fluid barrier function in patients with dementia of Alzheimer type and multiinfarct dementia. *J. Neurol. Sci.,* 60:465–472.
3. Anderton, B. H., Breinburg, D., Downes, M. J., Green, P. J., Tomlinson, B. E., Ulrich, J., Wood, J. N., and Kahn, J. (1982): Monoclonal antibodies show that neurofibrillary tangles and neurofilaments share antigenic determinants. *Nature,* 298:84–86.
4. Appel, S. H. (1981): A unifying hypothesis for the cause of amyotrophic lateral sclerosis, parkinsonism, and Alzheimer's disease. *Ann. Neurol.,* 10:499–505.
5. Arendt, T., Bige, V., Tennstedt, A., et al. (1985): Neuronal loss in different parts of the nucleus basalis is related to neuritic plaque formation in cortical target areas in Alzheimer's disease. *Neuroscience,* 14:1–14.
6. Armstrong, E. M., LeRoy, S., Shields, D., et al. (1985): Somatostatin immunoreactivity within neuritic plaques. *Brain Res.,* 338:71–80.
7. Ball, M. J. (1977): Neuronal loss, neurofibrillary tangles and granulovacuolar degeneration in the hippocampus with aging and dementia. *Acta Neuropathol. (Berl.),* 37:111–118.
8. Barde, Y. A., Edgar, D., and Theonen, H. (1982): Purification of a new neurotrophic factor from mammalian brain. *EMBO J.,* 1:549–553.
9. Berg, D. K. (1984): New neuronal growth factors. *Annu. Rev. Neurosci.,* 7:149–170.
10. Bjorklund, A., and Stenevi, U. (1979): Regeneration of monoaminergic and cholinergic neurons in the mammalian central nervous system. *Physiol. Rev.,* 59:62–100.
11. Bradshaw, R. A. (1978): Nerve growth factor. *Annu. Rev. Biochem.,* 47:191.
12. Candy, J. M., Oakley, A. E., Klinowski, J., et al. (1986): Aluminosilicates and formation in Alzheimer's disease. *Lancet,* 1:354–357.

13. Chan-Palay, V., Lang, W., Allen, Y. S., et al. (1985): Cortical neurons immunoreactive against NPY are altered in Alzheimer type dementia. *J. Comp. Neurol.*, 238:390–400.

14. Cohen, S. (1960): Purification of a nerve growth promoting protein from the mouse salivary gland and its neurocytotoxic antiserum. *Proc. Natl. Acad. Sci. USA*, 46:302–311.

15. Cowan, W. M. (1970): Anterograde and retrograde transneuronal degeneration in the central and peripheral nervous system. In: *Contemporary Research Methods in Neuroanatomy*, edited by W. J. Nauta and S. V. Ebbson, p. 217. Springer, New York.

16. Elovaara, I., Icen, A., Palo, J., et al. (1985): CSF in Alzheimer's disease—studies on blood-brain barrier function and intrathecal protein synthesis. *J. Neurol. Sci.*, 70:73–80.

17. Forno, L. S. (1978): The locus ceruleus in Alzheimer's disease. *J. Neuropathol. Exp. Neurol.*, 37:614.

18. Geddes, J. W., Monaghan, D. T., Cotman, C. W., et al. (1985): Plasticity of hippocampal circuitry in Alzheimer's disease. *Science*, 230:1179–1181.

19. Glenner, G. G. (1980): Amyloid deposits and amyloidosis. *N. Engl. J. Med.*, 302:1283–1291, 1333–1343.

20. Glenner, G. G., and Wong, C. W. (1984): Alzheimer's disease: initial report of the purification and characterization of a novel cerebrovascular amyloid protein. *Biochem. Biophy. Res. Commun.*, 120:885–890.

21. Gnahn, H., Hefti, F., Heumann, R., et al. (1983): NGF-mediated increase of choline acetyltransferase (ChAT) in the neonatal forebrain: evidence for a physiological role of NGF in the brain? *Dev. Brain Res.*, 9:45–52.

22. Goldman, J. E. (1983): The association of actin with Hirano bodies. *J. Neuropathol. Exp. Neurol.* 42:146–152.

23. Goldman, J. E., and Yen, S-H. (1986): Cytoskeletal protein abnormalities in neurodegenerative diseases. *Ann. Neurol.*, 19:209–223.

24. Hefti, F. (1985): Nerve growth factor (NGF) promotes survival of septal cholinergic neurons after injury. *Proc. Soc. Neurosci.*, 11:660.

25. Hefti, F. (1986): Nerve growth factor (NGF) promotes survival of septal cholinergic neurons after fimbrial transections. *J. Neurosci.*, 6:2155–2162.

26. Hefti, F., Hartikka, J., Eckenstein, S., et al. (1985): Nerve growth factor (NGF) increases choline acetyltransferase but not survival of fiber growth of cultured septal cholinergic neurons. *Neuroscience*, 14:55–68.

27. Herzog, A. G., and Kemper, T. L. (1980): Amygdaloid changes in aging and dementia. *Arch. Neurol.*, 37:625–629.

28. Kidd, M. (1964): Alzheimer's disease: an electron microscopic study. *Brain*, 87:307–320.

29. Kitt, C. A., Price, D. L., Struble, R. G., et al. (1984): Evidence for cholinergic neurites in senile plaques. *Science*, 226:1443–1445.

30. Kitt, C. A., Struble, R. G., Cork, L. C., et al. (1985): Catecholaminergic neurites in senile plaques in prefrontal cortex of aged non-human primates. *Neuroscience*, 16:691–699.

31. Korsching, S., Auburger, G., Heumann, R., et al. (1985): Levels of nerve growth factor and its mRNA in the central nervous system of the rat correlate with cholinergic innervation. *EMBO J.*, 4:1389–1393.

32. Kosik, K. S., Duffy, L. K., Dowling, M. M., et al. (1984): Microtubule-associated protein 2: monoclonal antibodies demonstrate the selective incorporation of certain epitopes into Alzheimer neurofibrillary tangles. *Proc. Natl. Acad. Sci. USA*, 81:7941–7945.

33. Kosik, K. S., Joachim, C. L., and Selkoe, D. J. (1986): Microtubule-associated protein, tau, is a major antigenic component of paired helical filaments in Alzheimer's disease. *Proc. Natl. Acad. Sci. USA*, 83:4044–4048.

34. Levy-Montalcini, R. (1982): Developmental neurobiology and the natural history of nerve growth factor. *Annu. Rev. Neurosci.*, 5:341–362.

35. Levi-Montalcini, R., and Hamburger, V. (1951): Selective growth stimulating effects of mouse sarcoma on the sensory nervous system of the chick embryo. *J. Exp. Zool.*, 116:321–361.

36. Lewis, P. R., and Shute, C. C. D. (1967): The cholinergic limbic system: projection to hippocampal formation, medial cortex, nuclei of the ascending cholinergic reticular system and the subfornical organ in the supraoptic crest. *Brain*, 90:521–540.

37. Mancardi, G. L., Perdelli, F., Rivano, C., et al. (1980): Thickening of the basement membrane of cortical capillaries in Alzheimer's disease. *Acta Neuropathol. (Berl.)*, 49:79–93.

38. Mann, D. M. A., Yates, P. O., and Marcyniuk, B. (1984): Alzheimer's presenile dementia,

senile dementia of Alzheimer type and Down's syndrome in middle age form an age-related continuum of pathological changes. *Neuropathol. Appl. Neurobiol.*, 10:185–207.

39. Mann, D. M. A., Yates, P. O., and Marcyniuk, B. (1985): Correlation between senile plaque and neurofibrillary tangle counts in cerebral cortex and neuronal counts in cerebral cortex and subcortical regions in Alzheimer's disease. *Neurosci. Lett.*, 56:51–55.

40. Mann, D. M. A., Yates, P. O., and Marcyniuk, B. (1987): Dopaminergic neurotransmitter systems in Alzheimer's disease and in Down's syndrome at middle age. *J. Neurol. Neurosurg. Psychiatry*, 50:341–344.

41. Marcyniuk, B., Mann, D. M. A., and Yates, P. O. (1986): Loss of cells from locus ceruleus in Alzheimer's disease is topographically arranged. *Neurosci. Lett.*, 64:247–252.

42. Marcyniuk, B., Mann, D. M. A., and Yates, P. O. (1986): The topography of cell loss from locus ceruleus in Alzheimer's disease. *J. Neurol. Sci.*, 76:335–345.

43. Masters, C. L., Multnaup, G., Simms, G., et al. (1985): Neuronal origin of cerebral amyloid: neurofibrillary tangles of Alzheimer's disease contain the same protein as the amyloid of plaque cores and blood vessels. *EMBO J.*, 4:2757–2763.

44. McKhann, G., Drachman, D., Folstein, M., et al. (1984): Clinical diagnosis of Alzheimer's disease: report of the NINCDS-ADRDA work group under the auspices of the Department of Health and Human Services Task Force in Alzheimer's disease. *Neurology*, 34:939–944.

45. Mill, J. F., Chao, M. V., and Ishii, D. M. (1985): Insulin, insulin-like growth factor II, nerve growth factor effects on tubulin mRNA levels and neurite formation. *Proc. Natl. Acad. Sci. USA*, 82:7126–7130.

46. Mobley, W. C., Rutkowski, J. L., Tennekoon, G. I., et al. (1986): Choline acetyltransferase activity in striatum of neonatal rats increased by nerve growth factor. *Science*, 229:284–287.

47. Morrison, J. M., Rogers, J. H., Scherr, S., Benoit, R., and Bloom, F. E. (1985): Somatostatin immunoreactivity in neuritic plaques of Alzheimer's patients. *Nature*, 314:90–92.

48. Morrison, R. S., Sharma, A., DeVellis, J., and Bradshaw, R. A. (1986): Basic fibroblast growth factor supports the survival of cerebral cortical neurons in primary culture. *Proc. Natl. Acad. Sci. USA*, 83:7537–7541.

49. Nadler, J. V., Matthews, D. A., Cotman, C. W., et al. (1974): Development of cholinergic innervation in the hippocampal formation of the rat. II. Qualitative changes in choline acetyltransferase and acetylcholinesterase activities. *Dev. Biol.*, 36:142–154.

50. Nieto-Sampedro, M., Lewis, E. R., Cotman, C. W., et al. (1982): Brain injury causes a time-dependent increase in neurotrophic activity at the lesion site. *Science*, 217:860–861.

51. Ojika, K., and Appel, S. H. (1984): Neurotrophic effects of hippocampal extracts on medial septal nucleus in vitro. *Proc. Natl. Acad. Sci. USA*, 81:2567–2571.

52. Oppenheim, R. W. (1981): Neuronal cell death and some related regressive phenomena during neurogenesis: a selective historical review and progress report. In: *Studies in Developmental Neurobiology*, edited by W. M. Cowan. Oxford University Press, New York.

53. Pearson, R. C. A., Esiri, M. M., Hiorns, R. W., et al. (1985): Anatomical correlates of the distribution of the pathological changes in the neocortex in Alzheimer's disease. *Proc. Natl. Acad. Sci. USA*, 82:4531–4534.

54. Perl, D. P., and Brady, A. R. (1980). Alzheimer's disease: x-ray spectrometric evidence of aluminum accumulation in neurofibrillary tangle-bearing neurons. *Science*, 208:197–199.

55. Perry, G., Rizzuto, N., Autilio-Gambetti, L., et al. (1984): Ultrastructural localization of cytoskeletal markers on Alzheimer's paired helical filaments. *J. Neuropathol. Exp. Neurol.*, 43:346.

56. Perry, R. H., Candy, J. M., Perry, E. K., et al. (1982): Extensive loss of choline acetyltransferase activity is not reflected by neuronal loss in the nucleus of Meynert in Alzheimer's disease. *Neurosci. Lett.*, 33:311–315.

57. Price, D. L., Struble, R. G., Altschuler, R. J., et al. (1985): Aggregation of tubulin in neurons in Alzheimer's disease. *J. Neuropathol. Exp. Neurol.*, 44:366.

58. Riopelle, R. J., Richardson, P. M., and Verge, V. M. K. (1985): Receptors for nerve growth factor in the rat central nervous system. *Proc. Soc. Neurosci.*, 11:1056.

59. Roher, A., Wolfe, D., Palutke, M., et al. (1986): Purification, ultrastructure and chemical analysis of Alzheimer's disease amyloid plaque core protein. *Proc. Natl. Acad. Sci. USA*, 83:2662–2666.

60. Ross, A. H., Grob, P., Bothwell, M., et al. (1984): Characterization of nerve growth factor

receptor in neural crest tumors using monoclonal antibodies. *Proc. Natl. Acad. Sci. USA,* 81:6681–6685.

61. Schechter, R., Yen, S-H., and Terry, R. D. (1981): Fibrous astrocytes in senile dementia of the Alzheimer's type. *J. Neuropathol. Exp. Neurol.,* 40:95–101.

62. Shelton, D. L., and Reichardt, L. F. (1986): Studies on the expression of beta-nerve growth factor (NGF) gene in the central nervous system: level and regional distribution of NGF mRNA suggest that NGF functions as a trophic factor for several distinct populations of neurons. *Proc. Natl. Acad. Sci. USA,* 83:2714–2718.

63. Sofroniew, M. V., Pearson, R. C. A., Eckenstein, F., et al. (1983): Retrograde changes in cholinergic neurons in the basal forebrain of the rat following cortical damage. *Brain Res.,* 289:370–374.

64. Terry, R. D. (1981): Neuronal and glial cell counts in senile dementia of the Alzheimer's type and in age-matched normal specimens. *Gerontology,* 27:115.

65. Terry, R. D., Peck, A., DeTeresa, R., Schechter, R., and Horoupian, D. S. (1981): Some morphometric aspects of the brain in senile dementia of the Alzheimer type. *Ann. Neurol.,* 10:184–192.

66. Tomozawa, Y., and Appel, S. H. (1986): Soluble striatal extracts enhance development of mesencephalic dopaminergic neurons in vitro. *Brain Res.,* 399:111–124.

67. Ullrich, A., Gray, A., Berman, C., et al. (1983): Human beta-nerve growth factor gene sequence highly homologous to that of mouse. *Nature,* 303:821–825.

68. Walicke, P., Cowan, W. M., Ueno, N., et al. (1986): Fibroblast growth factor promotes survival of dissociated hippocampal neurons and enhances neurite extension. *Proc. Natl. Acad. Sci. USA,* 83:3012–3016.

69. Walker, L. C., Kitt, C. A., Struble, R. G., et al. (1985): GAD-like immunoreactive neurites in senile plaques. *Neurosci. Lett.,* 59:165–169.

70. Whitehouse, P. J., Price, D. L., Clark, A. W., Coyle, J. T., and DeLong, M. R. (1981): Alzheimer disease: evidence for selective loss of cholinergic neurons in the nucleus basalis. *Ann Neurol.,* 10:122–126.

71. Will, B., and Hefti, F. (1985): Behavioral and neurochemical effects of chronic intraventricular injections of nerve growth factor in adult rats with fimbria lesions. *Behav. Brain Res.,* 17:17–24.

72. Wilmes, F., and Hossman, K. A. (1979): A specific immunofluorescence technique for the demonstration of vasogenic edema in paraffin embedded material. *Acta Neuropathol. (Berl.),* 45:47–51.

74. Wisniewski, K., Jervis, G. A., Moretz, R. G., and Wisniewski, H. M. (1979): Alzheimer neurofibrillary tangles in diseases other than senile dementia and presenile dementia. *Ann. Neurol.,* 5:288–294.

73. Wisniewki, H. M., and Kozlowski, P. B. (1982): Evidence for blood-brain barrier changes in senile dementia of the Alzheimer's type (SDAT). *Ann. N.Y. Acad. Sci.,* 396:119–130.

75. Yanker, B. A., and Shooter, E. M. (1982): The biology and mechanism of action of nerve growth factor. *Annu. Rev. Biochem.,* 51:845–868.

76. Yen, S-H., Gaskin, F., and Fu, S. M. (1983): Neurofibrillary tangles in senile dementia of the Alzheimer's type share an antigenic determinant with intermediate filaments of the vimentin class. *Am. J. Pathol.,* 113:373–381.

77. Yen, S-H., Gaskin, F., and Terry, R. D. (1981): Immunocytochemical studies of neurofibrillary tangles. *Am. J. Pathol.,* 104:77–89.

# Subject Index

*301*